The Recognition of Anti-Rheumatic Drugs

The Recognition of Anti-Rheumatic Drugs

Edited by

D. C. Dumonde

The Mathilda and Terence Kennedy Institute of Rheumatology, London

and

M. K. Jasani

CIBA Laboratories, Horsham, West Sussex

Proceedings of an International Symposium held in London in April, 1977

MTP

Published by
MTP Press Limited
St. Leonard's House
LANCASTER

ISBN 0 85200 192–4

Text set in 11/12 pt Photon Imprint, printed by photolithography, and bound in Great Britain at The Pitman Press, Bath

Contents

List of Contributors

C. S. BACH
Research Division
CIBA Laboratories
Horsham
West Sussex RH12 4AB

P.A. BACON
Royal National Hospital for Rheumatic Diseases
Upper Borough Walls
Bath BA1 1RL

EUGENE V. BARNETT
Department of Medicine
University of California at Los Angeles
School of Medicine
The Center for the Health Sciences
Los Angeles
California 90024, USA

ALAN BLACKHAM
Fisons Ltd
Pharmaceutical Division
Research & Development Laboratories
Bakewell Road
Loughborough
Leicestershire LE11 0CY

W. WATSON BUCHANAN
The Centre for Rheumatic Diseases
Baird Street
Glasgow G4 0EH

A. CASTRO
Universidade de Sao Paulo
Faculdade de Medicina de Ribeirao Preto
"Campus" De Ribeirao Preto
CEP 14 100
Ribeirao Preto
Estado de Sao Paulo
Brazil

R. R. A. COOMBS
Department of Pathology
University of Cambridge
Division of Immunology
Laboratory Block
Addenbrooke's Hospital
Hills Road
Cambridge CB2 2QQ

F. M. A. CORREA
Universidade de Sao Paulo
Faculdade de Medicina de Ribeirao Preto
"Campus" De Ribeirao Preto
CEP 14 100
Ribeirao Preto
Estado de Sao Paulo
Brazil

MAURICE F. CUTHBERT
Principal Medical Officer
Department of Health & Social Security
Medicines Division
Penderel House
287 High Holborn
London WC1V 7HT

W. CARSON DICK
Consultant Physician
The Centre for Rheumatic Diseases
Baird Street
Glasgow G4 0EH

D. C. DUMONDE
Immunology Division
The Mathilda and Terence Kennedy Institute of Rheumatology
Bute Gardens
Hammersmith
London W6 7DW

S. H. FERREIRA
Universidade de Sao Paulo
Faculdade de Medicina de Ribeirao Preto
"Campus" De Ribeirao Preto
CEP 14 100
Ribeirao Preto
Estado de Sao Paulo
Brazil

MARVIN B. GOLDLUST
Senior Research Investigator
Department of Experimental Pathology
E.R. Squibb & Sons Inc
The Squibb Institute for Medical Research
PO Box 4000
Princeton
New Jersey 08540, USA

F. HAY
Department of Immunology
Middlesex Hospital
Mortimer Street
London W1

M. K. JASANI
Research Division
CIBA Laboratories
Horsham
West Sussex RH12 4AB

M. G. JOHNSTON
Department of Pathology
University of Toronto
Division of General and Experimental Pathology
Medical Sciences Building
Toronto 5
Canada

MARGARET KOPANIAK
Department of Pathology
University of Toronto
Division General and Experimental Pathology
Medical Science Building
Toronto 5
Canada

ARVI LARSEN
The Mathilda and Terence Kennedy Institute of Rheumatology
Immunology Division
Bute Gardens
Hammersmith
London W6 7DW

A. J. LEWIS
Organon Laboratories Ltd
Newhouse
Lanarkshire ML1 5SH

G. P. LEWIS
Department of Pharmacology
Royal College of Surgeons of England
Institute of Basic Medical Sciences
35/43 Lincoln's Inn Fields
London WC2A 3PN

K. LOCKWOOD
Research Division
CIBA Laboratories
Horsham
West Sussex RH12 4AB

BERENICE LORENZETTI
Universidade de San Paulo
Faculdade de Medicina de Ribeirao Preto
"Campus" De Ribeirao Preto
CEP 14 100
Ribeirao Preto
Estado de Sao Paulo
Brazil

S. MONCADA
The Wellcome Research Laboratories
Langley Court
Beckenham
Kent BR3 3BS

H. Z. MOVAT
Department of Pathology
University of Toronto
Division of General and Experimental Pathology
Medical Sciences Building
Toronto 5
Canada

A. G. MOWAT
Rheumatology Unit
Nuffield Orthopaedic Centre
Headington
Oxford OX3 7LD

ALEXANDER W. PATTERSON
Department of Pharmacy
Heriot-Watt University
79 Graff Market
Edinburgh EH1 2HJ

CARL M. PEARSON
Division of Rheumatology
University of California at Los Angeles
School of Medicine
Los Angeles
California 90024 USA

ROBERT J. PERPER
Department of Pathology
The New York Hospital
Cornell Medical Center
525 East 68th Street
New York NY 10021 USA

A. R. POOLE
Joint Diseases Research Laboratory
Shriner's Hospital for Crippled Children
Cedar Avenue
Montreal
P. Quebec
Canada

J. M. ROBERTS
Research Division
CIBA Laboratories
Horsham
West Sussex RH12 4AB

MARIA SALETE
Universidade de Sao Paulo
Faculdade de Medicina de Ribeirao Preto
"Campus" De Ribeirao Preto
CEP 14 100
Ribeirao Preto
Estado de Sao Paulo
Brazil

J. SELDRUP
Geigy Pharmaceuticals
Hurdsfield Industrial Estate
Macclesfield
Cheshire SK10 2LY

J. L. TURK
Department of Pathology
The Royal College of Surgeons of England
35/43 Lincoln's Inn Fields
London WC2A 3PN

J. R. VANE
The Wellcome Research Laboratories
Langley Court
Beckenham
Kent BR3 3BS

K. WHALEY
University Department of Pathology
Western Infirmary
Glasgow G11 6NT

List of Discussants

In addition to the contributors listed on p. ix, the following took part in discussions I–VI and in the Round Table Discussion.

D. ALARCON-SEGOVIA
Department of Immunology and Rheumatology
Instituito Nacional de Nutrition
Mexico 22, D. F.
Mexico City
Mexico

Z. BENTWICH
Department of Medicine
and Unit of Clinical Immunology
Kaplan Hospital
Rehovot
P.O. Box 1
Israel

D. M. BURLEY
CIBA Laboratories
Wimblehurst Road
Horsham
West Sussex

A. T. A. DOBLE
Immunology Unit
Glaxo Research Ltd.
Greenford
Middlesex OHE UB6

P. H. EVANS
M.R.C. Pneumoconiosis Unit
Llandough Hospital
Penarth
Glamorgan CF6 1XW

L. E. GLYNN
The Mathilda and Terence
Kennedy Institute of Rheumatology
Bute Gardens
Hammersmith
London W6 7DW

A. A. J. GOLDBERG
Medical Consultant
Reckitt & Colman
c/o 37 Lyttleton Road
London N2 0DQ

JOHN G. HAWKES
Bedford General Hospital
South Wing
Kempston Road
Bedford MK42 9DJ

G. A. HIGGS
Wellcome Research Laboratories
Langley Court
Beckenham
Kent BR3 3BS

M. I. V. JAYSON
Department of Rheumatology
University of Manchester
Manchester M13 9PT

A. R. MACKENZIE
Department of Biochemistry
Allen and Hanbury's Research Ltd.
Ware
Herts SG12 0DJ

K. D. MUIRDEN
Department of Medicine
Royal Melbourne Hospital
Post Office
Parkville
Victoria 3050
Australia

S. ORLOFF
International League Against Rheumatism
Hospital Universitaire Brügmann
Place A. Van Gehucten 4
B-1020 Brussels
Belgium

R. E. PETTY
Department of Paediatrics
Rheumatic Disease Unit
The University of Manitoba
Health Sciences Center
80 Sherbook Street
Winnipeg
Manitoba
Canada

CYRIL SCHNEIDER
Research Department
Miles Laboratories Ltd.
Stoke Poges
Bucks SL2 4LY

I. F. SKIDMORE
Department of Biochemistry
Allen and Hanbury's Research Ltd.
Ware
Herts SG12 0DJ

K. TRNAVSKY
Research Institute of Rheumatic Diseases
921 01 Piestany
Kupelny Ostrov 932
Czechoslovakia

M. WEATHERALL
Wellcome Research Laboratories
Langley Court
Beckenham
Kent BR3 3BS

J. WEBB
Sutton Rheumatism Research Laboratory
Royal North Shore Hospital
St Leonards
New South Wales 2065
Australia

T. J. WILLIAMS
Department of Pharmacology
Royal College of Surgeons of England
35–43 Lincoln's Inn Fields
London WC2A 3PN

Foreword

Rheumatoid arthritis and allied inflammatory diseases represent a major challenge to medical practice and pharmaceutical enterprise. On the one hand, we now admit that the term 'rheumatism' is without aetiological or pathogenetic significance and that the recognition of inflammatory rheumatic disease relies largely upon our ability to assemble deviations from normality into certain patterns which may partly fulfil our notional classification criteria. On the other hand, we also admit that current treatment and control of inflammatory rheumatic disease, though increasingly more powerful, represents a 'halfway' stage of achievement. The adoption of 'stop-gap' palliation has become obligatory because the underlying mechanisms of disease remain largely unknown. How can we proceed rationally to the recognition of new and better drugs with a more selective action against the 'rheumatic' process whilst enduring the dual handicap of pathogenetic ignorance and nosological uncertainty? This symposium, convened by Dr Jasani, addresses itself to exactly this central question, without apology and without prejudice.

At various international meetings held during World Rheumatism Year 1977, rheumatoid arthritis has become accepted as the great inflammatory disease of our time: yet it is salutary to reflect upon changing ideas of the aetiology and pathogenesis of this remarkable syndrome. In the golden age of bacteriology, rheumatoid arthritis was once regarded as an infectious disease; and rheumatic inflammation was accepted as an illustration of the 'anthropocentric' activities of Metchnikov's leucocytes in attempting to expel (or merely imprison) foreign enemy agents. Interest in the microbial hypothesis gradually waned after the failure of many attempts to isolate micro-organisms from rheumatoid joints and after the failure of antibiotic therapy to ameliorate the disease. During the last two decades, advances in immunology, microbiology and genetics have combined with advances in molecular pharmacology to promote a greater understanding of the inflammatory process. There is now a growing view that rhematoid arthritis and allied diseases arise from subtle defects in the regulation of immunological and inflammatory responses upon which both genetic and environmental factors may find expression.

The idea that such diseases may arise from genetically based immunopathological responses to ubiquitous microbial and other stimuli focuses investigative attention upon the nature and localization of rheumatic inflammation and upon the laboratory study of the inflammatory process in experimental animal models chosen for their resemblance to features of the human disease. Sections IV and V of this book demonstrate how analysis of experimental immune complex disease and of lymphocyte-mediated inflammation are beginning to provide insight into pathogenetic mechanisms of rheumatic inflammation as well as yielding new models for the pre-clinical selection of potential anti-rheumatic agents. Sections I–III 'set the scene' for the derivation of these models by providing up-to-date information on the properties of mediators; the behaviour of leucocytes; and their respective roles in the development of vascular responses in so far as they appear relevant to processes of rheumatic inflammation.

The contents of this volume reflect closely an enjoyable and authoritative two-day symposium which Dr Jasani covened in London in April 1977 as part of the First WHO/ILAR Advanced Course on Investigative Rheumatology. However, many of the contributors to this volume wrote or revised their papers after the symposium itself and in this sense the volume represents 'more' than a mere record of what took place at the two-day meeting. In editing the work, Dr Jasani has ensured that the references are up-to-date and that the dual theme of the symposium itself is reflected in the order of published papers and in the edited discussions. We believe that this publication is distinctive in juxtaposing information on the standardization of clinical criteria for the assessment of rheumatic disease and the clinical problems of recognizing anti-rheumatic drug activity, against the background of current approaches to the study of inflammation and of immunologically mediated tissue damage. The recognition of anti-rheumatic drugs is clearly a multi-disciplinary problem in which pharmacologists, immunologists and other laboratory workers need to interact closely with those who take care of patients and with those who are responsible, as in the pharmaceutical industry, for the innovation of new therapeutic substances and for their control. We are grateful to the many sponsors that enabled this symposium to take place and to the initiatives from both the World Health Organization and the International League Against Rheumatism that enabled the convening of this symposium on the occasion of World Rheumatism Year.

D. C. Dumonde

Preface

During the past 25 years, anti-rheumatic drugs have been selected empirically either on the basis of clinical measurements or in accordance with pharmacological resemblance to cortisone or aspirin in a variety of experimental models of inflammation such as for example foot-pad oedema induced with kaolin or carrageenan, cotton pellet granuloma, ultra violet-induced erythema and adjuvant arthritis.

A rational choice has remained elusive, largely on account of lack of knowledge of the pathophysiological mechanisms underlying rheumatoid synovial inflammation. With the newly emerging insight into the biological properties of specifically sensitized, immune lymphocytes and circulating immune complexes (reviewed in the Foreword by Dr D. C. Dumonde), it seemed timely to assess both the usefulness of existing laboratory methods and standardization in disease assessment.

It is too early as yet to judge the long-term impact of the dual approach of this international symposium, held on the occasion of the First Advanced Workshop Course on Investigative Rheumatology convened by the World Health Organisation (WHO) and International League Against Rheumatism (ILAR). What should, however, be evident from the ensuing records of its proceedings is that to recognize anti-rheumatic drugs that could halt rheumatoid synovitis and prevent the progressive erosive articular damage which brings about bony deformities of the inflamed joints it is essential to select chemicals not by comparison with cortisone or aspirin but according to the degree of their effectiveness against inflammation caused by immune complexes and lymphocytes which release lymphokines. To do this, the readers will no doubt conclude, it is essential to have *in vivo* models which include a role for blood vessels and lymphatics in addition to polymorphonuclear leukocytes (PMNs), platelets, macrophages and a multiplicity of plasma constituents. Consequently attempts to characterize substances active against single components of immunological inflammation, e.g. through *in vitro* study of the inhibition of lymphokines, degradative enzymes, prostaglandin biosynthesis, chemotaxis of PMNs or the stabilization of lysosomes, are likely to provide drugs with limited therapeutic usefulness in RA. The *in vitro* approach may, however, prove advantageous when a better insight into the relative importance of various cellular and plasmatic factors to the development of rheumatoid inflammation becomes available.

The art of recognition of, and development of, better anti-rheumatic drugs is of course a technology, the success of which, however, depends upon two factors: first, the scientific foundation of our concepts in the field of rheumatoid inflammation and secondly the co-operation of clinicians and the patients they care for. This, I hope, will explain why the participants of this Symposium were drawn from such diverse disciplines as pharmacology, physiology, immunology, rheumatology, toxicology, bio-medical statistics, practice of medicine and rheumatology, and clinical trials practitioners.

The assembly of individuals from such diverse backgrounds and from most corners of the world has of course been possible only because of the unceasing encouragement given to us first by those who care for our health in general, and that includes especially the WHO and those who care for the health and well-being of rheumatic patients in particular, and here I would like to single out especially ILAR and the Arthritis and Rheumatism Council of Great Britain. The hard support for the Symposium was provided by members of the pharmaceutical industry. To the officials of all these organizations I wish to extend our sincere thanks for their invaluable support.

With much pleasure and satisfaction, I also wish to thank the following: all the contributors for their co-operation in providing abstracts for the Symposium and manuscripts for the Proceedings; Dr D. C. Dumonde for his constant encouragement and guidance; Dr Gillian R. Bullock for the electron micrograph of an activated lymphocyte and Dr June Almeida for that of a circulating immune complex (×220 000) comprising hepatitis B antigen and antibody—photographs which adorn this volume; Mr Roy Henderson, Miss Popeck, and Mr Murray of the Cunard International Hotel, Hammersmith, London; and last but not least, Mr David Bloomer and Mr Martin Lister of MTP Press Limited, as well as Miss Anne Bryant and Mrs Norma Knott for their unfailing co-operation and courtesy.

M. K. Jasani

Section I:

Mediator Concepts: Pain and Its Inhibition

Chairman: **G. P. LEWIS**

1
Nature of the Inflammatory Response with Special Reference to Mediators

G. P. LEWIS

INTRODUCTION

The problem we are dealing with today starts with the variable and largely unknown aetiology of inflammatory diseases. At the residential course which some of us attended during the last few weeks, it became painfully obvious from genetic and microbiological studies that our knowledge of the aetiology of rheumatic diseases was scanty. This aspect is of course vitally important to a pharmacological approach because as Carl Pearson pointed out at that meeting, the ideal anti-rheumatic drug would be an anti-aetiological agent. But it seems that at present such a possibility is not in the hands of pharmacologists and that we must wait for further efforts from the biologists before we can get to the real source of the problem. Therefore we have to search for other points in the inflammatory process which would be suitable targets for a therapeutic approach.

INFLAMMATION AND ANTI-INFLAMMATION

Figure 1.1 gives a view of some of the main steps in the inflammatory process. In the early studies of inflammation in which the noxious stimuli were non-immunological, the obvious signs of the acute inflammatory response produced were vasodilatation, increased vascular permeability and pain. These were regarded as the cardinal signs of inflammation and it was towards these signs that the search for anti-inflammatory drugs was directed. First, a search was made for the chemical substances which mediated these effects and I shall come back to these later. Then attempts were made to synthesize antagonists of these mediators; and thirdly, in order to test these antagonists, models were devised which embodied some or all of the cardinal signs of acute inflammation. It might have been rather unfortunate that the first group of chemical substances to be used as anti-inflammatory agents were found to be active in these simple laboratory tests like skin reddening, rat-paw oedema, turpentine pleurisy and so on, because subsequently these tests became the standard models in the search for new anti-rheumatic drugs. As we can see from Figure 1.1, this limited the search just to those pathways which are marked in heavy

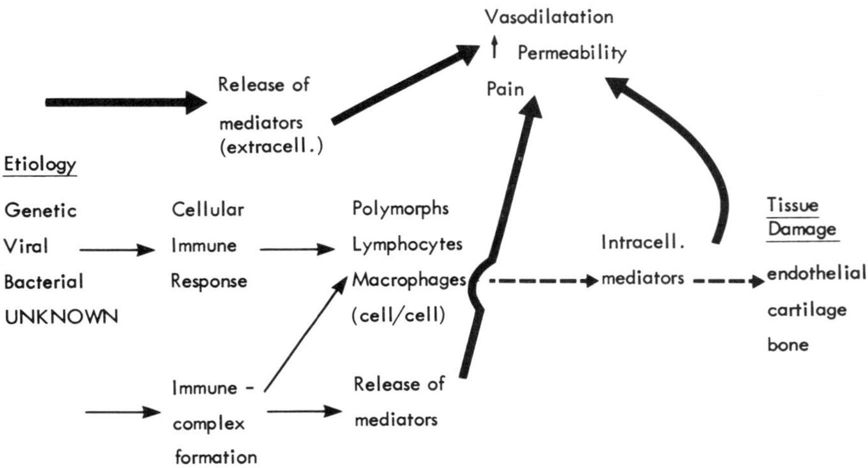

Figure 1.1 Some pathways involved in inflammation

type and thus to anti-inflammatory rather than anti-rheumatic drugs. Even nowadays some companies still rely on these simple tests as their main screen for anti-rheumatic compounds. It seems to me that they will only produce copies of the anti-inflammatory drugs already available bearing the same advantages and disadvantages. However, some investigators still believe that such tests are of value, for example Dr A. J. Lewis believes that the vascular response to u.v. irradiation is useful in the evaluation of anti-rheumatic drugs. One point of interest is that Dr Lewis has found that the anti-rheumatic drugs which have a delayed onset of action, i.e. gold and D-penicillamine reduce this u.v.-induced erythema, so we shall be watching closely for details of that finding.

Immunologists studied immune complex formation and cellular immune responses long before pharmacologists thought that these pathways should be pursued as targets for a therapeutic approach. And even then, these pathways were not examined in themselves but were incorporated into the models where we still measured the effects of agents on the vascular changes. Models which would allow us to examine the effects of potential therapeutic agents on single immunological pathways would be very useful. Would it, for instance, ever be possible to develop a drug acting to prevent an immune response and still retain sufficient specificity to avoid overwhelming toxicity? What does it mean for a drug to be active in an Arthus reaction or a Dumonde and Glynn model[1] in terms of its activity on individual pathways? To show that the drugs we have available are effective in these models is not enough because what we really want is a drug that proves fully active against inflammation in rheumatoid arthritis (RA).

One of the models most extensively used has been adjuvant arthritis and Carl Pearson, who did so much in the development of the model, will summarize for us what contribution he thinks this model has made and still is making. And finally a different kind of cell-mediated response will be described by Dr Jasani and that is the homograft reaction.

MEDIATORS OF CHRONIC INFLAMMATION

Biochemical changes in lymph during inflammation in rabbit skin homografts

Dr Jasani and I started to use the homograft reaction as a model for rheumatoid inflammation some years ago because so many of the features of skin graft rejection, both macroscopic and microscopic, resemble the changes which occur in the inflamed joints in RA and we wanted if possible to examine underlying mechanisms in the model[2]. At first we were particularly interested in the biochemical changes which occurred in lymph during the reaction. In order to study these changes we employed a technique which had been used to examine changes in the interstitial space after several kinds of injury[3]. We collected lymph directly from rabbit hind limbs bearing either autografts (which do not reject) or homografts (which do reject). We found that the pattern of intracellular enzymes leaking from the grafts into the lymph was different for autografts and homografts.

Figure 1.2 shows the activities of 6 intracellular enzymes in the lymph supernatant collected from a rabbit over a period of 17 days. At day −3 the cannula was implanted into the femoral lymphatic; at day 0 the skin was grafted onto the lower limb and at day 6 the process of rejection started. The first point we observed in this series of experiments was that there was an increase in the activity of some of the enzymes during the first 2–4 days after grafting, i.e. during the healing-in of the grafts. We saw an increase during this time of two transaminases GOT and GPT and small increases in acid phosphatase and cathepsin. It was usually these four enzymes which increased in the pre-rejection period. The main increase however, occurred just after rejection and at this time there was an increase in all the enzyme activities and particularly in LDH and β-glucuronidase (β-gluc).

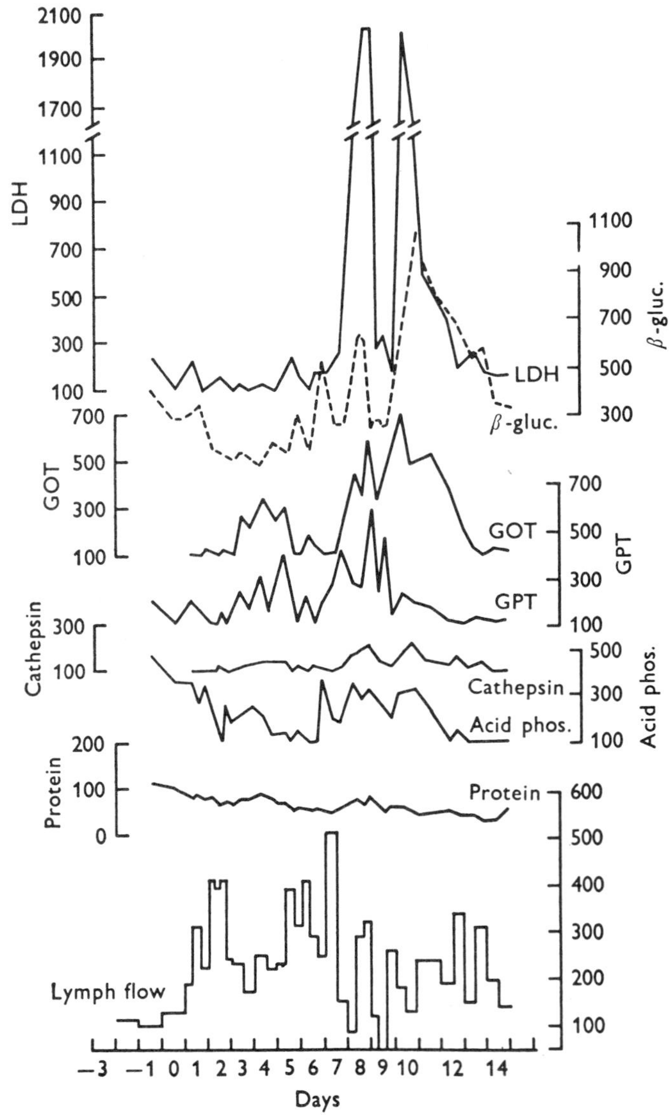

Figure 1.2 Composition of lymph and lymph flow from hind limb of NZW rabbit bearing six skin homografts. Rejection began on day 7. Enzymes and lymph flow are expressed as % of control values. Result of one experiment in which the collection of lymph was begun 3 days before grafting and lymph collected several times daily. Clotting occurred on day 7, at the onset of rejection, and on day 9, but once cleared it was possible to continue collections up to the 14th postoperative day. (Jasani and Lewis, 1971[2]: by permission of *Journal of Physiology*.)

Figure 1.3 illustrates the changes in enzyme activities in the femoral lymph collected from a limb bearing autografts. There are two experiments represented in this figure. One started 3 days before grafting and continued to

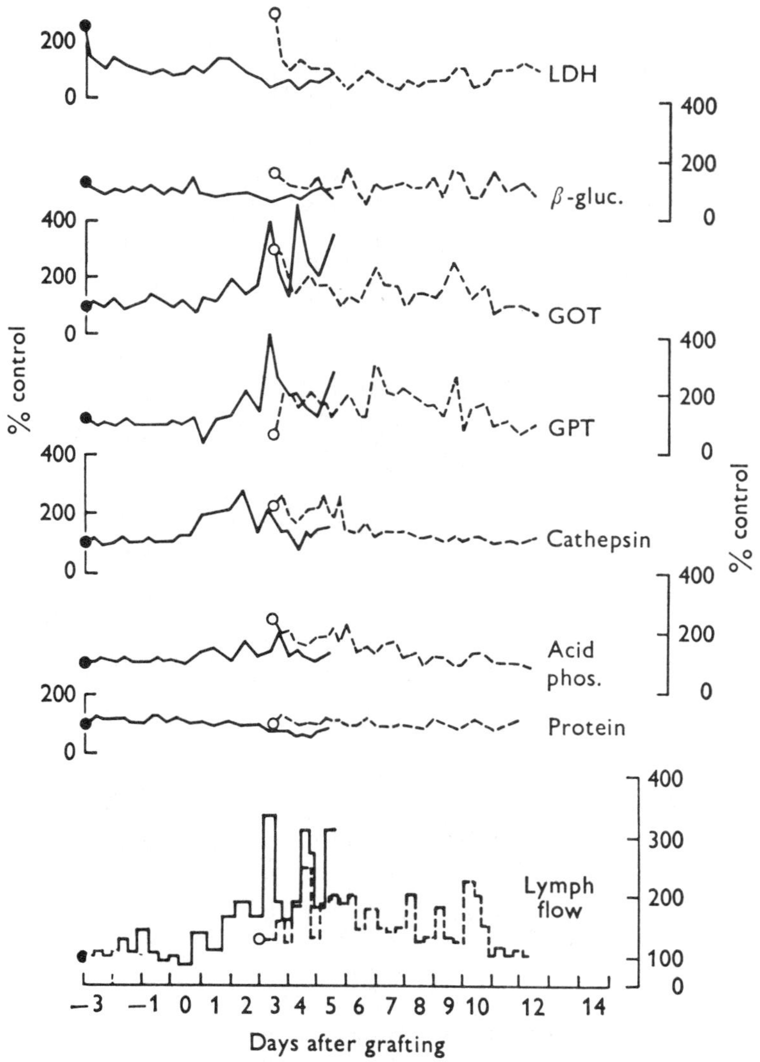

Figure 1.3 Composition of lymph and lymph flow from rabbit hind limb bearing six skin autografts. Enzymes and lymph flow are expressed as % of control values. Results of two experiments, one in which the collection of lymph was begun three days before grafting ●— and in the other on the third day after grafting, O---. Lymph was collected several times daily. (Jasani and Lewis, 1971[2]: by permission of *Journal of Physiology*.)

day 6 when the lymph clotted and the other in which cannulation was made three days after grafting the lymph was collected until day 11.

What we see is an increase in the same four enzymes during the period 2–4 days after grafting, but no later increase. Since rejection does not occur in the case of autografts, it seems likely that the main increases which were found in the homograft experiments are related to the specific immunological reaction of rejection. On the other hand, these early increases appear to be related to the non-specific reaction to the trauma of transplantation because it occurs in both homograft and autograft experiments.

A clue as to the origin of these enzymes in the homograft lymph came from experiments in which we examined the enzyme activities of the lymphocytes in the lymph. We found that there was an increase in the enzyme activities of the lymphocytes at the time of rejection; not an increase in the cell count but an increase in the activities per cell. In addition these cells were particularly rich in LDH and β-gluc — the two enzymes which increased most of all in the lymph supernatant during rejection. It appears therefore that the main increases which we find in supernatant homograft lymph originate in the lymphocytes which undergo necrosis around the graft tissue.

Dr Jasani will refer to another aspect of the homograft reaction, i.e. fibrin deposition which he thinks is another lymphocyte-induced effect. He also has some interesting information about the effect of anti-inflammatory drugs on this phenomenon. So here then we are dealing with mediators which play a role in chronic inflammatory reactions. The fact that they are enzymes does not, to my mind, exclude their being classified as mediators.

With regard to the scheme outlined in Figure 1.1, a suitable target for a therapeutic approach could be the selective reduction of an excess of hydrolytic and other enzyme activity either through enzyme inhibition or prevention of their release.

Lymph flow during inflammation in rabbit skin homografts

Another finding from our earlier experiments with homografts agreed very nicely with the work of Dudley Dumonde and his colleagues[4] on lymphocyte-activation products which they have called lymphokines. When we examined the lymphatic and vascular connexions of the graft, we found that in most high-dose homograft experiments a lymphatic connection was never established between the donor and the host. This is illustrated in Figure 1.4 which summarizes the results obtained from seventy-one homograft experiments and contrasts them with those obtained from fifty-three autograft experiments in which rejection does not occur. From day 7 onwards after grafting a lymphatic connexion was present in all autografts and it was independent of the number of grafts per animal. On day 6 after grafting, 7 out of 9 autografts had lymphatic connexions and even on day 5, 2 out of 9 autografts already had such connexions. On the other hand, no lymphatic connexion was established in

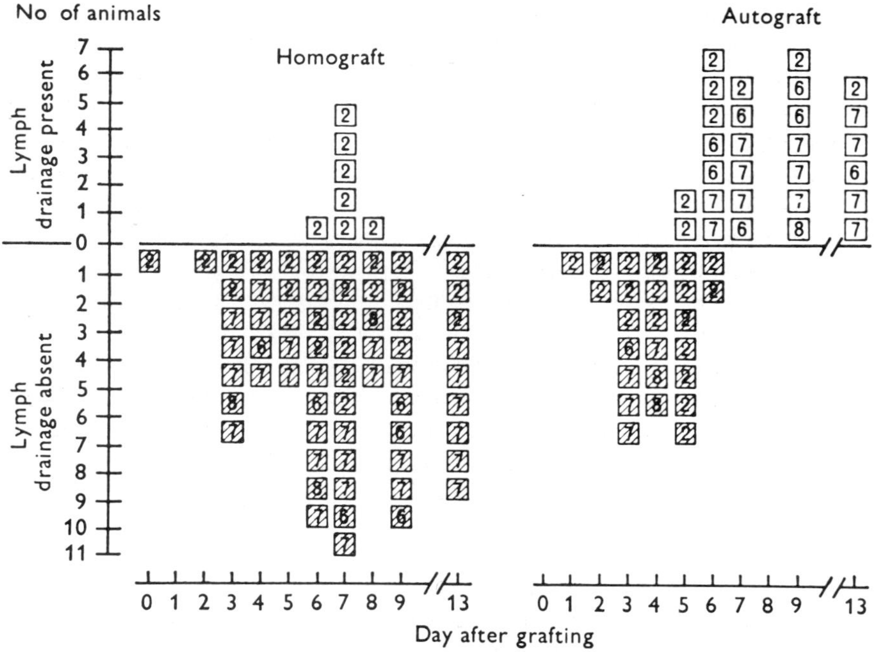

Figure 1.4 Presence or absence of lymph drainage in homografts and autografts as judged by the appearance in the lymphatic cannula of Evans blue dye injected into the graft tissue. Each square represents the result of one experiment obtained on the day indicated by the abscissae. The numeral in each square denotes the number of grafts per animal. The open squares above the line give the experiments in which lymph drainage occurred, the hatched squares below the line those in which it did not occur. (Jasani and Lewis, 1971[2]: by permission of *Journal of Physiology*.)

homografts after the 8th post-operative day. Lymphatic connexions were obtained in only seven out of the thirty-three experiments tested between days 6 and 8 and only in experiments with low dose of grafts per animal. Of these seven experiments with lymphatic drainage five occurred on day 7 and one each on day 6 and day 8. An explanation of this finding came when we examined the vascularization of the grafts (Figure 1.5).

Figure 1.5 summarizes results obtained from fifty-three experiments with autografts and seventy-six with homografts. In both groups vascularization between graft and host tissue occurred in about half the experiments on day 4 and it was present in all experiments on day 5. From day 6 onwards, the autografts and homografts behaved differently. All the autografts retained their vascularity whilst in an increasing number of homografts from day 6 onwards, the blood flow ceased as a result of the onset of rejection.

Although the establishment of vascularity of homografts is the same with animals receiving a low or a high dose of grafts, the time of vascular shut-down is influenced by the number of grafts transplanted. On day 6, all five animals

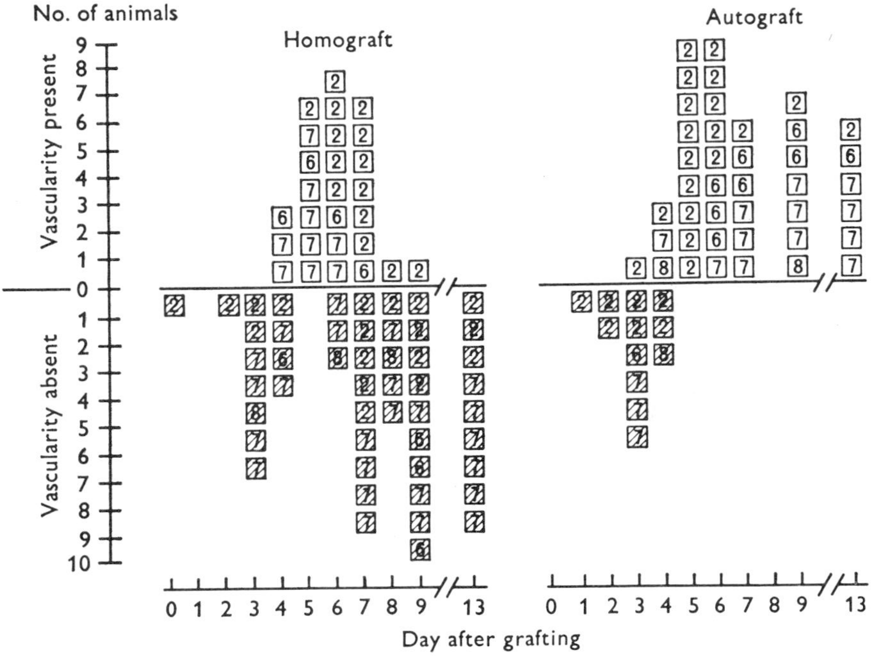

Figure 1.5 Presence or absence of vascularization in homografts and autografts as judged by blueing of the skin after intravenous injection of Evans blue. Each square represents the results of one experiment obtained on the day indicated by the abscissae. The numeral in each square denotes the number of grafts per animal. The open squares above the line give the experiments in which vascularity was present, the hatched squares below the line those in which it was absent. (Jasani and Lewis, 1971[2]: by permission of *Journal of Physiology*.)

with two grafts still retained blood flow as opposed to three out of six animals with 6–8 grafts. Further, on day 7, only one out of five animals with high dosage grafts retained vascular connexion while six out of eleven did so in the low dosage group. These findings parallel the observations concerning the appearance of the grafts in that the low dosage grafts remain pink and vascularized for about 24 hours longer than the high-dose grafts.

Even a slight retardation of the rejection process, of not more than 24 hours, as occurred in animals bearing the low-dose homografts therefore favours the development of a lymphatic connexion between the donor homograft and the recipient tissue. In animals bearing the high dose of homografts (6–8) daily treatment with the immunosuppressive agent, cyclophosphamide, delayed the vascular shut-down by up to 5–7 days. In all of them vascularity as well as lymphatic connexion developed and once established was retained as in the autografts.

According to these findings in animals bearing high-dose homografts a lymphatic connexion is not established between the host and the donor graft unless homograft rejection is delayed, the explanation being that the vascular shut-down accompanying the onset of rejection occurs before the lymphatics develop.

The reason for mentioning this finding is because of its wider implications in the mechanism of graft rejection. The sensitization that leads to rejection of the graft tissue takes place in two stages; first contact between the antigen of the graft tissue and lymphocytes entering the graft from the blood stream; and second, passage of the primed lymphocytes into the regional lymph node. To achieve the second stage it has been implied that there must be a lymphatic drainage of the graft itself to convey the primed lymphocytes to the regional lymph node. Our experiments show that this is not a pre-requisite of homograft rejection. However, a lymphatic drainage of the underlying graft bed does appear to be present and may constitute a third stage in the sensitization process, i.e. the migration of the primed cell, or a different cell like a macrophage, back into the recipient tissue before it is taken by the host's lymphatic system to the regional lymph node. So perhaps we must add to our list of chronic mediators diffusable substances which might bring about such cell-to-cell interactions (Table 1.1).

Table 1.1 Mediators of chronic inflammation

Kinins, prostaglandins?
Enzymes:
Hydrolases (acidic and neutral), cathepsin
Collagenases, etc.
Lymphokines: Mitogenic, cytotoxic, chemotactic, vasoactive
Complement factors: Chemotactic, vasoactive, anaphylotoxin, etc.
Cell-to-cell interactants: Helpers, suppressors, etc.

Alternatively, it is possible that the diffusable products from lymphocytes might help to provide an explanation of the effects seen in regional lymph nodes during the rejection reaction in a different way. Perhaps lymphocytes activated at the site of the graft produce lymphokines peripherally which diffuse into the host tissue, are taken up in the lymph as soluble substances and are transported to the regional lymph node, possibly together with primed lymphocytes to produce the changes observed. Dr Dumonde and his colleagues have already shown that injection of these lymphocyte-activation products into the afferent lymphatics produces effects in the regional lymph node that closely resemble the effects produced in the node by a cell-mediated response in the tissue.

Blood flow during inflammation in rabbit skin homografts

There is also evidence that some of the vascular changes which occur during chronic inflammation are mediated by lymphocytic mediators. Catherine Bach's chapter explains the theory that the fluid retention which occurs in homografts is lymphocyte-mediated. Beverley Young, Tim Williams and I[5] at the Royal College of Surgeons have also been looking at blood flow changes in grafts using the ^{133}Xe clearance technique by measuring the washout of radioactivity from each graft with a collimated γ-scintillation detector.

Figure 1.6 shows that the clearance plot of a homograft 1 day after grafting is monoexponential. On days 5, 6 and 7, the curves contained in addition a faster component which could be derived by curve-peeling. Figure 1.6 shows the curve on day 6 with its two derived exponentials. Biexponential curves were also produced in normal skin. On day 8, homograft curves returned to monoexponentials (Figure 1.6) corresponding to visible signs of rejection,

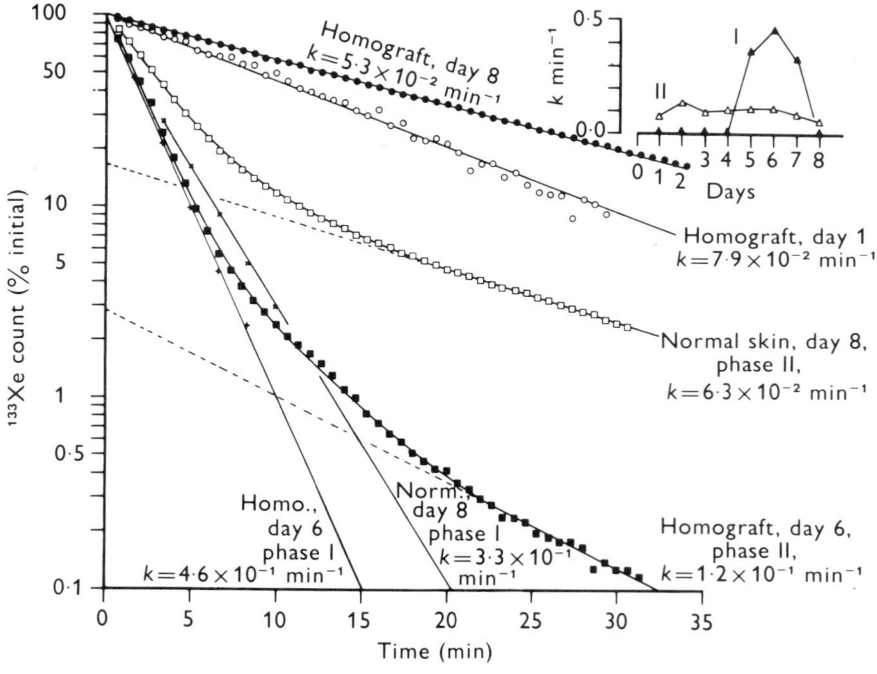

Figure 1.6 ^{133}Xe clearance curves in one homograft 1, 6 and 8 days after grafting. Inset shows the changes in rate constants for the homograft, phases I and II. (From Lewis *et al.*, 1971[5]: by permission of *Journal of Physiology (London)*.)

whereas autograft curves remained biexponential. Changes in slope of the slow phase (phase II) reflect changes in graft thickness and vascularity of the subcutaneous graft bed and the slope of the fast component (phase I) of the ^{133}Xe clearance curve provides a measure of blood flow in grafted skin.

When the blood flow changes which occur in homografts were compared with those in autografts, we found that although blood flow developed during day 3–4 in both types of graft, the vascular connexion remained only in autografts; at the onset of rejection of homografts there was a sharp shut-down of blood vessels. We are interested now in finding out the mediator of this effect, but as yet we have only been able to show that it is probably not an 'acute' mediator.

It is interesting that in these experiments we found that changes in exudation of plasma proteins did not correspond to the blood flow, changes being less pronounced in the homografts than one would expect. This agrees very well with Catherine Bach's findings and with the fact that we[2] did not find an increase in the protein concentration in the lymph draining homografts.

This interesting relationship between increased vascular permeability, hyperaemia and stasis is going to be discussed, although not in homografts by Dr Movat.

Concluding remarks

All these models which I have mentioned represent an attempt to embody as many of the features of chronic inflammation as possible, but generally little attempt was made to analyse the mechanisms of each step of the reaction. The alternative approach is to dissect the reaction into its components and to examine each of these pathways in isolation. Researchers into the immune complex and cell-mediated responses will explain simple procedures to examine the effects of potential anti-rheumatic drugs on these central pathways. Several factors found in the pathways outlined in Figure 1.1 influence the migration and accumulation of cells, but it is now obvious that not all inflammatory cells are influenced in the same way or at the same time and Dr Perper's chapter deals with the way in which various cell types are influenced and what procedures we can use to evaluate the effects of drugs on these pathways.

MEDIATORS OF ACUTE INFLAMMATION

Returning to the subject of acute mediators (Table 1.2) we can still regard histamine and bradykinin as two of the primary mediators of acute inflammation. Histamine is stored in mast cells and generally produces the immediate response which lasts until the kinin-forming system is activated and kinins are produced as a result of enzyme action. 5-Hydroxytryptamine probably plays a role in reactions which involve platelets and this will be discussed in the section on the Arthus reactions and in Dr Movat's chapter on thrombosis in the microcirculation.

Prostaglandins must now also be considered as mediators in acute and possibly in chronic inflammation, but it seems that they are not primary mediators but modulators of the actions of other mediators. The next two chapters by Salvador Moncada and Sergio Ferreira deal with the role of prostaglandins (PGs) in inflammation and I shall just briefly discuss two points

Table 1.2 Mediators of acute inflammation

Histamine	stored in mast cells
Bradykinin	formed in body fluids
5-Hydroxytryptamine	taken up and stored
Prostaglandins	synthesized from cell membranes
SRS-A	formed in allergic reactions in lung

from the work going on in our department, in which PGs interact with the other mediators.

First, Williams[6–8] has been studying the potentiating action of PGs on the effect of histamine and bradykinin on vascular permeability. Figure 1.7 shows the effect of increasing doses of PGE_2 on exudation of labelled albumin (above) and on blood flow measured by ^{133}Xe clearance (below). Even at 300 ng, PGE_2 did not cause increased vascular permeability although as little as 0.3 ng produced vasodilatation. When these doses of PG were mixed with a standard

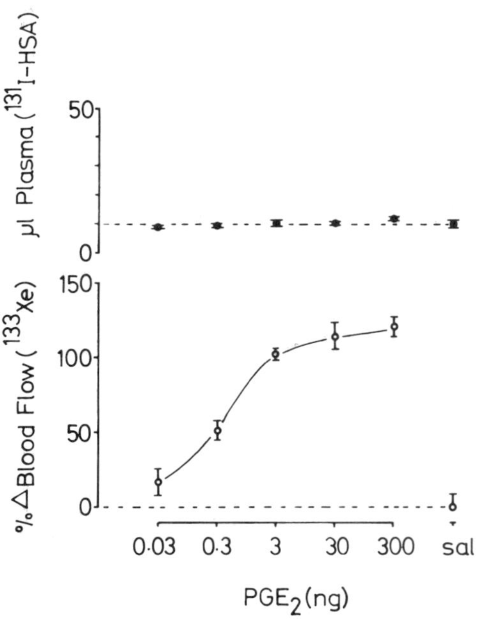

Figure 1.7 Dose-response curve to PGE_2 in rabbit skin. Top trace shows that increasing doses of PGE_2 (in 100 μl injections) produced little evidence of exudation, as measured by [^{131}I] albumin accumulation. Dotted line represents plasma volume in saline-injected control sites. Lower trace shows increasing blood flow in response to increasing doses of PGE_2, as measured by ^{133}Xe clearance. Blood flow is expressed as percentage of flow in saline-injected sites. (Results are expressed as: mean ± SE mean, $n = 6$.) (Williams, 1976[8]: by permission of *Postgraduate Medical Journal.*)

dose of histamine (Figure 1.8) there was not only an increasing vasodilatation but an increasing enhancement of the effect that the standard dose of histamine has on exudation of plasma protein. The evidence collected so far supports the view that this potentiation is due to the vasodilatation produced by the PG.

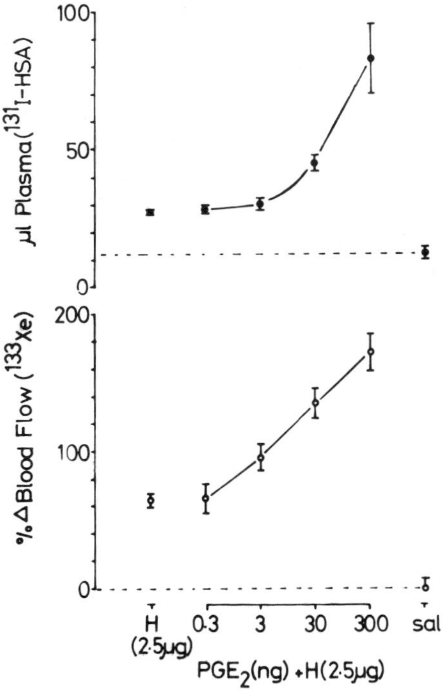

Figure 1.8 Potentiation of plasma exudation produced by a fixed dose of histamine and increasing doses of PGE_2. (Results expressed as in Figure 1.7.) (Williams, 1976[8]: by permission of *Postgraduate Medical Journal*.)

Figure 1.9 shows that endogenously produced PGs can act in the same way[7]. Although no potentiation was observed with bradykinin/*Bordetella pertussis* mixture, it was found that intradermal injection of *B. pertussis* (2.5×10^8 organisms/site) greatly potentiated the exudation produced by an injection of bradykinin given some time later. It appears therefore that time is required for the potentiating agent to be formed, and the optimum is usually obtained when the *B. pertussis* is injected 60 min before the bradykinin. Furthermore, it is abolished by PG-synthetase inhibitor indomethacin, although the potentiating effect of PG itself is not affected by indomethacin[8]. I think that this is the first demonstration of potentiation by endogenously produced PGs.

That is one kind of modulation by PGs but finally I would like to show you

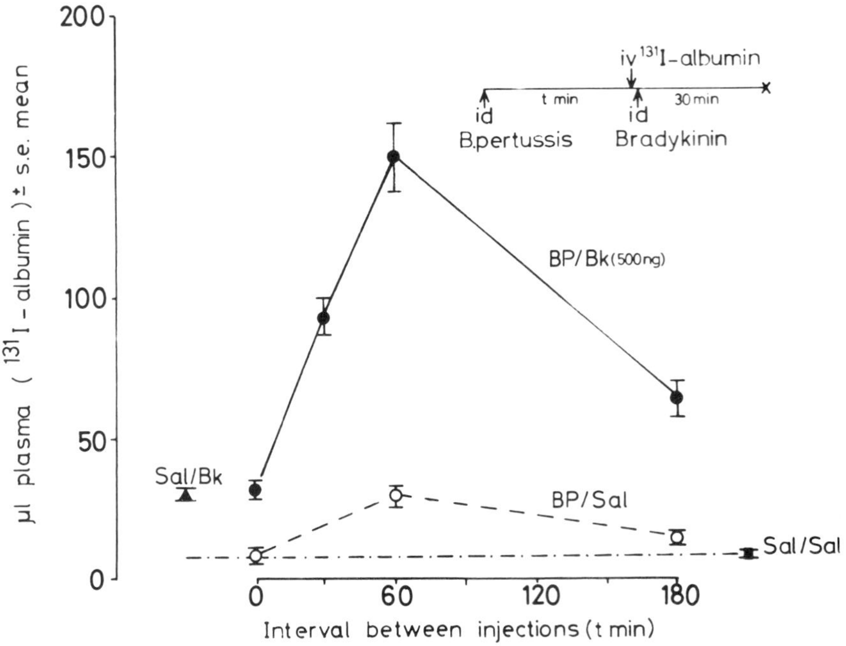

Figure 1.9 Time-course of potentiation of bradykinin (500 ng)-induced exudation by a preceding intradermal injection of *B. pertussis* (2.5×10^8 organisms) in rabbit skin. ● 1st injection of *B. pertussis*/2nd injection of bradykinin. ▲ saline/bradykinin, ○ *B. pertussis*/saline, ■ saline/saline. Abscissa is interval between 1st and 2nd injections. Exudation was measured for 30 min following 2nd injection. $n = 6$. (Williams, 1977[7]: by permission of *British Journal of Pharmacology*.)

how PGs can exert a modulating effect in the opposite direction. It has been shown that some inflammatory cells have receptors which when stimulated cause an increase in intracellular cAMP, which in some way inhibits the release of mediators [9,10]. It has also been shown that PGs stimulate such a receptor and cause a reduction in the release of other mediators. Engineer, Piper and Sirois[11] at the Royal College of Surgeons have shown this to occur in an immunological response in sensitized guinea-pig lungs. The amount of prostaglandin and SRS-A released after challenge of perfused sensitized guinea-pig lungs was observed in controls and compared with a series of sensitized lungs treated with different concentrations of indomethacin. Indomethacin reduced the amount of PGs synthesized and therefore the amount released, whilst at the same time the amount of SRS-A release was increased. It certainly looks as if this is an inhibition of a negative feed-back mechanism.

It seems likely that these sort of interactions of mediators might well play an important role both in acute and chronic inflammation.

References

1. Dumonde, D. C. and Glynn, L. E. (1962). The production of arthritis in rabbits by an immunological reaction to fibrin. *Br. J. Exp. Path.*, **43**, 373
2. Jasani, M. K. and Lewis, G. P. (1971). Lymph flow and changes in intracellular enzymes during healing and rejection of rabbit skin grafts. *J. Physiol. (Lond.)*, **219**, 525
3. Lewis, G. P. (1975). A lymphatic approach to tissue injury. *New Engl. J. Med.*, **293**, 287
4. Dumonde, D. C. (1970). Lymphokines: mediators and regulators of cellular immune responses. *Ann. Immunol.*, **2**, 129
5. Lewis, G. P., Peck, M. J., Williams, T. J. and Young, Beverley, A. (1975). Measurement of blood flow in rabbit skin homografts and autografts using a ^{133}Xe clearance technique. *J. Physiol. (Lond.)*, **254**, 32
6. Williams, T. J. (1976). Simultaneous measurement of local plasma exudation and blood flow changes induced by intradermal injection of vasoactive substances, using ^{131}I albumin and ^{133}Xe. *J. Physiol. (Lond.)*, **254**, 4
7. Williams, T. J. (1976). Potentiation of bradykinin-induced exudation following intradermal injection of particulate or colloidal materials in the rabbit: evidence for prostaglandin release and action in inflammation. *Br. J. Pharmacol.* (in press)
8. Williams, T. J. (1976). Oedema and vasodilatation in inflammation: the relevance of prostaglandins. *Postgraduate Med. J.* (in press)
9. Orange, R. P., Austen, W. G. and Austen, K. F. (1971). Immunological release of histamine and SRS-A from human lung. *J. Exptl. Med.*, **134**, 136
10. Bourne, H. R., Lichtenstein, L. M., Melmon, K. L., Henney, C. S., Weinstein, Y. and Shearer, G. M. (1974). Modulation of inflammation and immunity by cyclic AMP. *Science*, **184**, 19
11. Engineer, D., Piper, P. J. and Sirois, P. (1976). Interaction between the release of SRS-A and of prostaglandins. *Br. J. Pharmacol*, **57**, 460

2
Metabolic Products of Arachidonic Acid in Inflammation

S. MONCADA

1. INTRODUCTION

Inflammation is a complex response during which chemical mediators such as histamine, 5-hydroxytryptamine (5HT), slow reacting substance in anaphylaxis (SRS-A), various chemotactic factors, bradykinin and prostaglandins of the E and F series may be liberated locally. Known anti-inflammatory substances have little or no antagonistic activity towards the direct effects of at least four types of mediators released during inflammation, namely histamine, 5HT, bradykinin and the prostaglandins. Similarly, potent antagonists of 5HT or histamine have little or no value in inflammation. Consequently, one must question the importance of these long-standing mediators in the maintenance of inflammation. Moreover, it is fundamentally important to clarify the way in which all mediators interact to bring about the signs and symptoms of the inflammatory reaction in order to understand the process.

As a consequence of the discovery that aspirin-like drugs inhibit the biosynthesis of prostaglandins[1–3], our knowledge of the inflammatory process has increased, and the way in which prostaglandins participate in this process has been clarified[4–6].

In the last few years new products of arachidonic acid metabolism (Figure 2.1) have been discovered. Their role during the inflammatory process is being currently studied and information is still incomplete.

2. THE EFFECTS OF OTHER PRODUCTS OF ARACHIDONIC ACID METABOLISM

Prostaglandin endoperoxides (PGG_2 and PGH_2) cause pronounced biological

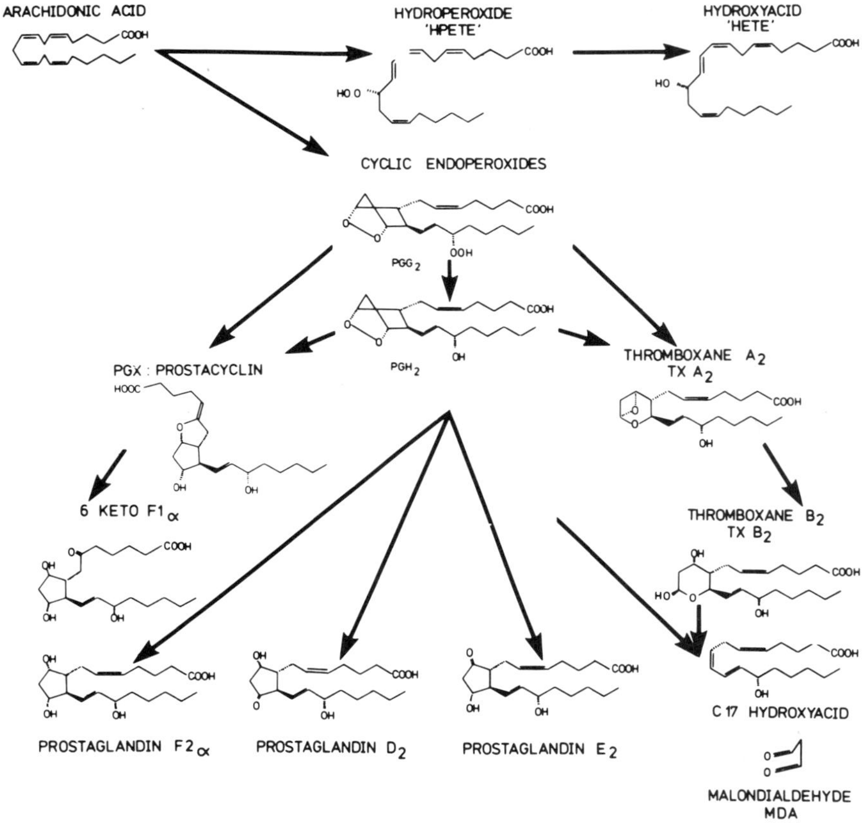

Figure 2.1 Metabolic pathway of arachidonic acid

effects, such as contraction of the rabbit aorta and guinea pig trachea. In both these tissues the endoperoxides are more potent than the stable prostaglandins. They also increase airway resistance in guinea pigs and induce platelet aggregation[7]. Some of the actions of endoperoxides might be due to their conversion into thromboxane A_2 (TXA_2). Furthermore, stable analogues of the endoperoxides (which exhibit thromboxane-like activity) are among the most powerful pulmonary pressor agents in the dog[8] and inducers of platelet aggregation *in vitro*[9]. Figure 2.1 shows the structures of the products of arachidonic acid metabolism.

As far as the pro-inflammatory activity of these compounds is concerned, Willis *et al.*[10] reported that LASS (later characterized chemically as PGH_2) did not show any pain-producing activity in mice and had very little pro-inflammatory activity when injected into the paws of rats. More recent reports have indicated that prostaglandin endoperoxides or their stable analogues have similar effects to PGE_2, potentiating the pro-inflammatory effect of other mediators[11,12].

It is not yet clear whether the effects of prostaglandin endoperoxides are direct or due to their conversion into other substances. However, an interesting proposition has been advanced by Kuehl *et al.*[13]. They suggest that the conversion from PGG_2 to PGH_2 gives rise to an oxygen radical which might be responsible for some of the signs and symptoms of inflammation. Our own experiments do not support this hypothesis since the pro-inflammatory effects of PGH_2 and PGG_2 are not different[14].

So far there are no reports on the effect of TXA_2 on inflammation and its role will be difficult to assess in view of its very short half life ($\simeq$ 30 sec). However, phagocytosing white cells[15] and aggregating platelets[16,17] produce TXA_2, and thromboxane B_2 (TXB_2) the stable end product of TXA_2 has been reported to be chemotactic[18]. Moreover, fluid obtained from carrageenan-induced granuloma converts arachidonic acid into TXB_2 *in vitro*[19]. In view of this, selective inhibition of TXA_2 formation could modify the inflammatory process.

Selective inhibition of thromboxane formation has been attempted using benzydamine[20], a phenyl phosphonate derivative of phloretin phosphate designated as N-0164 [21], and imidazole or 1-methyl imidazole[22]. Imidazole has very little activity on cyclo-oxygenase ($IC_{50} > 800$ μg/ml) but has anti-inflammatory activity[23]. Whether this effect is a result of inhibition of thromboxane synthetase or any other action remains to be clarified. It is also important to clarify the participation of other unstable intermediates in arachidonic acid metabolism in the inflammatory process.

The biological activity of the products of the lipoxygenase pathway of arachidonic acid metabolism is not well documented but recent work[24] has shown that HETE is chemotactic for polymorphonuclear leukocytes and it is possible that HPETE, the hydroperoxide intermediate in the formation of HETE, might contribute to the production of pain in the same way as other fatty acid peroxides[25]. Drugs which inhibit the lipoxygenase as well as the cyclo-oxygenase would reduce both chemotaxis and prostaglandin production. This could represent a significant advantage in terms of anti-inflammatory activity over the aspirin-like drugs, which only inhibit the cyclo-oxygenase pathway and have little or no effect on the migration of PMN leukocytes.

Recently, an unstable product of arachidonic acid metabolism has been discovered[26–28]. This substance, which was called PGX, is formed by the vessel wall and is a potent inhibitor of platelet aggregation and a vasodilator. Its chemical structure has been characterized and the compound renamed as prostacyclin or PGI_2 [29]. The generation of prostacyclin is inhibited by a lipid peroxide, 15-hydroperoxy arachidonic acid[27,28] and other fatty acid hydroperoxides[30]. As a result of these findings it has been suggested[31] that lipid peroxides generated during the early stages of the inflammatory process could, by inhibiting prostacyclin formation, divert prostaglandin endoperoxide metabolism to the pro-inflammatory prostaglandin E_2 and TXA_2. If this concept is substantiated, part of the inflammatory process could be considered as a lipid peroxide disease, since lipid peroxides mimic some of the signs and symptoms of inflammation[25] and besides, they would re-direct the arachidonic acid metabolism towards pro-inflammatory products.

Although the study of its pharmacology is still limited, prostacyclin seems a more selective and specific substance than the stable prostaglandins E_1 or E_2. An example of this is that although prostacyclin is a much more potent inhibitor of platelet aggregation than PGE_1 (20–40 times) its pro-inflammatory activity or the pro-inflammatory activity of its stable metabolite 6-keto $PGF_{1\alpha}$ [29,32] are less apparent[33].

References

1. Vane, J. R. (1971). Inhibition of prostaglandin synthesis as a mechanism of action for aspirin-like drugs. *Nature (London),* **231,** 232
2. Ferreira, S. H., Moncada, S. and Vane, J. R. (1971). Indomethacin and aspirin abolish prostaglandin release from the spleen. *Nature (London),* **231,** 237
3. Smith, J. B. and Willis, A. L. (1971). Aspirin selectively inhibits prostaglandin production in human platelets. *Nature (London),* **231,** 235
4. Vane, J. R. (1974). Mode of action of aspirin and similar compounds. In H. J. Robinson and J. R. Vane (eds.) *Prostaglandin Synthetase Inhibitors,* pp. 155–163. (New York: Raven Press)
5. Ferreira, S. H. and Vane, J. R. (1974). New aspects of the mode of action of non-steroid anti-inflammatory drugs. *Ann. Rev. Pharmacol.,* **14,** 57
6. Ferreira, S. H., Moncada, S. and Vane, J. R. (1974). Prostaglandins and signs and symptoms of inflammation. In H. J. Robinson and J. R. Vane (eds.) *Prostaglandin Synthetase Inhibitors,* pp. 175–187. (New York: Raven Press)
7. Hamberg, M., Hedqvist, P., Strandberg, K., Svensson, J. and Samuelsson, B. (1975). Prostaglandin endoperoxides. IV. Effects on smooth muscle. *Life Sci.,* **16,** 451
8. Kadowitz, P. (1976). In: 1976 Winter Prostaglandin Conference Report, Vail, Colorado. *Prostaglandins,* **11,** 437
9. Malmsten, C. (1976). Some biological effects of prostaglandin endoperoxide analogues. *Life Sci.,* **18,** 169
10. Willis, A. L., Vane, F. M., Kuhn, D. C., Scott, C. G. and Petrin, M. (1974). An endoperoxide aggregator (LASS) formed in platelets in response to thrombotic stimuli. *Prostaglandins,* **8,** 453
11. Vane, J. R. (1976). Prostaglandins as mediators of inflammation. In B. Samuelsson and R. Paoletti (eds.) *Advances in Prostaglandin and Thromboxane Research,* pp. 791–802. (New York: Raven Press)
12. Hagermark, O., Strandberg, K. and Hamberg, M. (1976). Potentiating effects of prostaglandin E_2 and the prostaglandin endoperoxide PGH_2 on cutaneous responses in man. *J. Invest. Derm.,* **66,** 266
13. Kuehl, Jr., F. A., Hules, J. L., Egan, J. W., Ham, E. A., Beveridge, G. C. and van Arman, C. G. (1977). Role of prostaglandin endoperoxide PGG_2 in inflammatory processes. *Nature (London),* **265,** 170
14. Ferreira, S. H., Moncada, S. and Vane, J. R. (1977). Are prostaglandins or their unstable endoperoxide intermediates the primary inflammatory mediators affected by aspirin-like drugs? (In preparation)
15. Higgs, G. A., Bunting, S., Moncada, S. and Vane, J. R. (1976). Polymorphonuclear leukocytes produce thromboxane A_2-like activity during phagocytosis. *Prostaglandins,* **12,** 749
16. Svensson, J., Hamberg, M. and Samuelsson, B. (1975). Prostaglandin endoperoxides, IX.

Characterization of rabbit aorta contracting substance (RCS) from guinea-pig lung and human platelets. *Acta Physiol. Scand.*, **94,** 222

17. Needleman, P., Moncada, S., Bunting, S., Hamberg, M. and Vane, J. R. (1976). Identification of an enzyme in platelet microsomes which generates thromboxane A_2 from prostaglandin endoperoxides. *Nature (London),* **261,** 558
18. Boot, J. R., Dawson, W. and Kitchen, E. A. (1976). The chemotactic activity of thromboxane B_2: a possible role in inflammation. *J. Physiol.*, **257,** 47
19. Chang, W–C., Murota, S. I. and Tsurufuji, S. (1977). Thromboxane B_2 transformed from arachidonic acid in carrageenin-induced granuloma. *Prostaglandins,* **13,** 17
20. Moncada, S., Needleman, P., Bunting, S. and Vane, J. R. (1976). Prostaglandin endoperoxide and thromboxane generating systems and their selective inhibition. *Prostaglandins,* **12,** 323
21. Kulkarni, P. S. and Eakins, K. E. (1976). N-0164 inhibits generation of thromboxane A_2-like activity from prostaglandin endoperoxides by human platelet microsomes. *Prostaglandins,* **12,** 465
22. Moncada, S., Bunting, S., Mullane, K., Thorogood, P., Vane, J. R., Raz, A. and Needleman, P. (1977). Imidazole: A selective inhibitor of thromboxane synthetase. *Prostaglandins,* **13,** 611
23. Puig Muset, P., Puig Parellada, P. and Martin Esteve, J. (1972). *Biochemical and Pharmacological Aspects of Imidazole.* 177p. (Barcelona: Editorial Jims)
24. Turner, S. R., Tainer, J. A. and Lynn, W. S. (1976). Biogenesis of chemotactic molecules by the arachidonate lipoxygenase system of platelets. *Nature (London),* **257,** 680
25. Ferreira, S. H. (1972). Prostaglandins, aspirin-like drugs and analgesia. *Nature (London),* **240,** 200
26. Moncada, S., Gryglewski, R. J., Bunting, S. and Vane, J. R. (1976). An enzyme isolated from arteries transforms prostaglandin endoperoxides to an unstable substance that inhibits platelet aggregation. *Nature (London),* **263,** 663
27. Gryglewski, R. J., Bunting, S., Moncada, S., Flower, R. J. and Vane, J. R. (1976). Arterial walls are protected against deposition of platelet thrombi by a substance (prostaglandin X) which they make from prostaglandin endoperoxides. *Prostaglandins,* **12,** 685
28. Moncada, S., Gryglewski, R. J., Bunting, S. and Vane, J. R. (1976). A lipid peroxide inhibits the enzyme in blood vessel microsomes that generates from prostaglandin endoperoxides the substance (prostaglandin X) which prevents platelet aggregation. *Prostaglandins,* **12,** 715
29. Johnson, R. A., Morton, D. R., Kinner, J. H., Gorman, R. R., McGuire, J. R., Sun, F. F., Whittaker, N., Bunting, S., Salmon, J. A., Moncada, S. and Vane, J. R. (1976). The chemical characterization of prostaglandin X (prostacyclin). *Prostaglandins,* **12,** 915
30. Salmon, J. A., Smith, D., Flower, R. J., Moncada, S. and Vane, J. R. (1977). Characterization of prostacyclin synthesizing enzyme in the arterial wall. (In preparation)
31. Moncada, S. and Vane, J. R. (1977). The discovery of prostacyclin (PGX); a fresh insight into arachidonic acid metabolism. *Proc. of the Interscience Foundation Meeting,* Santa Monica, California. Dec. 1–3, 1976. (In press)
32. Pace-Asciak, C. (1976). Isolation, structure and biosynthesis of 6-keto prostaglandin $F_{1\alpha}$ in the rat stomach. *J. Am. Chem. Soc.*, **98,** 2348
33. Higgs, E. A., Moncada, S. and Vane, J. R. (1977). Inflammatory effects of prostacyclin (PGI_2) and 6-oxo-$PGF_{1\alpha}$ in the rat paw. (In preparation)

3
Antialgic effect of Aspirin-like Drugs and the Inhibition of Prostaglandin Synthesis

S. H. FERREIRA, BERENICE B. LORENZETTI, MARIA SALETE, A. CASTRO and F. M. A. CORREA

INTRODUCTION

Salicylates, in common with other non-steroidal anti-inflammatory drugs (NSAIDs), do not depress the pain threshold of non-injured tissue as is the case with narcotic analgesics such as morphine, or local anaesthetics. Instead, they lower the pain threshold of only inflamed tissues; and this is why their pain-relieving effect is referred to as antialgic rather than analgesic.

Woodbury[1] considered that salicylates alleviated certain types of pain, including that associated with inflammation, by virtue of their selective depressant effect on the CNS. Although experimental evidence in support of his idea is still weak, the notion remains attractive in view of a general relationship that exists between the antialgic and antipyretic effect of most NSAIDs. Antipyresis is most probably due to the central action of salicylate-like drugs on the hypothalamus[2].

In the past 10 years the observations of Lim and associates[3,4] have been followed by reports, including our own[5–10], showing that aspirin-induced antialgesia may be due to an action of the drug locally at the site of inflammation. If so, the questions which concern us today are (a) is the antialgic effect of aspirin secondary to its anti-inflammatory action, i.e. depression of oedema and chemotaxis and migration of inflammatory cells? and (b), is it due to a direct inhibitory effect of aspirin-like drugs on the peripheral or central neural tissue? or is it the end result of the inhibition of the formation and release of specific mediators that produce pain or hyperalgesia?

Hyperalgesia denotes a state of sensitization of pain receptors in which pain can be evoked with mechanical stimuli, e.g. pressure, of a severity inadequate for the production of pain in non-inflamed tissue, or tissues not subjected to chemical substances such as prostaglandins.

The evidence reviewed below indicates that aspirin-like drugs provide antialgesia through a dual action, namely prevention of hyperalgesia in the inflamed site and also by an as yet ill-defined physiological effect on the CNS. Their antialgic action at both the sites appears to be related to their ability to inhibit the biosynthesis of prostaglandins, rather than to their anti-inflammatory action. In fact, as indicated by data reviewed in the first section there is no clear-cut inter-relationship between inflammatory pain and oedema or infiltration of leukocytes.

DISSOCIATION OF OEDEMA, CELL MIGRATION AND INFLAMMATORY PAIN

The antialgic activity of aspirin-like drugs and corticosteroids has been widely regarded to be the indirect consequence of their anti-inflammatory action[11–13]. In the rat though, paw oedema can be elicited by 5-hydroxytryptamine, egg white, dextran or passive cutaneous anaphylaxis without hyperalgesia[14–16]. Furthermore doses of aspirin (50–400 mg/kg) which markedly reduce hyperalgesia caused by subplantar injection of Brewer's yeast (0.1 ml) do not significantly reduce the degree of attendant oedema[17]. Likewise, indomethacin administered into dog knee joint together with sodium urate inhibited hyperalgesia without a significant effect on cell migration[18].

DISSOCIATION OF HYPERALGESIA FROM OEDEMA

Striking examples of dissociation between these two manifestations of the inflammatory response, recently observed in our laboratory, are illustrated in Figure 3.1.

In these experiments oedema was measured plethismographically and hyperalgesia by a modification of the Randall and Selitto method[11]. In our modification a constant pressure (20 mmHg) is applied by means of a piston to the rat foot, using an apparatus similar to that described by Mezey and van Arman[19]. The criteria for hyperalgesia were met when the rat carried out an escape movement following an increase in respiratory frequency. The time for the reaction was measured and the hyperalgesia was quantified by subtracting either the initial reaction time measured at the beginning of the experiments or the result obtained with the non-inflamed contralateral paw.

The results (Figure 3.1) show first that rats treated daily for one week with insulin (IU, NPH) developed the expected oedematous response to carrageenan (100 μg; Marine Colloids), but showed virtually no hyperalgesia. In contrast rats rendered leukopenic (more than 50%, but less than 70% of basal leukocyte counts) using methotrexate (2, 1 and 1 mg/kg dose given on consecutive days)

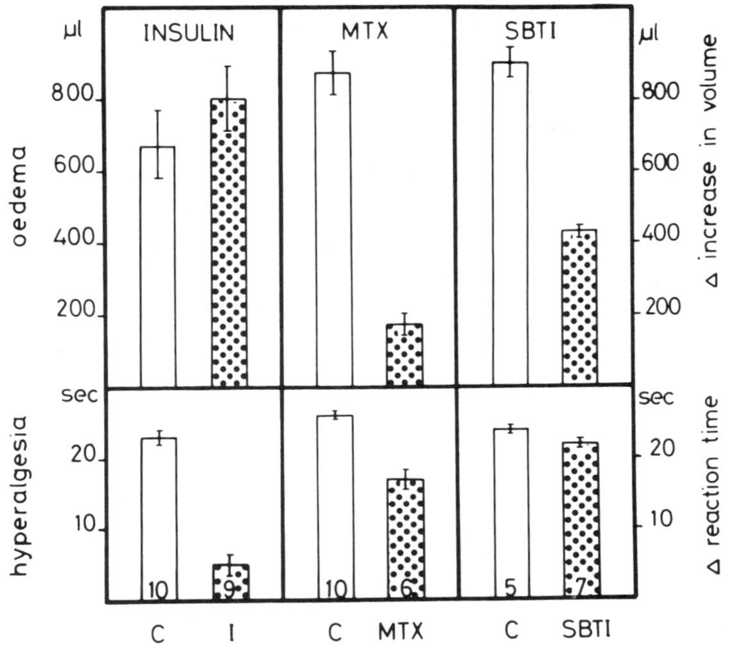

Figure 3.1 Dissociation between oedema and hyperalgesia. The measurements were made four hours after inflammation was induced by an intraplantar injection of 100 μg of carrageenan. Details of the treatment with insulin, methotrexate (MTX) and soybean trypsin inhibitor (SBTI) are given in the text. The control group for each experiment is indicated by C and the number of animals for each group is given inside the columns

showed a pronounced reduction of carrageenan oedema with only a small, though statistically significant, reduction of hyperalgesia. Thirdly, late treatment (two hours after carrageenan) with soybean trypsin inhibitor (SBTI) was found to reduce by almost 50% the carrageenan-induced oedema but influenced hardly at all the accompanying hyperalgesia. The SBTI results partially confirm previous observations[20].

DISSOCIATION OF HYPERALGESIA FROM MIGRATION OF INFLAMMATORY CELLS

The results of methotrexate experiments illustrated in Figure 3.1 show also that in leukopenic rats the oedema is reduced but the animals still show hyperalgesia in response to carrageenan. The results imply that migrating cells are not critically important for the development of hyperalgesia in this model as in the avian standing and temperature test of Brune *et al.*[21]. The conclusion differs, however, from those of the investigators who have studied urate-induced synovitis in the dog[22–24].

We believe that the inter-relationship between hyperalgesia and the presence of PMNs in the inflamed site depends upon the nature of inflammatory stimulus. The results shown in Figure 3.2 support this suggestion. They show that although intra-articular instillation of glycogen or endotoxin (75 μg) in the dog promotes migration of similar numbers of leucocytes by the fourth hour, incapacitation results only with endotoxin. In addition, they show that a lower dose of endotoxin (0.5 μg), harmless if injected by itself, causes marked hyperalgesia if instilled into a joint which had been treated with glycogen 4 hours previously. The experiments establish that migration of PMNs, or simply the presence of leukocytes in an exudate, is not the 'cause' of incapacitation. For incapacitation to occur it is necessary that the stimulus be capable of releasing pain mediators or pro-mediators (enzymes which generate mediators).

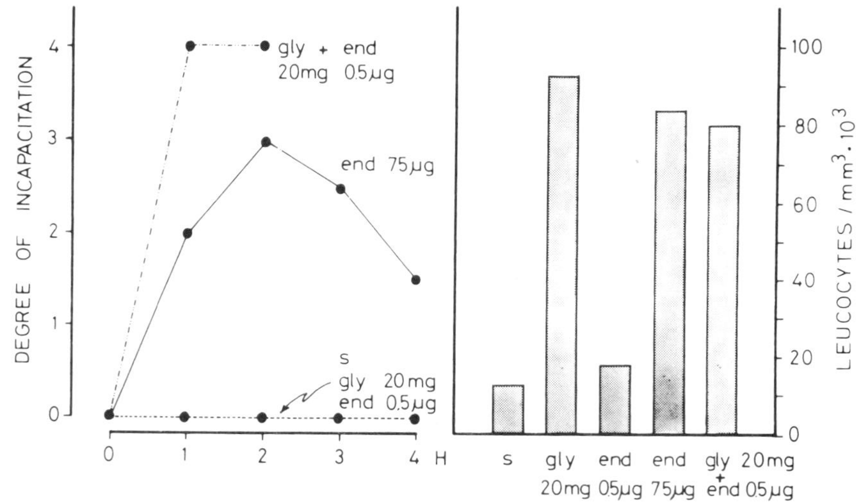

Figure 3.2 Cell migration and incapacitation induced by glycogen and/or endotoxin injected into the dog knee joint. Left panel shows the development of incapacitation evaluated by the following scale: 0, normal; 1 mild and 2, pronounced limping during walk; 3, dog walks with affected leg; 4, dog does not use the affected leg when walking. Administration of saline (s) glycogen (gly) or 0.5 μg of endotoxin (end) caused no incapacitation. An injection of 0.5 μg of endotoxin indicated by (●·· – ··–●) given 4 hours after an injection of glycogen induced an incapacitation greater than that caused by an injection of 75 μg of endotoxin (full line). The right panel shows the leukocyte count of the exudate at the end of the experiment. For saline, glycogen, endotoxin (0.5 and 75 μg) this corresponds to the 4 hours time point on the left panel. For 20 mg glycogen followed by 0.5 μg of endotoxin this corresponds to six hours after the glycogen injection which is indicated by the two hours time point, on the left panel

It seems clear therefore that neither oedema nor migrating cells per se account for the development of inflammatory pain. We believe that pain develops following the release of chemical mediators from local or migrating cells, and that of the known mediators prostaglandins play a key role in the production of pain because they sensitize pain receptors to the noxious effect of mechanical or chemical trauma. Evidence in support of this view is reviewed below.

PROSTAGLANDINS, LIPOPEROXIDES, HYPERALGESIA AND OVERT PAIN

The ability of prostaglandins to cause hyperalgesia in man[25] was known two years prior to the observations in 1971, at the Royal College of Surgeons of England, of Vane[26], Smith and Willis[27], Ferreira, Moncada and Vane[28] that aspirin-like drugs inhibit the synthesis and release of prostaglandins both *in vitro* and *in vivo*. But the possibility that aspirin-like drugs relieved pain through their ability to inhibit the bio-synthesis of prostaglandins could not be seriously entertained until it was shown[5] that whereas bradykinin, histamine, and acetylcholine (i.d.) produce short-lasting overt pain, equimolar amounts of prostaglandins (i.d.) cause long-lasting hyperalgesia (as tested by pressure). Prostaglandins do not cause overt pain even if applied to a cantharidine blister[29].

When subdermal infusion of prostaglandins was employed in man[5] to mimic their continuous release in an inflammatory condition, it was found that the hyperalgesia was time-dependent. Thus amounts which were ineffective if infused over 30 min proved to be hyperalgesic when infused over 2 hours. These experiments revealed also that in contrast to the effect of intradermal injections, subdermal infusions of bradykinin, histamine, or a mixture of bradykinin and histamine, did not cause overt pain. Yet, when PGE_1 was added to infusions of bradykinin or histamine (or a mixture of both) strong pain developed. Furthermore, in areas made hyperalgesic by an infusion of prostaglandins a second infusion of either histamine or bradykinin caused overt pain; though at sites where bradykinin, or histamine, had been previously infused, a subsequent infusion of the prostaglandin did not evoke overt pain.

This unique ability of prostaglandins to sensitize pain receptors is also observed in the rat. Carrageenan, when injected into the rat paw, causes marked hyperalgesia after four hours. Bradykinin, histamine or 5-hydroxytryptamine cause little or no hyperalgesia when given alone or together with carrageenan. Prostaglandins cause a mild effect but when added to carrageenan cause intense hyperalgesia[30].

Another important observation concerns pruritus. Neither histamine, bradykinin nor PGE_1 infusions by themselves caused itch[5]. However, when PGE_1 was infused with histamine, itching was always obtained (when PGE_1 was infused with bradykinin, there was pain rather than itch). This role of prostaglandins in potentiating the effects of histamine has recently been confirmed[31]. The sensitizing action of prostaglandins to pain induced by bradykinin can also be shown to occur in the dog's spleen and knee joint.

Lim and his colleagues[32,33] used nociception induced by intra-arterial injections of bradykinin into the spleen to show that aspirin-like drugs act peripherally as analgesics. In order to test whether bradykinin induces pain through prostaglandin release, we injected bradykinin into the spleen of the dog[34]. Prostaglandins were released in similar amounts, both *in vitro* and *in vivo* by injections of adrenaline or bradykinin. As adrenaline is a much weaker pain-producing substance than bradykinin in this system, it was clear that a prostaglandin could not be the *mediator* of the pain-producing activity of bradykinin.

In another series of experiments[34], we used the reflex rise in blood pressure induced by intra-arterial bradykinin injections into the spleen of lightly anaesthetized dogs as an indication of sensory stimulation. Doses of bradykinin which released prostaglandin from the spleen caused reflex increases in blood pressure, in proportion to the dose used and these were reduced by indomethacin. When PGE_1 was given with bradykinin in the indomethacin-treated dogs, the reflex-increase in blood pressure was restored, sometimes to greater than control values.

Measurement of this reflex rise in blood pressure has also proved useful for studying the effect of prostaglandins on the nociceptive reflex induced by bradykinin injected into dog knee joints[8]. Increasing doses of bradykinin induced a dose-dependent rise in blood pressure. Local treatment with aspirin or indomethacin partially inhibited the bradykinin responses, probably by inhibiting the local formation of prostaglandins generated by the trauma caused by the manipulation of the joints. Infusion of prostaglandins produced a long lasting potentiation of the algogenic effect of bradykinin. When local generation of prostaglandins was blocked by indomethacin and the enhanced sensitivity of the joints brought back by an infusion of prostaglandins, further injection of indomethacin did not alter the responses of the injection of bradykinin into the joints. This observation indicates that aspirin-like drugs do not affect the sensitivity of the receptors to the action of bradykinin.

The pain potentiating action of prostaglandins on the effect of chemical stimulation has also been shown on the isolated perfused ear[9,10] and on mice writhing response[35]. Staszewska-Barezak *et al.*[36] measured the reflex rise in blood pressure induced by topical application of bradykinin to the exposed left ventricle of the anaesthetized dog. This, too, is decreased by indomethacin and increased again by prostaglandins; prostaglandin release may, therefore, contribute to the pain associated with cardiac ischaemia. All these results, taken together, suggest that sensitization by prostaglandins of the sensory nerves to chemical stimulation by other substances is a general phenomenon.

Lipoperoxides

At this stage we would like to comment on rabbit aorta contracting substance (RCS) which has strong pharmacological activity in that it contracts rabbit aorta and many other arterial muscle strips[37,38] as do lipoperoxides generated by lipo-oxidase acting on fatty acids such arachidonic, linoleic and linolenic[39,40].

The possibility that fatty acid hydroperoxides can contribute to the production of pain in man has been previously explored[5]. Intensity of pain produced by intradermal injections of hydroxyperoxides of arachidonic, linoleic and linolenic acids was greater than that induced by either the parent fatty acids or acetylcholine, bradykinin, histamine or prostaglandin E_1. Recently[41] it has been shown that another substance, thromboxane, generated by oxidation of arachidonic acid and which is similar to endoperoxide intermediates of prostaglandin synthesis, causes contraction of rabbit aorta and platelet aggnegation and these effects are blocked by aspirin-like drugs. Thromboxane has been identified as the most important component of RCS.

From all these results we can draw three conclusions: (a) lipoperoxide intermediates in the prostaglandin biosynthetic pathway may have pain-producing properties, as do prostaglandin E_1 and E_2 at high concentrations; depending on the intensity of activation of the prostaglandin generating system by a trauma, the generation of the intermediate could exceed its conversion to prostaglandin, thus causing an acute type of pain. (b) In low concentrations, prostaglandin E_1 (and prostaglandin E_2) sensitize the pain fibres to mechanical and chemical stimuli. (c) The effects of prostaglandins E_1 and E_2 are cumulative and long-lasting. Thus, continual generation of minute amounts of prostaglandin at a site of injury will sensitize the nerves, so that mechanical stimulation or mediators such as bradykinin and histamine can cause pruritus or pain.

PROSTAGLANDIN RELEASE IN INFLAMMATION

To further support the importance of prostaglandins in the development of inflammatory pain it is essential to review the evidence indicating: (a) that prostaglandins are released during the inflammatory process, (b) that agents which inhibit biosynthesis of prostaglandins relieve inflammatory pain, i.e. provide antialgesia.

Cells do not store prostaglandins but have the capacity to synthesize and release them upon stimulation. Distortion of the cell membrane seems to be a common feature of different prostaglandin-producing stimuli. Prostaglandins have been found in most inflammatory exudates and many forms of skin damage, in man and animals (for a review, see[42]).

The presence of prostaglandins in exudates depends upon the balance between release by local or migrating cells and removal. It is possible that the rate of accumulation in most mild inflammation is so low (due to its rapid rate of disappearance) that prostaglandins cannot be detected with the methods now available. Furthermore, it is possible that the prostaglandins relevant to the symptoms may be generated by the structures upon which they act (i.e. sensory nerves and vessels). The ability to detect prostaglandin in an exudate may reflect a very quick and intense tissue damage, which possibly is not the case in chronic human diseases. The point I would like to make here is that the absence of prostaglandin in an exudate cannot exclude the contribution of prostaglandins to the process. However, in other cases depending on the type of trauma and the animal species, it is possible that prostaglandins do not play a role, or play only an insignificant role, in inflammation such as that accompanying passive cutaneous anaphylaxis in the rat[16].

INHIBITION OF PROSTAGLANDIN BIOSYNTHESIS BY ANTIALGICS

The ability of aspirin-like NSAIDs to inhibit the synthesis of prostaglandins has been demonstrated in almost all laboratory animals as well as man (see reviews[42,43]). Such compounds are therefore also referred to as cyclo-oxygenase inhibitors. Several investigators have compared the anti-inflammatory activity of aspirin-like drugs with their activity against prostaglandin synthetase. A general correlation is observed, even when the comparison is based on oral administration of the drug on the one hand and direct inhibition of an *in vivo* microsomal enzyme preparation on the other. The rank order was the same against carrageenan rat paw oedema as against spleen synthetase, except that indomethacin was out of the rank order for the rat paw test[44]. Even more striking is the correlation demonstrable by comparing pairs of enantiomers: this has been done for naproxen and for indomethacin analogues. In each case, the isomer of each pair with anti-inflammatory activity also strongly inhibited prostaglandin synthetase, whereas the one with weak anti-inflammatory activity was also weak against the synthetase[45,46].

Recently, we described a method in which inflammatory exudates were induced in rats by subcutaneous implantation of sponges impregnated with carrageenan[47]. With this test it was possible to correlate inhibition *in vivo* of prostaglandin synthesis and anti-inflammatory activity. Drugs without anti-inflammatory activity, like phenelzine, chlorpromazine and desimipramine, failed to show any activity *in vivo* even though they caused inhibition of PG synthesis *in vitro*. To our knowledge, there is no drug that inhibits synthesis of prostaglandins *in vivo* which blocks anti-inflammatory or antialgic properties.

There are some agents such as paracetamol or novalgine which, in man, are anti-pyretic analgesics without conspicuous anti-inflammatory activity (although they may show an anti-oedema effect in experimental animals). This observation is frequently raised as an argument against our interpretation of the mechanism of analgesia of aspirin-like drugs[48]. However, aspirin-like drugs show a differential sensitivity towards prostaglandin synthetase enzymes from different tissues[44]. Paracetamol is equivalent to aspirin, and novalgine is more potent than aspirin against prostaglandin synthetase in nervous tissue[49]. One may thus suggest that a prostaglandin synthetase inhibitor like paracetamol is an analgesic displaying only small anti-oedema properties because of this differential sensitivity of the cyclo-oxygenase and also possibly owing to its preferential distribution in the nervous tissues (of which sensory nerves are a part).

SYNERGISM BETWEEN LOCAL AND CENTRAL EFFECT

Because paracetamol is considered to have more antialgic than anti-oedema effect we decided to investigate the effect of its administration into the cerebral ventricle of the rat on the hyperalgesia caused by an intra-plantar injection of carrageenan. We used the method described above (see section on dissociation between pain and oedema) but in these experiments the measurements of hyperalgesia were made by a person who ignored the drug treatment of the rat.

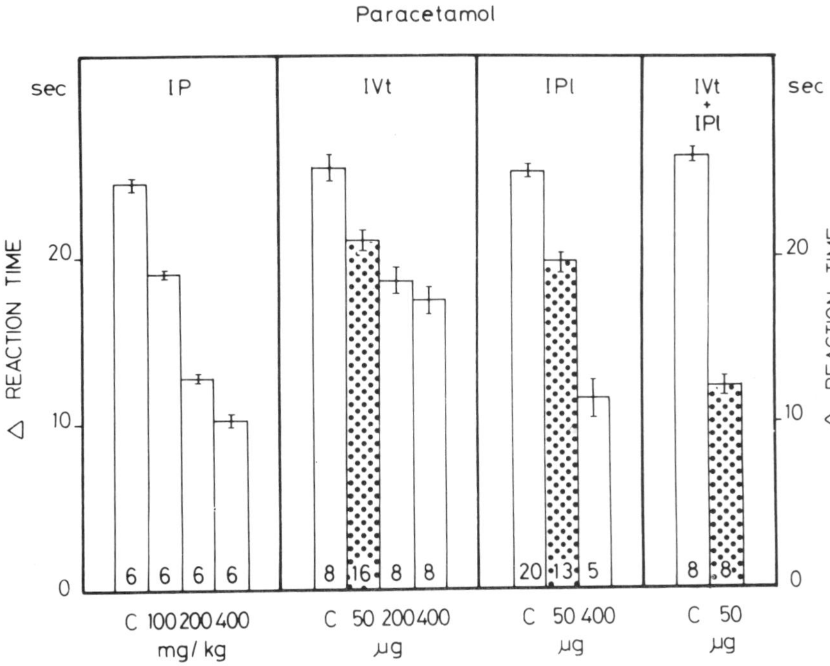

Figure 3.3 Synergism between central and local injection of paracetamol on the hyperalgesia caused by carrageenan. The four panels show the results obtained with intraperitoneal (IP), intraventricular (IVt), intraplantar (IPl) and the combined IVt and IPl administration of paracetamol. Paracetamol was given two hours after 100 μg of carrageenan was injected into the rat paw

Morphine given centrally (50 μg) was able to increase the threshold of response for both inflamed and non-inflamed paws. Paracetamol, up to 400 μg, given into the ventricles or into a normal paw had no effect.

However, intraventricular injections of paracetamol made 2 hours after the intraplantar injection of 100 μg of carrageenan induced, as is shown in Figure 3.3, a dose-related inhibition of hyperalgesia. The degree of hyperalgesia induced by intraventricular paracetamol was similar to that observed after its administration into the paw itself (Figure 3.3); though less than that seen following injection into the peritoneal cavity. Interestingly, however, administration of paracetamol simultaneously into both the ventricle and the inflamed paw gave an effect equivalent to a dose eight times greater than that injected into the paw alone. Similar synergism was also observed with indomethacin (10 μg), observations which suggest that other members of the family of NSAIDs that inhibit cyclo-oxygenase may also provide antialgesia through a dual mechanism.

SUMMARY AND CONCLUSIONS

Evidence reviewed in this paper shows that:

1. Hyperalgesia, and consequently pain, can be dissociated from oedema or inflammatory cell migration. The presence or absence of hyperalgesia in inflammatory conditions characterized by infiltration of leukocytes depends upon the nature of the inflammatory stimulus. Glycogen induces infiltration of PMNs but does not induce hyperalgesia; whereas endotoxin and carrageenan induce both leukocyte emigration and hyperalgesia concurrently.

2. Prostaglandins do not cause overt pain but when slowly infused, or when slowly released over long periods of time (as during an inflammatory reaction) they produce prolonged hyperalgesia, and so intensify the painful effects of other mediators.

3. Inhibition of the synthesis and release of prostaglandins and lipoperoxides results in the relief, but not abolition, of inflammatory pain. In the case of aspirin-like NSAIDs, such relief appears to originate not only from the pharmacological effect of the drug at the site of inflammation but also from that in the CNS. Relief of pain can occur without concurrent depression of other signs of inflammation such as swelling or leukocyte migration.

Acknowledgements

We thank FAPESP (Brazil, 75/0296) and the Wellcome Foundation for research grants.

References

1. Woodbury, D. M. (1965). Analgesics and antipyretics salicylates and congeners; phenacetin and congeners; antipyrine and congeners; colchicine. In L. S. Goodman and A. Gilman (eds.) *The Pharmacological Basis of Therapeutics*, 3rd edition. (New York: Macmillan)
2. Wit, A. and Wang, S. C. (1968). Temperature-sensitive neurons in preoptic/anterior hypothalamic region: actions of pyrogen and acetylsalicylate. *Am. J. Physiol.*, **215**, 1160
3. Lim, R. K. S., Guzman, F., Rodgers, D. W., Goto, K., Braun, G., Dickerson, G. D. and Engle, R. J. (1964). Site of action of narcotic and non-narcotic analgesics determined by blocking bradykinin-evoked visceral pain. *Arch. Int. Pharmacodyn.*, **152**, 25
4. Lim, R. K. S. (1968). Neuropharmacology of pain and analgesia. In R. K. S. Lim, D. Armstrong and E. G. Pardo (eds.) *Pharmacology of Pain*. p. 169. (London: Pergamon)
5. Ferreira, S. H. (1972). Prostaglandins, aspirin-like drugs and analgesia. *Nature, New Biology*, **240**, 200
6. Ferreira, S. H., Moncada, S. and Vane, J. R. (1973). Prostaglandins and the mechanism of analgesia produced by aspirin-like drugs. *Br. J. Pharmacol.*, **49**, 86
7. Ferreira, S. H., Moncada, S. and Vane, J. R. (1974). Prostaglandins and the signs and symp-

toms of inflammation. In H. J. Robinson and J. R. Vane (eds.) *Prostaglandin Synthetase Inhibitors.* p. 175. (New York: Raven Press)

8. Moncada, S., Ferreira, S. H. and Vane, J. R. (1975). Inhibition of prostaglandin biosynthesis as the mechanism of analgesia of aspirin-like drugs in the dog knee joint. *Eur. J. Pharmacol.,* **31,** 250
9. Juan, H. and Lembeck, F. (1974). Inhibition of action of E-prostaglandins (PGs) on paravascular pain receptors. *Naunyn-Schmiedebergs Arch. Pharmacol.* **285, R**36
10. Juan, H. and Lembeck, F. (1976). Release of prostaglandins from the isolated perfused rabbit ear by bradykinin and acetylcholine. *Agents Actions,* **6**(5), 642
11. Randall, L. O. and Selitto, J. J. (1957). A method for measurement of analgesic activity on inflamed tissue. *Arch. Int. Pharmacodyn.,* **111,** 409
12. Smith, P. K. (1960). The pharmacology of salicylates and related compounds. *Ann. N.Y. Acad. Sci.,* **86,** 38
13. Vinegar, R., Traux, J. F. and Selph, J. L. (1976). Quantitative comparison of the analgesic and anti-inflammatory activities of aspirin, phenacetin and acetaminophen in rodents. *Eur. J. Pharmacol.,* **37,** 23
14. Gilfoil, T. and Klavins, J. (1965). 5-Hydroxytryptamine, bradykinin and histamine as mediators of inflammatory hyperesthesia. *Am. J. Physiol.,* **208**(5), 867
15. Van Arman, C. G. Nuss, G. W., Winter, C. A. and Flataker, L. (1968). Proteolytic enzymes as mediators of pain. In R. K. S. Lim, D. Armstrong and E. G. Pardo (eds.) *Pharmacology of Pain.* p. 25. (Oxford: Pergamon Press)
16. Ferreira, S. H. (1976). Prostaglandins and the immunological trauma. In G. P. Lewis (ed.) *The Role of Prostaglandins in Inflammation.* p. 83. (Bern: Hans Huber)
17. Gilfoil, T. M., Klavins, I. and Grumbach, L. (1963). Effects acetylsalicylic acid on the oedema and hyperesthesia of the experimentally inflamed rat's paw. *J. Pharmacol. Exp. Ther.,* **142,** 1
18. van Arman, C. G., Carlson, R. P., Risley, E. A., Thomas, R. H. and Nuss, G. W. (1970). Inhibitory effects of indomethacin, aspirin and certain drugs on inflammation induced in rat and dog by carrageenan, sodium urate and ellagic acid. *J. Pharmacol. Exp. Ther.* **175,** 459
19. Mezey, K. C. and van Arman, C. G. (1974). Methodology of testing new anti-inflammatory drugs. In G. Katona and José R. Blengio (eds.) *Inflammation and Anti-inflammatory Therapy.* p. 279. (New York: Spectrum Publications)
20. Van Arman, C. G., Begany, A. J., Miller, L. M. and Pless, H. H. (1965). Some details of the inflammations caused by yeast and carrageenan (with appendix on kinetics of the reaction). *J. Pharmacol. Exp. Ther.* **150**(2), 328
21. Brune, K., Minder, Brigite, Glatt, M. and Schmid, L. (1974). Do polymorphonuclear leucocytes function as mediators in acute inflammation? In G. P. Velo, D. A. Willoughby and J. P. Giroud (eds.) *Future Trends in Inflammation.* p. 289. (Padua and London: Piccin Medical Books)
22. McCarthy, D., Phelps, P. and Pyenson, J. (1966). Crystal-induced inflammation in canine joints. I. An experimental model with quantification of the host response. *J. Exp. Med.,* **124,** 99
23. Chang, Y. H. and Gralla, E. J. (1968). Suppression of urate crystal-induced canine joint inflammation by heterologous anti-polymorphonuclear leukocyte serum. *Arthr. Rheum.,* **11,** 145
24. Van Arman, C. G. and Carlson, R. P. (1974). Anti-inflammatory drugs and the behaviour of leucocytes. In G. P. Velo, D. A. Willoughby and J. P. Giroud (eds.) *Future Trends in Inflammation.* p. 159. (Padua and London: Piccin Medical Books)
25. Juhlin, S. and Michaelsson, G. (1969). Cutaneous vascular reactions in healthy subjects and patients with urticaria and atopic dermatitis. *Acta Derm. Vener. (Stockholm),* **49,** 251
26. Vane, J. R. (1971). Inhibition of prostaglandin synthesis as a mechanism of action for aspirin-like drugs. *Nature New Biol.,* **231,** 232

27. Smith, J. B. and Willis, A. L. (1971). Aspirin selectively inhibits prostaglandin production in human platelets. *Nature New Biol.*, **231**, 236
28. Ferreira, S. H., Moncada, S. and Vane, J. R. (1971). Indomethacin and aspirin abolish prostaglandin release from the spleen. *Nature New Biol.*, **231**, 237
29. Horton, E. W. (1963). Action of prostaglandin E_1 on tissues which respond to bradykinin. *Nature (London)*, **200**, 892
30. Ferreira, S. H., Harvey, E. A. and Vane, J. R. (1975). Hyperalgesia, inflammatory oedema and prostaglandin. In: *Proc. VI Intern. Pharmacol. Congr., Abstr.* 1001, Helsinki, Finland
31. Greaves, M. W. and McDonald-Gibson, W. (1973). Itch: Role of prostaglandins. *Br. Med. J.*, **3**, 608
32. Guzman, F., Braun, C. and Lim, R. K. S. (1962). Visceral pain and the pseud-affective response to intra-arterial injection of bradykinin and other algesic agents. *Arch. Int. Pharmacodyn.*, **136**, 353
33. Guzman, F., Braun, C., Lim, R. K. S., Potter, G. D. and Rodgers, D. W. (1964). Narcotic and non-narcotic analgesics which block visceral pain evoked by intra-arterial injection of bradykinin and other algesic agents. *Arch. Int. Pharmacodyn.*, **149**, 571
34. Ferreira, S. H., Moncada, S. and Vane, J. R. (1973). Some effects of inhibiting endogenous prostaglandin formation on the responses of the cat spleen. *Br. J. Pharmacol.*, **47**, 48
35. Church, M. K. and James, G. W. L. (1977). Hyperalgesia after treatment of mice with prostaglandins and arachidonic acid and its antagonism by anti-inflammatory analgesic compounds. *Arch. Int. Pharmacodyn.*, (in press)
36. Staszewska-Barezak, J., Ferreira, S. H. and Vane, J. R. (1976). An excitatory nociceptive cardiac reflex elicited by bradykinin and potentiated by prostaglandins and myocardial ischemia. *Cardiovasc. Res.*, **10**, 314
37. Piper, P. J. and Vane, J. R. (1969). Release of additional factors in anaphylaxis and its antagonism by anti-inflammatory drugs. *Nature (London)*, **223**, 20
38. Palmer, M. A., Piper, P. J. and Vane, J. R. (1973). Release of rabbit aorta contracting substance (RCS) and prostaglandins induced by chemical or mechanical stimulation of guinea pig lungs. *Br. J. Pharmacol.*, **49**, 226
39. Gryglewski, R. and Vane, J. R. (1972). The generation from arachidonic acid of rabbit aorta contracting substance (RCS) by a microsomal enzyme preparation which also generates PGs. *Br. J. Pharmacol.*, **46**, 449
40. Ferreira, S. H. and Vargaftig, B. B. (1974). Inhibiting by non-steroid anti-inflammatory agents of rabbit aorta contracting activity generated in blood by slow reacting substance C. *Br. J. Pharmacol.*, **50**. 543
41. Hamberg, M., Svensson, J. and Samuelsson, B. (1975). Thromboxanes: A new group of biologically active compounds derived from prostaglandin endoperoxides. *Proc. Nat. Acad. Sci.*, **72**, 2994
42. Ferreira, S. H. and Vane, J. R. (1974). New aspects of the mode of action of non-steroid anti-inflammatory drugs. *Ann. Rev. Pharmacol.*, **14**, 57
43. Ferreira, S. H. and Vane, J. R. (1974). Aspirin and prostaglandins. In P. W. Ramwell (ed.) *The Prostaglandins II*. (New York, London: Plenum Press)
44. Flower, R. J., Gryglewski, R., Herbaczynska, C. K. and Vane, J. R. (1972). The effects of anti-inflammatory drugs on prostaglandin biosynthesis. *Nature New Biol.*, **238**, 107
45. Tomlinson, R. V., Ringold, H. J., Qureshi, M. C. and Forchielli, E. (1972). Relationship between inhibition of prostaglandin synthesis and drug efficacy: support for the current theory on mode of action of aspirin-like drugs. *Biochem. Biophys. Res. Commun.*, **46**, 552
46. Ham, E. A., Cirillo, V. J., Zanetti, M., Shen, T. Y. and Kuehl, F. A. Jr. (1972). Studies on the mode of action of non-steroidal anti-inflammatory agents. In P. W. Ramwell and B. B. Pharris (eds.) *Prostaglandins in Cellular Biology*. p. 342. (New York: Plenum Press)
47. Higgs, G. A., Harvey, E. A., Ferreira, S. H. and Vane, J. R. (1976). The effects of anti-inflammatory drugs on the production of prostaglandins *in vivo*. In Samuelsson, B. and Paoletti, R.

(eds.) *Advances in Prostaglandin and Thromboxane Research.* Vol. 1 p. 105. (New York: Raven Press)

48. Smith, M. J. H. (1975). Prostaglandins and aspirin: An alternative view. *Agents Actions,* **5**(4), 315
49. Dembinska-Kiec, A., Zmuda, A. and Krupinska, J. (1976). Inhibition of prostaglandin synthetase by aspirin-like drugs in different microsomal preparations. In B. Sammuelsson and R. Paoletti (eds.) *Advances in Prostaglandin and Thromboxane Research.* Vol. 1, p. 99. (New York: Raven Press)

Discussion I

Nature of Inflammatory Response with Special Reference to Mediators and Lipid Peroxides in Inflammation (Chapters 1 and 2)

G. P. LEWIS: Arachidonic acid metabolism would appear to be a really exciting field, with lots of possibilities for the future. Dr Moncada, I only hope that the metabolic pathways (Figure 1, Chapter 2) do not get further complicated, otherwise we shall need two projectors!

R. J. PERPER: Is there any reason to believe, or any data to support the possibility, that complete suppression of prostaglandin (PG) synthesis would benefit chronic inflammation. Or does anyone know whether that might aggravate chronic inflammation?

S. MONCADA: The role of PGs in acute inflammatory reaction is well established and the inhibition of their formation is associated with depression of some manifestations of the inflammatory response.

However, the role of PGs in chronic inflammation such as rheumatoid arthritis still remains to be clarified.

J. R. VANE: If I might comment on Dr Perper's question, an area that might be worth investigating is whether PGE_2 causes bone resorption in RA as is claimed by several laboratories on the basis of *in vitro* observations.

G. P. LEWIS: We do know that potent inhibitors of Pg-synthetase do not alter the underlying cause in RA, so in that particular sense at least, they are not really fully effective in RA.

W. CARSON DICK: I deal with patients and not pathways. Therefore, interesting though the pathways are, the questions that matter to me are: Would the inhibition of PG-synthesis in a whole variety of organs harm the patient? Do the relative potencies of the PG-synthetase inhibitors detected in laboratory correspond with their clinical efficacy? Thirdly, what is the clinical relevance of studies on individual components of the inflammatory process made in isolation of the remaining factors? Finally, is it not true that clinical suppression of at least some parts of the arachidonic acid metabolic pathway shows little clinical improvement in RA, but increased incidence of side-effects, especially with prolonged use?

I would be grateful for answers to these questions.

M. F. CUTHBERT: With regard to Dr Dick's comments I would like to point out that in my experience indomethacin does no harm to patients with asthma even when administered in quite large doses over many months. The trials, both acute and chronic, were made in collaboration with Dr Peter Smith (*see* Br. J. Clin. Pharmacol. **2,** 293–295; 307–309; 1975) and involved asthmatics who were known to be tolerant to aspirin.

M. K. JASANI: Would Dr Moncada specify the experiments he made to test the hypothesis of Kuehl et al. (Ref. 13, Chapter 2) that the conversion from PGG_2 to PGH_2 gives rise to an oxygen radical that is responsible for some of the signs and symptoms of inflammation.

S. MONCADA: They were very simple experiments in which we compared the pro-inflammatory activity of PGG_2 and the pro-inflammatory activity of PGH_2 using a previously described method (Nature, **246,** 217; 1973). If the mechanism proposed by Kuehl worked, then certainly PGG_2 should potentiate carrageenin-induced foot-pad oedema more than could PGH_2; but in our experiments we found no significant differences between the effects of the two compounds.

G. P. LEWIS: There are two places where free oxygen radical can be formed during the metabolism of arachidonic acid (p. 20); one when PGG_2 is converted to PGH_2 and the other when HPETE is converted to HETE. Would both conversions result in free radical formation?

S. MONCADA: Yes.

T. J. WILLIAMS: With regard to the Kuehl hypothesis, we found both PGG_2 and PGE_2 to be vasodilators and also potentiators of vasodilatation. Interestingly though, we found PGG_2 to be less potent than PGE_2 and that to my mind stresses the greater importance of PGE_2 as a mediator of vasodilatation. Dr Moncada, if prostacycline PGI is a vasodilator, why is it not pro-inflammatory in the same way as PGG_2 or PGE_2?

S. MONCADA: We have found prostacycline (PGI) can produce erythema, and in high concentrations it can also induce oedema formation, but unlike PGE_2 it does not sensitize pain receptors.

E. V. BARNETT: Is there any evidence to support the possibility that the imidazole moiety of imuran (imidazole-6-mercaptopurine) is freed *in vivo* and accounts for part of the anti-inflammation effect of imuran? I raise such a possibility as it could explain why it is easier to maintain RA patients satisfactorily on alternate-day steroid therapy when they are receiving a low dose of imuran.

Antialgic Effect of Aspirin-like Drugs and the Inhibition of Prostaglandin Synthesis (Chapter 3)

T. J. WILLIAMS: Dr Ferreira, does the fact that you found oedema to occur without hyperalgesia during the PCA reaction imply that Pgs are not produced during this type of inflammatory response?

S. H. FERREIRA: May be they are produced but only in too small an amount. Also indomethacin does not prove effective against oedema of PCA reaction, not at least in my hands.

M. I. V. JAYSON (Royal Infirmary, Bristol): I am a little concerned about the use of the word 'pain' in the context of these experiments. Pain is a subjective sensation. It is something that is felt in the mind, and without the mind pain does not exist.

In this regard, and especially in regard to the hyperalgesia experiments, it is worth mentioning some work that we did measuring pain threshold — sensitivity to some form of noxious stimulus — in patients with painful arthritis. When pain threshold was measured in these patients in a site that was in no way affected by the arthritis they were found to have a lower pain threshold — they were more sensitive to the pain.

After removal of the painful site by operation, their pain thresholds returned to normal. There was a general alteration in sensitivity to pain felt within the mind due to removal of a peripheral painful stimulus.

This might well be analogous to Dr Ferreira's own experiments where he is altering the inflammatory response. He might be altering the subject's or the animal's sensitivity to pain purely by this combination of stimuli rather than by any specific effect on nerve endings.

S. H. FERREIRA: I believe that to be correct. As you would have noted advisedly I restricted use of the term 'pain' to only the human experiments. For experiments on the rat I prefer the term hyperalgesia, whereas for those on the dog I use incapacitation to describe the neural response to inflammation. All I should now like to stress is that tranquilizers which have no effect on inflammation have no effect on physiological responses such as the mean reaction time in this rat, or the reflex rise in blood pressure of the dog.

Section II:
Chemotaxis and Activation of Complement

Chairman: **R. J. PERPER**

4
The Rheumatological Significance of Chemotaxis

R. J. PERPER

INTRODUCTION

The accumulation of circulating leukocytes in the interstitial space can be caused by many factors, including chemical attraction (chemotaxis), vascular permeability changes secondary to physical or chemical stimuli, and the immobilization of leukocytes which had migrated to the area in a random way. Not all stimuli which increase vascular permeability necessarily cause the accumulation of leukocytes. For instance, noxious stimuli such as turpentine and carrageenan[1,2], initially induce extensive oedema without a concomitant accumulation of cells during the first several hours after their subcutaneous instillation.

Although leukocytes are attracted directionally to various chemical stimuli *in vitro*, a clear distinction must be made between *in vitro* observations and *in vivo* phenomena. In a discussion of chemotaxis, most authors concentrate on the description and characterization of the various factors which cause the directional migration of leukocytes *in vitro*. More recently attempts have been made to study the effect that these factors have on the responding cell in terms of positive or negative effects[3,4] and the nature of the interaction with the cell membrane[5]. Such studies are designed to dissect the underlying mechanisms responsible for the chemotactic response with the understanding that such information will eventually lead to a rational approach for modifying the chemotactic response *in vivo*. Studies of this kind eventually involve the injection of the chemotactic stimuli *in vivo* in order to demonstrate the biological relevance of the system.

Studies to be presented in this paper are limited to those experiments which pertain directly to the question of the rheumatological significance of chemotaxis. In this context only data concerning what induces the local accumulation of leukocytes at the site of arthritic conditions and what physiological conditions or pharmacological agents are capable of altering this accumulation of leukocytes are strictly relevant. In rheumatoid arthritis accumulations of neutrophils, monocytes, and lymphocytes occur in various proportions depending upon the severity of the disease and other as yet ill-defined factors operative in individual patients.

Various chemotactic stimuli have been found in the influenced joints. These include complement components, by-products of the kinin and clotting system, tissue degradation products, etc. In addition, increase in vascular permeability and effusions are usual. Thus, the local accumulation of leukocytes in arthritis is accompanied by the presence of chemotactic factors, increased vascular permeability and the usual signs of inflammation which include margination of leukocytes. The rheumatological significance of chemotaxis cannot be limited to any one of the various factors which contribute to the local accumulation of leukocytes, but must take into account all of the various parameters which influence the final result.

A critical question related to the significance of chemotaxis in rheumatology is whether or not the leukocytes which accumulate in synovial effusions are responsible for the resultant tissue damage. Certainly leukocytes in juxtaposition with immune complexes can induce acute inflammatory reactions by releasing neutral proteinases which activate the kinin and complement systems[6,7]. Whether collagenase, elastase and cathepsin G [8,9] present in these cells can produce tissue injury in the presence of synovial fluid remains a matter of speculation. Most authors favour the concept that tissue injury is produced by the advancing pannus in which the fibroblasts and machrophages arise to a large extent by local proliferation. In this case chemotaxis would be of small import. Regardless of one's viewpoint it is clear that there occurs an immigration of neutrophils, monocytes and lymphocytes which do no good to the patient and their elimination would be a desirable end point.

The data I now present were obtained using a method of separately quantifying the local accumulation *in vivo* of either the rat neutrophil, mononuclear phagocyte, or lymphocyte to a locally induced inflammatory stimulus.

METHODS

The method involves adoptively transferring rat ^{51}Cr-labelled isologous peritoneal exudate neutrophils, monocytes or lymphocytes to normal recipient rats in which acute or chronic paw inflammation was induced by subplantar instillation of carrageenan or Freund's complete adjuvant. The local accumulation of cells was quantified by direct scintillation counting of the amputated inflamed and non-inflamed contralateral paws, as well as an aliquot of circulating cells. The number of cells in the inflammatory reaction was estimated by subtracting the radioactivity in the inflamed extremity from that in the normal paw and relating these counts to the number of cells by determining the specific activity of the circulating leukocytes. The small amount of radioactivity in the plasma and in the oedematous fluid was corrected for by reference to previously prepared standard curves in which the plasma radioactivity was found to be directly related to that in a given amount of oedema. The cell type accumulated in the inflammation was predetermined by adoptively transferring selected ^{51}Cr-labelled cell suspensions in which only neutrophils, monocyte/macrophage or lymph node lymphocytes were capable of remaining in circulation. The methods used were previously described in detail[2] and have been shown to accurately represent the number of the specific cell type in the inflammation, independent of oedema formation, changes in haemodynamics and free plasma radioactivity. In all cases the histological findings were compatible with the estimate of cell numbers and cell types determined by the radioactivity method.

Two types of experiment will be described here; firstly those in which an acute inflammatory reaction was induced by the injection of carrageenan and the effect of various pharmacological agents was determined. Secondly, a series of studies in which the kinetics of the accumulation of various cell types to the secondary lesions of adjuvant arthritis will be described in detail.

RESULTS AND DISCUSSION

The effect of pharmacological agents on the accumulation of various cell types to the site of acute carrageenan reactions *in vivo*

Various drugs were given to rats one hour prior to the adoptive transfer of isologous peritoneal neutrophils and a simultaneously administered subplantar injection of carrageenan. Five hours later the animals, in groups of seven, were sacrificed and the number of neutrophils accumulated in the inflammatory reaction was calculated as described and compared with the number of cells in the paws of animals which were non-drug treated but subjected to the same experimental procedures. The results given in Table 4.1 indicate that the non-steroidal anti-inflammatory agents such as indomethacin, phenylbutazone, mefenamic acid, or aspirin had no effect on the accumulation of peritoneal neutrophils to the site of the acute carrageenan induced inflammatory reaction. This result was confirmed histologically. It should be noted that each of these agents was capable of significantly inhibiting oedema formation. Colchicine, however, significantly inhibited cell accumulation as well as oedema formation. The diuretic furosemide and the hypotensive agent clonidine did not affect cell accumulation which indicated that our quantification methods were independent of local haemodynamic effects.

The glucocorticosteroid, paramethasone, significantly inhibited both oedema formation and cell accumulation. In order to determine whether this was a local or a systemic effect, ^{51}Cr-labelled neutrophils were pre-incubated with hydrocortisone or buffer prior to adoptively transferring the cells to non-drug treated recipients. An aliquot of this same cell preparation was added to the up-

Table 4.1 Effects of various agents on the accumulation of adoptively transferred ^{51}Cr-labelled rat peritoneal neutrophils to a carrageenan-induced inflammatory reaction*

Agent	*Dose† mg/kg*	*Percentage inhibition‡ neutrophil accumulation*	*Swelling*
Paramethasone	1	61§	52§
Indomethacin	5	57**	31§
Phenylbutazone	100	0	35§
Mefenamic Acid	300	0	34§
Aspirin	300	0	38§
Colchicine	10	79§	55§
Furosemide	10	0	20
Clonidine	1	0	10

* Animals sacrificed 5 hours after adoptive transfer and carrageenan injection. The number of labelled circulating cells one hour after adoptive transfer did not differ between drug treated and control rats.

† Given orally one hour before subplantar injection of carrageenan and i.v. adoptive transfer of 70×10^6 ^{51}Cr-labelled isologous peritoneal neutrophils.

‡ $\% \text{ inhibition} = 100 - \frac{\text{cells in injected paw} - \text{cells in non-injected paw [Drug Treated]}}{\text{cells in injected paw} - \text{cells in non-injected paw [Control]}} \times 100$

§ $P < 0.05$ compared with a group of seven rats not drug treated.

** Significant increase in cell accumulation as compared with control.

per chamber of a modified Boyden system and their chemotactic movement to immune complexes placed in the lower chamber was determined using previously described methods[10]. The results given in Table 4.2 indicate that this steroid significantly inhibited both the *in vitro* chemotactic response as well as the ability of the same cells to accumulate at the carrageenan reaction *in vivo* after adoptive transfer.

In the studies in which cells were adoptively transferred the number of labelled cells in circulation was quantified by direct scintillation counting of the formed elements of the blood. This figure was used in the calculation of the number of cells accumulated in the lesion in order to relate counts to cell numbers. The number of counts in the formed elements of the blood also served as a measure of cell viability since each animal received the same number of ^{51}Cr-labelled leukocytes (70×10^6). In no case in which results are reported in this paper, did the number of cells in the circulation of the drug treated animals differ significantly from the number circulating in those animals not treated with drugs, indicating that at the dosage used, the drugs were not toxic to the cells. This is a good estimate of cell viability since we are measuring a functional characteristic of the cells rather than simply dye exclusion, which is a terminal event. We therefore conclude from the results in Tables 4.1 and 4.2 that glucocorticosteroids given systemically are capable of directly modifying the ability

Table 4.2 Effect of pre-incubating rat ^{51}Cr-labelled neutrophils with hydrocortisone on their ability to accumulate at an acute carrageenan reaction after adoptive transfer or to migrate to antigen/antibody complexes *in vitro**

	Pre-incubation (20′ – 20 °C)	
	Vehicle	*Hydrocortisone hemisuccinate* (5×10^{-4} M)
In vivo		
% injected cells in circulation† after adoptive transfer	3.1	2.9
Number of ^{51}Cr cells/g carrageenan swelling	47 150 ± 6200	25 250 ± 10 000
Size of carrageenan swelling (g)	1.24 ± 0.03	1.16 ± 0.03
In vitro		
Viability (Dye exclusion)	>99%	>99%
Number of cells migrating through filter‡	63	4

† 70×10^6 ^{51}Cr cells per animal i.v. 7 rats per group.
* Average of 4 microscopic fields ($\times$ 320) of the lowermost surface of each of 3 individual filters following incubation for 3 hours at 37 °C (3μ pore size). ^{51}Cr labelled cells used were an aliquot of the same cells which were adoptively transferred.
‡ Chemotactic stimulus was fresh rabbit serum activated with a bovine serum albumin (BSA) — Anti-BSA immune complex made at equivalence and then diluted to a final concentration of 10%

of the neutrophil to migrate to a site of inflammation, independent of their known effects on the vascular system.

Monocytes/macrophages

In these experiments the drug was administered one hour prior to the adoptive transfer of peritoneal macrophage/monocytes and the injection of carrageenan. A further dose of the drug was given six hours later and the animals were not sacrificed until eighteen hours following the adoptive transfer. This protocol was employed since we had previously shown[2] that between 0 and 1 hour following the injection of carrageenan, cells did not accumulate in the lesion, whilst between 1 and 5 hours, only the neutrophils accumulated. Monocytes did not appear until 5–18 hours after the injection of carrageenan.

The results given in Table 4.3, show that, with the exception of aspirin, non-steroidal anti-inflammatory drugs significantly inhibited mononuclear cell accumulation as compared with cells transferred into non-drug treated animals. In addition, the membrane active agent chlorpromazine also inhibited accumulation of monocytes. Colchicine on the other hand, had no effect on mononuclear cell accumulation to a carrageenan inflammation. Glucocorticosteroids inhibited both cell accumulation and oedema formation.

Table 4.3 Effect of various agents on the accumulation of adoptively transferred ^{51}Cr-labelled rat peritoneal mononuclear phagocytes to a carrageenan induced inflammatory reaction

Agent	*Dose** *mg/kg*	*Percentage inhibition† cell‡ accumulation*	*Swelling*
Paramethasone	1	64§	69§
Indomethacin	5	46§	37§
Phenylbutazone	100	38§	31§
Mefenamic acid	300	41§	25§
Aspirin	300	8	36§
Colchicine	10	0	0
Furosemide	10	0	0
Clonidine	1	0	0
Chlorpromazine	100	46§	37§

* Given twice orally 1 hour before and 5 hours after adoptive transfer and subplantar injection of carrageenan
† See Table 4.1 for calculation
‡ When a three day caseinate induced peritoneal exudate cell suspension is adoptively transferred only ^{51}Cr-labelled mononuclear phagocytes are present in circulation
§ $P < 0.05$ compared with a non-treated group (7 rats/group)

These results suggest that agents which interact with cell membranes, such as the non-steroidal anti-inflammatory agents and chlorpromazine, inhibit mononuclear cell accumulation perhaps on the basis of reducing the negative surface charge which is important in keeping cells from adhering to vascular walls during the margination process secondary to stasis. Alternatively, the smaller neutrophil which tends to remain in 'midstream' might depend more heavily on active motility for emigration. Alteration of its well-developed microtubular system with colchicine would have a profound inhibiting effect on its egress from the vasculature.

Regardless of the explanation it is significant that certain pharmacological agents can interact with specific cell types so as to modify their ability to selectively accumulate at the site of an inflammatory reaction. As mentioned previously, there was no reduction in the number of circulating cells in those animals treated with drugs or those cells pre-incubated before adoptive transfer. We feel therefore that under normal conditions, drugs can adversely affect cell accumulation *in vivo*, without altering their viability. Whether this effect is sufficient to modify the various rheumatological processes is as yet unknown. It is known that colchicine is active in acute gouty conditions where neutrophils are predominant and is less active in more chronic diseases where mononuclear phagocytes predominate.

The fact that glucocorticosteroids inhibit the migration of both cell types only reinforces the many mechanisms of action which this class of compounds is capable of exerting.

KINETICS AND THE EFFECT OF SERUM ON LYMPHOCYTE AND MONOCYTE ACCUMULATION TO THE SECONDARY LESIONS OF ADJUVANT DISEASE

The results given so far were concerned with acute inflammation whereas the usual rheumatological problems are chronic in nature. We therefore turned our attention to studying cell accumulation in the secondary lesions (non-adjuvant injected extremity) of adjuvant-induced arthritis in the rat. Chronic inflammation predominates in this disease which is characterized by the influx of lymphocytes and mononuclear phagocytes. Isologous ^{51}Cr-labelled peritoneal mononuclear phagocytes or lymph node lymphocytes were adoptively transferred to rats at various times after induction of adjuvant arthritis. In all cases each rat in groups of seven received 70×10^6 cells given intravenously. In these experiments we were therefore measuring the ability of normal cells to accumulate at the site of a developing arthritic lesion. Cell accumulation measured under these conditions would be an estimate of either the generation of selected chemotactic factors or the effect of serum upon the migration of the adoptively transferred cells.

The kinetics of cell accumulation in adjuvant disease is given in Figure 4.1. It can be seen that 3 or 6 days after adjuvant injection clinical disease had not developed in the non-injected extremity, as estimated by paw swelling. However, at 6 days there was a significant number of lymphocytes, but not monocytes, in the extremity in which the disease was eventually to develop. Histologically only lymphocytes could be found in the developing lesion at this time. At 12 and 20 days both lymphocytes and monocytes were capable of accumulating at the site where the inflammatory reaction was by then clinically manifest.

To determine whether serum factors were responsible for the selective migration of either lymphocytes or monocytes, we pre-incubated ^{51}Cr-labelled lymphocytes or peritoneal exudate mononuclear cells taken from normal rats with serum prior to transfer. The cells were exposed to serum taken from rats at various times after the induction of adjuvant disease. Incubation was for 30 min at 37 °C. After incubation the cells were washed once then transferred to other rats which were injected with carrageenan. Carrageenan was used as the phlogistic agent in order to test whether serum from the adjuvant animals would modify the accumulation of normal cells to a non-specific inflammatory reaction. The accumulation of cells in the carrageenan injected paw was measured 18 hours after adoptive transfer.

The results given in Figure 4.2 show that when pre-incubated with normal serum (0) lymphocytes did not accumulate in the carrageenan reaction, whereas a significant number of mononuclear phagocytes did. It was previously reported[2] that mononuclear cells but no lymphocytes accumulate during acute carrageenan reactions measured 18 hours after injection.

In contrast, lymphocytes from the same donor pool once incubated with

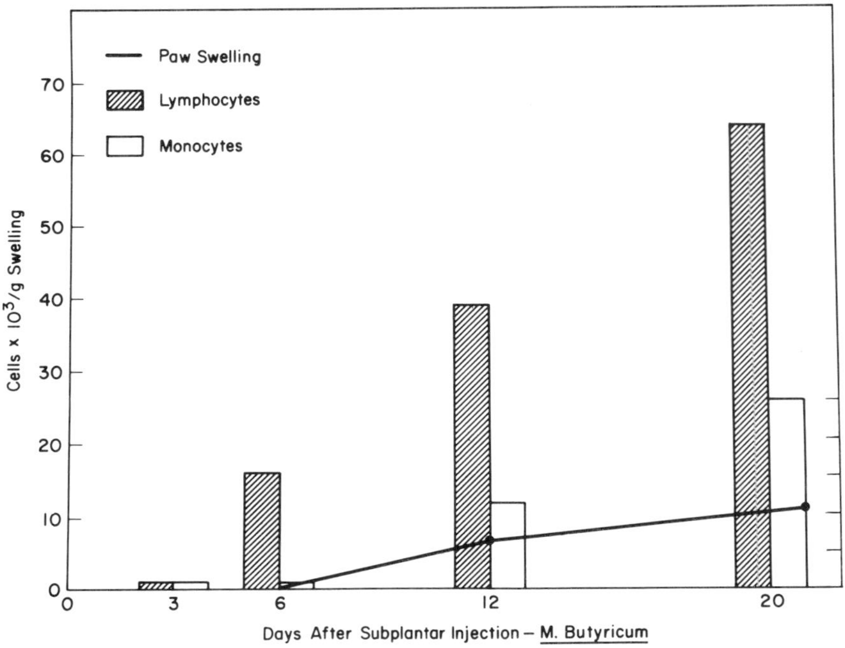

Figure 4.1 Normal ^{51}Cr-labelled Lewis rat peritoneal exudate mononuclear phagocytes, or lymph node lymphocytes, were adoptively transferred to groups of 7 to 10 isologous rats at various times after induction of adjuvant disease. Cell accumulation in the non-injected extremity was determined by direct scintillation counting using appropriate controls. The swelling is the weight (g) of the non-adjuvant injected, arthritic paw minus the average weight of the rear paw of a group of 20 rats of the same body weight

serum taken from rats injected with Freund's complete adjuvant 6 days previously, were found to accumulate in the carrageenan lesion. However, serum of adjuvant rats did not increase the number of mononuclear phagocytes. Thus, serum taken 6 days after adjuvant injection had the specific effect of inducing the accumulation of lymphocytes. This result was confirmed histologically.

Interestingly enough, serum taken from animals 12 and 21 days after injection of the adjuvant enhanced the accumulation of both lymphocytes and mononuclear phagocytes (Figure 4.2).

This unusual finding was confirmed *in vitro* by testing aliquots of the same cell populations used in *in vivo* studies. The cells after serum pre-incubation were placed in the upper compartments of modified Boyden chambers and their chemotactic activity to antigen–antibody complexes in the lower chamber was determined using previously published methods[10]. The results given in Figure 4.3, that lymphocytes pre-incubated with 6 day serum (and to a lesser extent

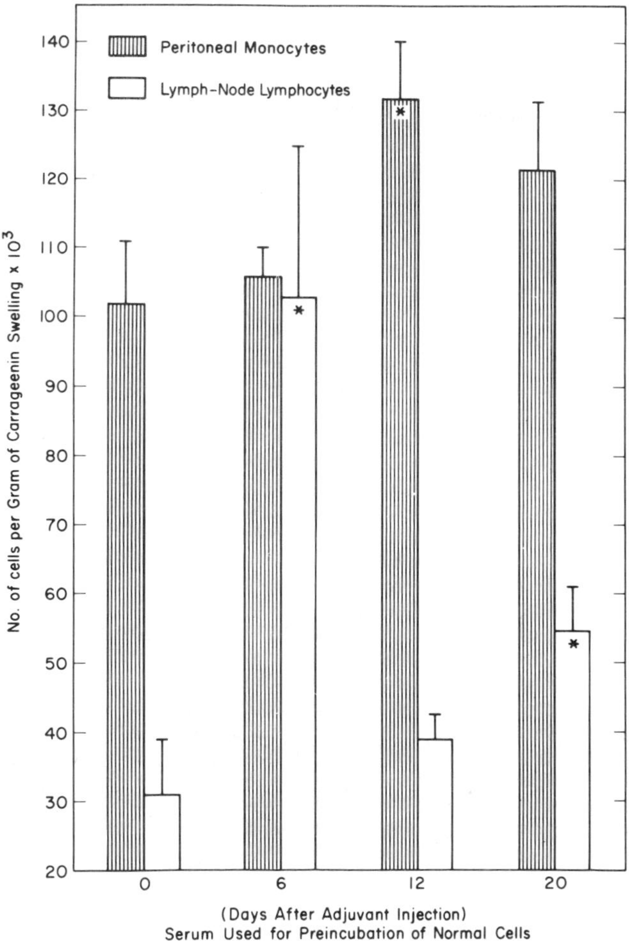

Figure 4.2 Normal ^{51}Cr-labelled Lewis rat peritoneal mononuclear phagocytes, or lymph node lymphocytes, were pre-incubated with serum from isologous rats taken at various times after the induction of adjuvant disease. After incubation the cells were transferred (i.v.) into other rats which received a simultaneously administered subplantar injection of carrageenan. Cell accumulation was determined 18 hours later by direct scintillation counting of the inflamed paw. (0) is normal serum. Each bar is the average of 7 rats/group ± SEM. * = $P < 0.05$

those incubated with 12 and 20 day serum) exhibited chemotactic activity *in vitro*. It should be noted that the quantitative effect of 6, 12 and 20 day serum was the same whether the chemotactic activity of the pre-incubated lymphocytes was tested *in vivo* or *in vitro*. (Compare Figures 4.2 and 4.3.)

The results of these experiments clearly indicate that lymphocytes treated with serum from rats injected 6 days previously with adjuvant would 'home' to non-specific inflammatory reactions *in vivo*, and to antigen–antibody complexes *in vitro*. Monocytes also were influenced by serum factors in that serum taken later in the course of the disease would induce monocytes to accumulate in greater numbers than normal, to a non-specific inflammatory reaction. The nature of the serum factors causing these effects is currently unknown.

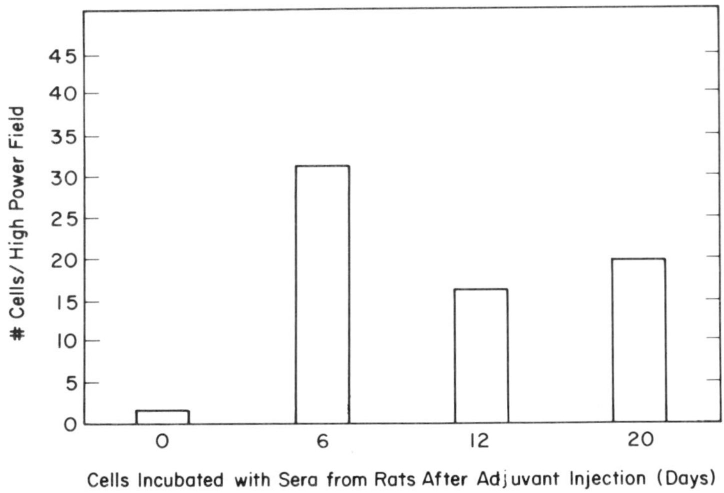

Figure 4.3 Chemotactic activity *in vitro* of aliquots of the same lymphocytes used in Figure 4.2 (lymph node cells pre-incubated with serum from rats taken at various times after induction of adjuvant disease). *In vitro* conditions were the same as detailed in the legend of Table 4.2. (0) is normal Lewis rat serum. Note that pre-incubation with serum from arthritic rats induced migration of lymphocytes to immune complexes

There are few if any publications indicating that serum factors will enhance chemotactic activity of leukocytes, though there are several reports indicating that tumour cell products, which can be found in serum, have inhibitory effects on leukocyte chemotaxis. Snyderman and his co-workers[11], and Normann and Sorkin[12] have reported that low molecular weight factors are produced by tumour cells which will inhibit monocyte chemotaxis *in vitro*. The first group also demonstrated that such factors when injected parenterally would inhibit macrophage cell accumulation to an inflammatory site four days after the injection of the extract. In this regard North and co-workers[13] previously had shown that tumours produce low molecular weight factors which are present in serum and which would inhibit the rate of migration of blood leukocytes into sterile inflammatory peritoneal exudates. Of importance to our studies is that in an accompanying publication[14], the same group have shown also that although initially there is a defect in macrophage-mediated anti-bacterial resistance after tumour implantation, subsequently there is enhancement of the anti-bacterial effect.

Thus it is possible that there is a sequential release first of inhibitors and then of stimulating factors during either the development of tumour resistance, or an inflammatory reaction. Regardless of these speculative interpretations, our data clearly indicate that serum taken 12 or 20 days after adjuvant injection will enhance the ability of adoptively transferred mononuclear cells to accumulate at a non-specific inflammatory reaction.

The effect of 6 day serum on enhancing lymphocyte accumulation to a non-specific inflammatory reaction *in vivo* and chemotaxis *in vitro* is somewhat surprising and requires further explanation. There is a paucity of data related to how chemotactic factors perturb the cell membrane so as to cause directional migration. It is generally assumed that perturbation of a portion of the membrane is followed by movement in the direction of the stimulus. It is possible that adjuvant serum contains factors (not present in normal serum) which perturb the cell membrane and cause a generalized irritability, which results in an increase in the cellular response to defined stimuli.

CONCLUDING REMARKS

The biological significance of these findings to the rheumatologist is that during the course of arthritis, it is possible that serum factors are generated which stimulate selective cell types to migrate to arthritic areas. This is in accord with clinical findings in which different cell types predominate in synovial effusions at different times during the course of the disease, even though the chronicity remains reasonably stable. The sequential generation of different chemotactic factors could also explain this observation.

Of equal importance to the rheumatologist is the availability of pharmacological agents which can inhibit the large-scale migration of leukocytes into the inflamed joint. Our data, in the rat, indicates that steroidal and non-steroidal anti-inflammatory agents delay the accumulation of mononuclear phagocytes to inflammatory reactions, and colchicine delays the appearance of neutrophils whereas the glucocorticosteroids inhibit the migration of both neutrophils and monocytic macrophages. Whether these agents have similar effects in man can only be answered when controlled trials become available.

References

1. DiRosa, M., Papadimitriou, J. M. and Willoughby, D. A. (1971). *J. Pathol.*, **105**, 239
2. Perper, R. J., Sanda, M., Chinea, G. and Oronsky, A. L. (1974). *J. Lab. Clin. Med.*, **84**, 378
3. Gigli, I. and Nelson, R. A. (1968). *Exp. Cell Res.*, **51** 45
4. Goetzl, E. J. and Austen, K. F. (1972). *J. Exp. Med.*, **136**, 1564
5. Jensen, J. A. and Esquenazi, V. (1975). *Nature (London)*, **256**, 213
6. Movat, H. Z., Steinberg, S. G., Habal, F. M. and Ranadive, N. S. (1973). *Lab. Invest.*, **29**, 669

7. Goldstein, I. M. and Weissmann, G. (1974). *J. Immunol.,* **113,** 1583
8. Oronsky, A. L., Perper, R. J. and Schroder, H. C. (1973). *Nature (London),* **246,** 417
9. Malemud, C. J. and Janoff, A. (1975). *Arth. Rheum.,* **18,** 361
10. Stecher, V. J. and Sorkin, E. (1969). *Immunology,* **16,** 231
11. Snyderman, R., Pike, M. C., Blaylock, B. L. and Weinstein, P. (1976). *J. Immunol.,* **116,** 585
12. Normann, S. J. and Sorkin, E. (1977). *Cancer Res.,* **37,** 705
13. North, R. J., Kirsten, D. P. and Tuttle, R. L. (1976). *J. Exp. Med.,* **143,** 559
14. North, R. J., Kirsten, D. P. and Tuttle, R. L. (1976). *J. Exp. Med.,* **143,** 574

5
Modulation of Complement Activation: a Pharmacotherapeutic Goal?

K. WHALEY

INTRODUCTION

The complement system (Figure 5.1) comprises a group of plasma proteins, which, when activated, provide some of the major mediators of the inflammatory response. Activation of the classical pathway usually results from the interaction of the first component (C1) with immune complexes[1]. As a consequence of this interaction, the precursor form of C1 is converted to an active enzyme, $C\bar{1}$* which has esterolytic and proteolytic activities[2,3]. $C\bar{1}$ catalyses the limited proteolysis of its two natural substrates, the fourth (C4)[4] and second (C2)[5] components of complement. C4 and C2 interact to form a complex $C\overline{42}$, which itself has proteolytic activity, the third component (C3) being its natural substrate[5]. Cleavage of C3 by C42 results in the formation of a low molecular weight product, C3a (anaphylotoxin), and C3b, the major cleavage product. Following the formation of C3b, C5 is cleaved into C5a (anaphylotoxin) and C5b, which subsequently complexes with C6, C7, C8 and C9, with resulting cell lysis[6] (Figure 5.1).

An alternative, or properdin pathway of complement activation, which has been partly characterized, is in many ways analogous to the classical pathway. Although it is triggered indirectly by certain immunoglobulin complexes, and possibly directly by polysaccharides found on certain yeasts or bacteria[7,8], the exact initiating mechanism is as yet undefined. However, activation requires the participation of properdin factor $\bar{D}$, an active serum esterase which also exists in precursor form in plasma[9]. $\bar{D}$ cleaves properdin factor B, a plasma

* A bar over the symbol indicates that the complement(s) is (are) in activated form.

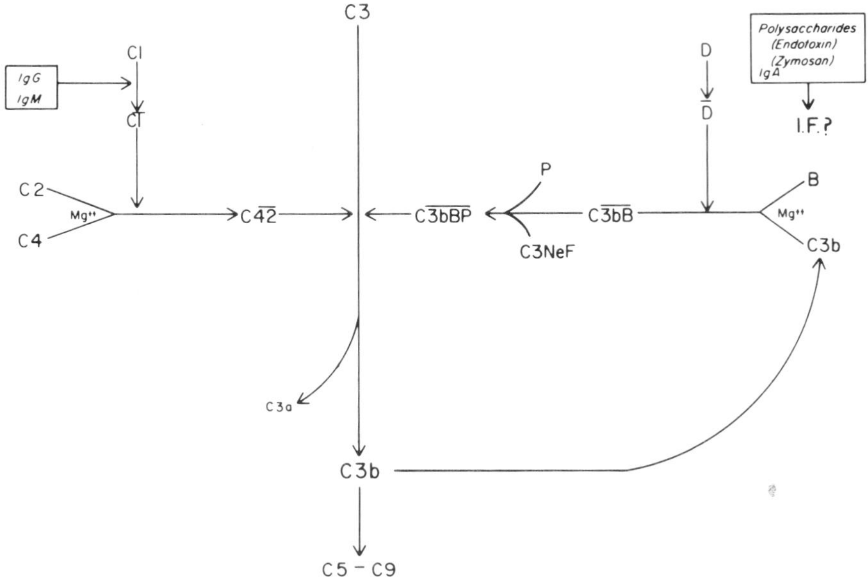

Figure 5.1 Molecular interactions occurring during classical and alternative pathway complement activation. Nomenclature is described in the text

glycoprotein, after the latter has complexed with C3b, the major cleavage product of C3[10]. The result is the formation of a bimolecular complex, $C\overline{3bB}$, the alternative pathway C3 convertase, which cleaves C3 in the same manner as $C\overline{42}$. Properdin stabilizes $C\overline{3bB}$ by preventing decay of factor B[11] as does C3 nephritic factor (C3NeF)[12].

Implicit in this scheme of alternative pathway activation is the requirement for C3b to form the initial $C\overline{3bB}$. In the properdin amplification loop, C3b, generated by classical pathway activation can complex with factor B and thus form the alternative pathway convertase. However, it has also been shown that the alternative pathway can be initiated in the absence of C3b, when properdin factors B and $\overline{D}$ and native C3 are simultaneously present[13,14].

PHLOGISTIC PRODUCTS OF COMPLEMENT ACTIVATION

As a result of complement activation, anaphylotoxins are generated (from C3 and C5) which cause histamine release from mast cells, smooth muscle contraction and increased vascular permeability[15,16]. Fragments with chemotactic properties also result from C3 and C5 cleavage[17,18]. The trimolecular complex $C\overline{567}$ [19] is also reputed to be chemotactic for macrophages. C-kinin is a low molecular weight fragment released from C2 during its cleavage by $C\bar{1}$[20]. C3b, the major cleavage product of C3 also has important phlogistic properties, apart from being responsible for the continuation of the cytolytic sequence via interaction with C5-C9 and triggering the properdin amplification loop, it is capable of interacting with cells bearing C3b receptors, a phenomenon known as immune adherence[21], and if these cells are phagocytic then phagocytosis is facilitated[22].

MODULATION OF COMPLEMENT ACTIVATION

Two processes exist whereby the complement system is modulated, the intrinsic decay of enzymes, and the presence of circulating inhibitors or inactivators (Table 5.1). Rapid decay of C2b, C5b, and Bb from C$\overline{42}$ [23] C$\overline{423b5b}$ [24] and C$\overline{3bB}$, and C$\overline{3bBP}$ [25] respectively, occurs linearly in a temperature-dependent fashion. Following decay, these enzymes can be regenerated by fresh C2, C5 or factor B (Table 5.1).

Table 5.1 Control mechanisms of the complement system

A. *Decay of enzymes*
(1) Loss of C2 from C$\overline{42}$
(2) Loss of C5 from C$\overline{423b5}$
(3) Loss of Bb from C$\overline{3bBb}$ and C$\overline{3bBbP}$
B. *Naturally occurring inhibitors and inactivators*
(1) C$\bar{1}$-Inhibitor
(2) C3b Inactivator
(3) C6 Inactivator
(4) Anaphylotoxin Inactivator
(5) β1H globulin

Other regulatory influences are the presence of naturally occurring inhibitors and inactivators which are plasma proteins capable of combining with or enzymatically destroying certain complement components. Five such proteins have been described C$\bar{1}$-inhibitor (C$\bar{1}$-INH), C3b inactivator (C3bINA), Cb inactivator (CbINA), anaphylotoxin inactivator and β1H globulin.

C$\bar{1}$-INH

This α_2-globulin inhibits not only enzymes of the complement system, but also the kinin-forming, coagulation and fibrinolytic systems. Specifically, these include C$\bar{1}$ and its subcomponents C$\overline{1r}$ and C$\overline{1s}$[26–30], kallikrein[30–33], PF/dil (permeability factor of dilution)[30–33], plasmin[30,34], Hageman factor[35] and its active fragments[34]. C$\bar{1}$-INH, reacts with C$\bar{1}$ in a temperature dependent fashion[35] and forms a molar complex with C$\overline{1s}$[36]. It appears therefore that C$\bar{1}$-INH stoichiometrically binds with the C1 enzyme on, or near its active site, to form an inactive complex.

C3bINA

C3bINA is a trace protein of human plasma. It was first shown to make cell bound C3b reactive with bovine conglutinin[37], hence the name conglutinogen activating factor (KAF). It has since been shown to enzymatically cleave C3b into two smaller fragments C3c and C3d, neither of which apparently possesses biological activity[38]. As a result of this interaction the participation of C3b in the classical[39] and alternative[40] pathways is blocked, as is immune adherence[37].

Purified C3bINA is far less effective than C3bINA in plasma in inactivating C3b [39], and it has been suggested that other C3b inactivating proteins or coenzymes are present in plasma. To date two factors have been identified, C3b inactivator accelerator[41] now identified as β1H globulin[42], and a 10S globulin which, in the presence of C3bINA, results in full enzymatic expression of C3bINA[43]. C3bINA also cleaves C4b[44], but the reaction is far less efficient than its action on C3b[42].

C6INA

This regulatory protein was first demonstrated in the sera of C6-deficient rabbits[45]. It inactivates cell-bound but not fluid-phase C6 blocking the haemolytic sequence by stopping the participation of C7. It effects upon the generation of the chemotactic factor, $C\overline{567}$, and reactive haemolysis are unknown. C6INA has been shown to be present in guinea-pig and human sera[33], but its biological significance is far from clear.

Anaphylotoxin inactivator

Anaphylotoxin inactivator is a plasma pseudoglobulin with α mobility on electrophoresis at pH 8.6, with a sedimentation coefficient of 10S[47]. It is a carboxypeptidase, cleaving the carboxyterminal arginine residue from C3a and C5a, rendering them biologically inactive[48].

β1H globulin

That β1H globulin was an important regulatory protein of the complement system stemmed from the search for a second C3b inactivating principle in human plasma. An activity which potentiated the inactivation of C3b by C3bINA was found and tentatively designated as C3b inactivator Accelerator[39]. This factor appeared to act in a non-enzymatic fashion, and both C3bINA and its accelerator had to be simultaneously present for potentiation to be observed[40]. Following purification of the activity and the production of antisera, it became obvious that C3b inactivator Accelerator was identical with a protein previously designated β1H-globulin on the basis of its electrophoretic

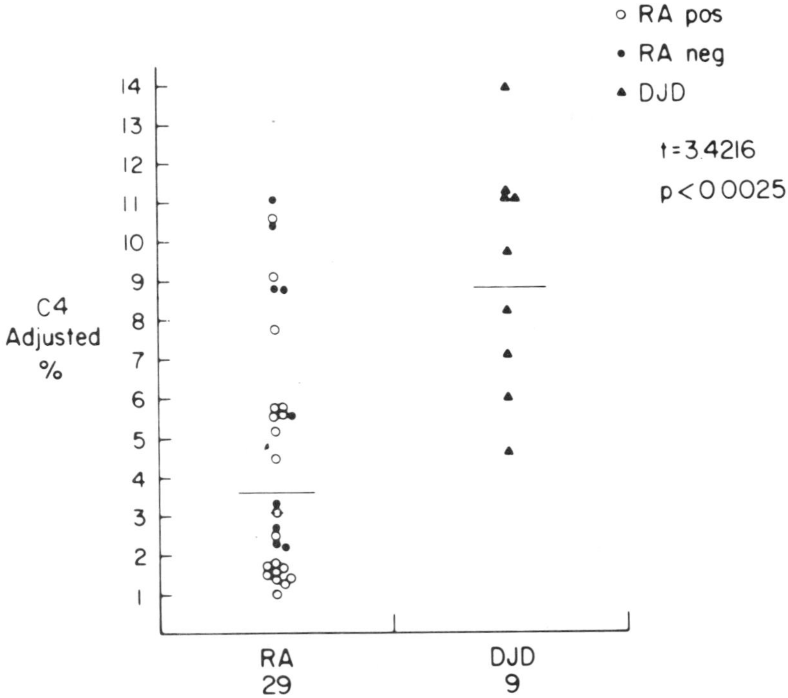

Figure 5.2 C4 concentrations in synovial fluid

mobility[42]. The purified protein was shown to have two further important regulatory functions. It possesses the ability to block the participation of C3b in both the classical and alternative pathways, by interacting with cells bearing C3b [40], although this interaction does not block immune adherence[49]. In contrast to C3bINA, β1H globulin also increases the decay of the alternative pathway C3 convertase, $\overline{\text{C3bB}}$ increasing the rate of decay of the enzyme[40] the loss of activity being associated with loss of radiolabelled factor B [50]. It acts on the unstable and properdin stabilized enzymes in a dose dependent fashion[40], but not on the nephritic factor stabilized enzyme[50]. The molecular interactions of this fascinating protein are currently unknown (Figure 5.3).

ACTIVATION OF THE COMPLEMENT SYSTEM IN RA AND SLE

Activation of the complement system in RA and SLE has been shown by the demonstration of lowered total haemolytic complement levels and reduced individual component levels[51–62] in serum and synovial fluid respectively (Figure 5.2 and Figure 5.3), the presence of C3 cleavage products[63,64], immunofluorescence[65–69], and hypercatabolism of radiolabelled components[70–73]. That activation of the alternative pathway occurs has been demonstrated by the fin-

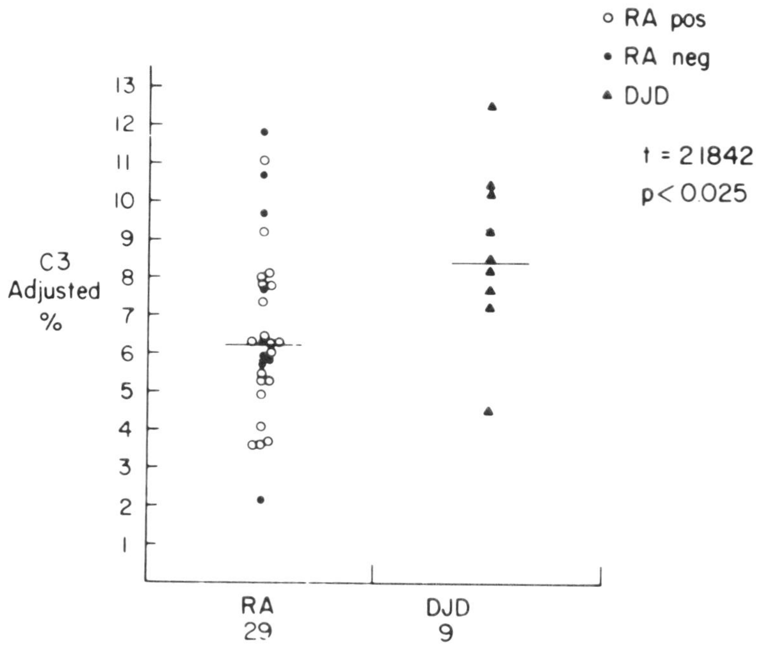

Figure 5.3 C3 concentrations in synovial fluid

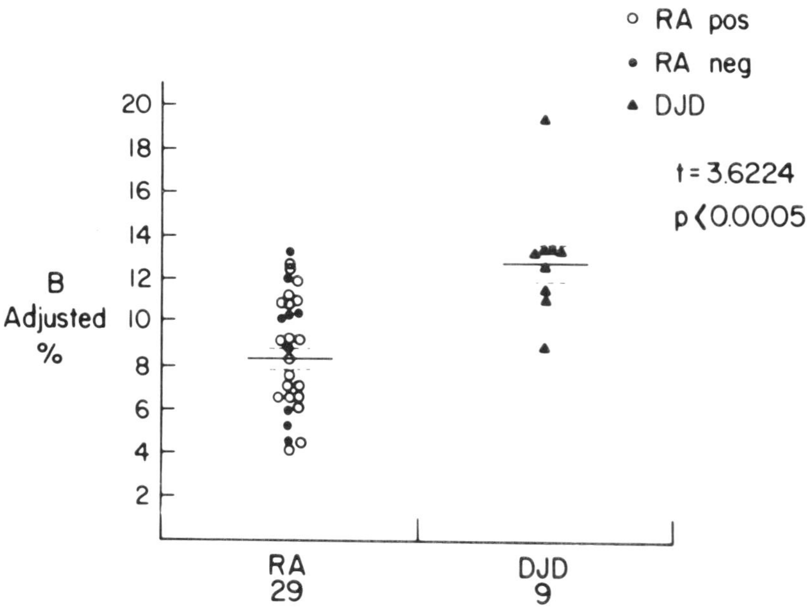

Figure 5.4 Factor B concentrations in synovial fluid

ding of cleavage products of factor B [74,75], reduced serum and synovial fluid concentrations of factor B (Figure 5.4) and properdin[62,76–78]. Immunofluorescence studies show deposition of properdin and factor B [69,79], and metabolic studies show increased catabolism of properdin and factor B [80–82]. In SLE there is evidence to suggest that immune complexes may activate the alternative pathway directly[83], but most of the activation represents recruitment by the C3b-amplification loop.

Reduced levels of C3bINA[40] and β1H globulin[84] occur in the synovial fluid in RA and serum in SLE, and appear to be related to the extent of alternative pathway activation as shown by the correlation of C3bINA or β1H concentrations with factor B, properdin and C3 but not C4 levels (Figure 5.5–5.8).

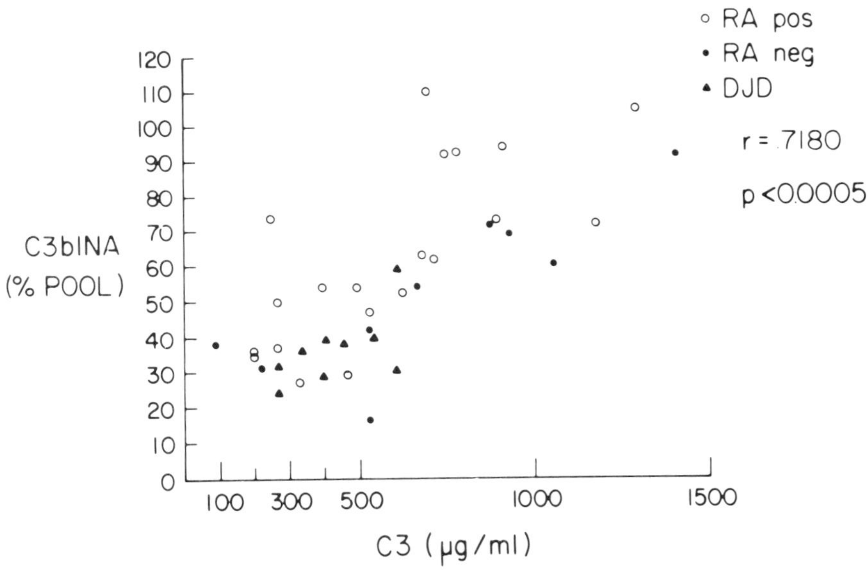

Figure 5.5 Correlation between C3bINA and C3 concentrations in synovial fluid

These findings can be explained by assuming that reduced levels of these regulatory proteins allow C3b to persist and form $\overline{C3bB}$ or $\overline{C3bBP}$ which would cleave further C3. Thus low levels of C3bINA or β1H would be associated with reduced concentrations of factor B properdin and C3. To explain why reduced concentrations of C3bINA and β1H occur metabolic studies using radiolabelled purified components are essential (Figures 5.5–5.8).

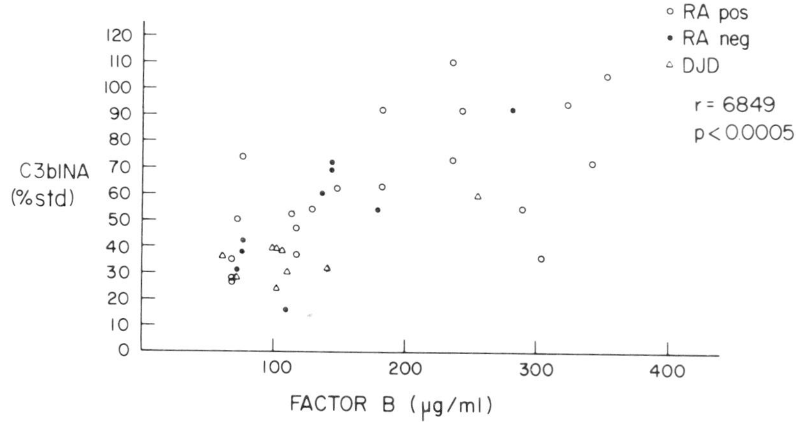

Figure 5.6 Correlation between C3bINA and factor B concentrations in synovial fluid

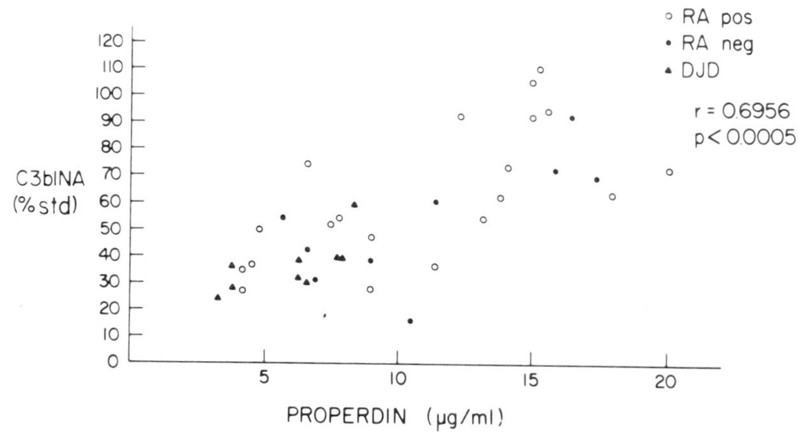

Figure 5.7 Correlation between C3bINA and properdin concentrations in synovial fluid

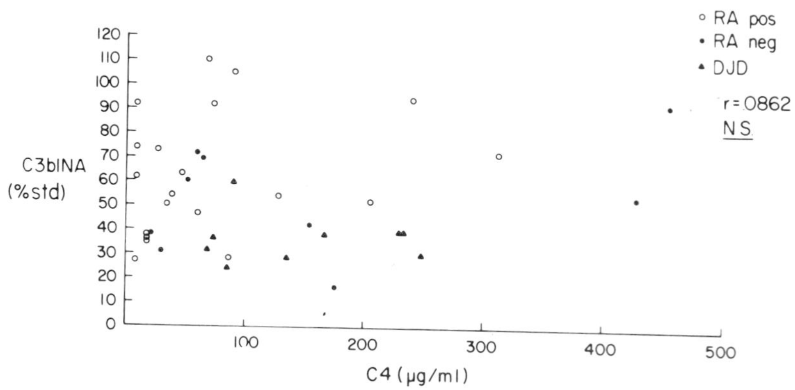

Figure 5.8 Lack of correlation between C3bINA and C4 concentrations in synovial fluid

PHARMACOLOGICAL MODULATION OF THE COMPLEMENT SYSTEM

When proposing pharmacological modulation of the complement system one can consider both long term and short term approaches.

Long term approach

(1) Studies of the synthesis of complement components in tissue culture need to be undertaken, and the mechanisms of control of synthesis need to be clearly delineated. The information should enable the development of a rational approach for inhibition of the synthesis of complement components.

(2) The synthesis of the regulatory proteins also needs to be studied, and mechanisms whereby selective stimulation of these proteins may be achieved is a desirable objective.

(3) Characterization of molecular interactions of the inhibitors and inactivators of the complement system, and the determination of means of pharmacological manipulation. If active oligopeptide fragments of the stoichiometric inhibitors can be identified, then these may possibly be synthesized in the laboratory and used during acute exacerbations of disease.

(4) Purification of large quantities of regulatory proteins and their infusion during the acute phase may be beneficial. Certainly this approach works in C3bINA deficiency.

Short term approach

Certain drugs are already known to act on the complement system inhibiting the formation of C3 and C5 convertases. These include:

1. Epsilon aminocaproic acid (EACA) and its analogue tranexamic acid, have both been successfully used to prevent attacks of hereditary angioedema in patients with $C\bar{1}$-INH deficiency[85,86]. They prevent the conversion of plasminogen to plasmin which can activate precursor C1.

2. Antrypol (Suramin), an anti-trypanosomal agent inhibits the binding of C1 to IgG aggregates[87], and blocks the enzymatic catalysis of C4 and C2 to form $C\overline{42}$, and also inhibits the enzymatic catalysis of C3 by $C\overline{42}$ [88]. It has been used to treat hereditary angioedema[89].

3. Liquoid (Sodium polyanethol sulphonate), a heparin-like drug, blocks the activation of C1s by $C\bar{1}r$ and inhibits the formation of $C\overline{42}$ by $C\bar{1}$ [90,91].

Using this information, and the already detailed knowledge of the immunochemistry of the complement system, it should be possible for the pharmacologists to produce non-toxic potent anticomplementary drugs which perhaps will have a beneficial effect on the chronic rheumatic diseases.

References

1. Borsos, T. and Rapp, H. (1965). Hemolysin titration based on fixation of the activated first component of complement. Evidence that one molecule of hemolysin suffices to sensitize an erythrocyte. *J. Immunol.*, **95,** 559
2. Sakai, K. and Stroud, R. M. (1973). Purification of molecular properties and activation of C1 proesterase, C1s. *J. Immunol.*, **110,** 1010
3. Valet, D. and Cooper, N. R. (1974). Isolation and characterization of the proenzyme form of the C1s subunit of the first complement components. *J. Immunol.*, **112,** 339
4. Muller-Eberhard, H. J. and Lepow, I. H. (1965). C1 esterase effect on activity and physical chemical properties of the fourth component of complement. *J. Exp. Med.*, **121,** 819
5. Muller-Eberhard, H. J., Polley, N. J. and Calcott, M. A. (1976). Formation and functional significance of a molecular complex derived from the second and fourth component of human complement. *J. Exp. Med.*, **125,** 359
6. Kolb, W. P., Haxby, J. A., Arroyave, C. and Muller-Eberhard, H. J. (1972). Molecular analysis of the membrane attack mechanism of complement. *J. Exp. Med.*, **135,** 549
7. Marcus, R. L., Shin, H. S. and Mayer, M. M. (1971). An alternate complement pathway: C3 cleaving activity, not due to $C\overline{4}$, $\overline{2a}$, on endotoxic lipopolysaccharide after treatment with guinea pig serum: Relation to properdin complement components. *Proc. Nat. Acad. Sci. (USA)*, **68,** 1351
8. Palmer, L., Schenberg, M. D., Bloom, L. and Wurz, L. (1955). Properdin system and immunity, II. Interaction of the properdin system with polysaccharides. *Science*, **122,** 505
9. Fearon, D. T., Austen, K. F. and Ruddy, S. (1974). Properdin factor D: Characterization of its active site and isolation of the precursor form. *J. Exp. Med.*, **139,** 355
10. Muller-Eberhard, H. J. and Götze, O. (1972). C3 proactivator convertase and its mode of action. *J. Exp. Med.*, **135,** 1003
11. Fearon, D. T. and Austen, K. F. (1975). Properdin: Binding to C3b and stabilization of the C3b-dependent C3 convertase. *J. Exp. Med.*, **142,** 856
12. Daha, M. R., Fearon, D. T. and Austen, K. F. (1976). C3 nephritic factor (C3NeF): Stabilization of fluid phase and cell-bound alternative pathway convertase. *J. Immunol.*, **116,** 1
13. Götze, O. and Muller-Eberhard, H. J. (1974). The role of properdin in the alternative pathway of complement activation. *J. Exp. Med.*, **139,** 44
14. Fearon, D. T. and Austen, K. F. (1975). Properdin: Initiation of the alternative complement pathway. *Proc. Nat. Acad. Sci. (USA)*, **72,** 3220
15. Bolish, V. A. and Muller-Eberhard, H. J. (1970). Anaphylotoxin inactivator of human plasma. Its isolation and characterization as a carboxypeptidase. *J. Clin. Invest.*, **49,** 2427
16. Cochrane, G. C. and Muller-Eberhard, H. J. (1968). The derivation of two distinct anaphylotoxin activities from the third and fifth component of human complement. *J. Exp. Med.*, **127,** 371
17. Jensen, J., Snyderman, R. and Mergenhagen, S. E. (1969). Chemotactic activity, a property of guinea pig C5 anaphylotoxin. In H. Z. Movat (ed.) *Cellular and Humoral Mechanisms of Anaphylaxis and Allergy*, pp. 265–278 (Basel: Karger)
18. Ward, P. A. and Newman, L. J. (1969). A neutrophil chemotactic factor from human C5. *J. Immunol.*, **102,** 93
19. Ward, P. A., Cochrane, C. G. and Muller-Eberhard, H. J. (1966). Further studies on the chemotactic factors of complement and its formation in vivo. *Immunology (London)*, **11,** 141
20. Klemperer, M. R., Rosen, F. S. and Donaldson, V. H. (1969). A polypeptide derived from the second component of complement (C2) which increases vascular permeability. *J. Clin. Invest.*, **48,** 44a
21. Nelson, R. A. (1953). The immune adherence phenomenon. An immunologically specific reaction between microorganisms and erythrocytes leading to enhanced phagocytosis. *Science*, **118,** 733

22. Gigli, I. and Nelson, R. A. Jr. (1968). Complement dependent immune phagocytosis. I. Requirements for C′1, C′4, C′2, C′3. *Exp. Cell Res.*, **51,** 45
23. Borsos, T., Rapp, H. J. and Mayer, M. M. (1961). Studies on the second component of complement. II. The nature of the decay of EAC′ 142. I. *Immunology,* **87,** 326
24. Cooper, N. R. and Muller-Eberhard, H. J. (1970) The reaction mechanism of human C5 in immune haemolysis. *J. Exp. Med.*, **132,** 775
25. Fearon, D. T., Austen, K. F. and Ruddy, S. (1973). Formation of a hemolytically active cellular intermediate by the interaction between properdin factors B and D and the activated third component of complement. *J. Exp. Med.*, **138,** 1305
26. Levy, L. R. and Lepow, I. H. (1959). Assay and properties of serum inhibitor of C′1-esterase. *Proc. Soc. Exp. Biol. Med.*, **101,** 608
27. Pensky, J., Levy, L. R. and Lepow I. H. (1961). Partial purification of serum inhibitor of C81-esterase. *J. Biol. Chem.*, **236,** 1674
28. Lepow, I. H. and Leon, M. A. (1962). Interaction of a serum inhibitor of C′1-esterase with intermediate complexes of the immune haemolytic system. I. Specificity of inhibition of C′1 activity associated with intermediate complexes. *Immunology,* **5,** 222
29. Gigli, I., Ruddy, S. and Austen, K. F. (1968). The stoichiometric measurement of the serum inhibitor of the first component of complement by the inhibition of immune hemolysis. *J. Immunol.*, **100,** 1154
30. Ratnoff, O. D., Pensky, J., Ogston, D. and Naff, G. B. (1969). The inhibition of plasmin, plasma kallikrein, plasma permeability factor, and the C1r subcomponent of the first component of complement by serum C81 esterase inhibitor. *J. Exp. Med.*, **129,** 315
31. Landerman, N. S., Webster, M. E., Becker, E. L. and Ratcliffe, H. E. (1962). Hereditary angioneurotic edema. II. Deficiency of inhibitor for serum globulin permeability factor and/or plasma kallikrein. *J. Allergy,* **33,** 330
32. Kagen, L. J. and Becker, E. L. (1963). Inhibition of permeability globulins by C′1-esterase inhibitor. *Fed. Proc.*, **22,** 613
33. Gigli, I., Mason, J. W., Colman, R. W. and Austen, K. F. (1970). Interaction of plasma kallikrein with the C1 inhibitor. *J. Immunol.*, **104,** 574
34. Schreiber, A. D., Kaplan, A. P. and Austen, K. F. (1973). Inhibition by C1INH of Hageman factor fragment activation of coagulation, fibrinolysis and kinin generation. *J. Clin. Invest.*, **52,** 1402
35. Forbes, C. D., Pensky, J. and Ratnoff, O. D. (1970). Inhibition of activated Hageman factor and activated plasma thromboplastin antecedent by purified serum C1 inactivator. *J. Lab. Clin. Med.*, **76,** 809
36. Harpel, P. C. and Cooper, N. R. (1975). Studies on human plasma $C\bar{1}$ inactivator enzyme interactions. I. Mechanisms of interaction with $C\bar{1}\bar{s}$, plasmin, and trypsin. *J. Clin. Invest.*, **55,** 593
37. Lachmann, P. J. and Muller-Eberhard, H. J. (1968). The demonstration in human serum of "conglutinogen activating factor" and its effect on the third component of complement. *J. Immunol.*, **100,** 691
38. Ruddy, S. and Austen, K. F. (1971). C3b inactivator of man. II. Fragments produced by C3b inactivator cleavage of cell-bound or fluid phase C3b. *J. Immunol.*, **107,** 742
39. Whaley, K. and Ruddy, S. (1976). C3b inactivator Accelerator a serum co-factor for C3b inactivator activity. Necessary for the full expression of its activity. *J. Immunol.*, **116,** 1754
40. Whaley, K. and Ruddy, S. (1976). Modulation of C3b hemolytic activity by a plasma protein distinct from C3b inactivator. *Science,* **193,** 1011
41. Whaley, K., Schur, P. H. and Ruddy, S. (1976). C3b inactivator in the rheumatic diseases. Measurement by radial immunodiffusion and by inhibition of formation of properdin pathway C3 convertase. *J. Clin. Invest.*, **57,** 1554
42. Whaley, K. and Ruddy, S. (1976). Modulation of the alternative complement pathway by β1H globulin. *J. Exp. Med.*, **144,** 1147

43. Shirishai, S. and Stroud R. M. (1975). Cleavage products of C4b produced by enzymes in human serum. *Immunochemistry,* **12,** 935
44. Cooper, N. R. (1975). Isolation and analysis of the mechanism of action of an inactivator of C4b in normal human serum. *J. Exp. Med.,* **141,** 890
45. Nelson, R. A. and Biro, C. E. (1968). Complement components of a hemolytically deficient strain of rabbits. *Immunology,* **14,** 527
46. Tamura, N. and Nelson, R. A. (1967). Three naturally occurring inhibitors of components of complement in guinea pig and rabbit serum. *J. Immunol.,* **99,** 582
47. Bokisch, V. A., Muller-Eberhard, H. J. and Cochrane, C. G. (1969). Isolation of a fragment (C3a) of the third component of human complement containing anaphylotoxin and chemotactic activity, and description of an anaphylotoxin inactivator of human serum. *J. Exp. Med.,* **129,** 1109
48. Bokisch, V. A. and Muller-Eberhard, H. J. (1970). Anaphylotoxin inactivator of human plasma. Its isolation and characterisation as a carboxypeptidase. *J. Clin. Invest.,* **49,** 2427
49. Whaley, K. and Ruddy, S. (1971). Unpublished observation
50. Weiler, J. M., Daha, M. D., Austen, K. F. and Fearon, D. T. (1976). Control of the amplification convertase of complement by the plasma protein β1H. *Proc. Nat. Acad. Sci.,* **73,** 3268
51. Pekin, T. J. Jr. and Zvaifler, N. J. (1964). Hemolytic complement in synovial fluid. *J. Clin. Invest.,* **43,** 1372
52. Fostiropoulos, F., Austen, K. F. and Bloch, K. J. (1965). Total hemolytic complement (CH50) and second component of complement ($C'2^{hu}$) activity in serum and synovial fluid. *Arthr. Rheum.,* **8,** 219
53. Hedberg, H. (1967). Studies on synovial fluid in arthritis. I. The total complement activity. *Acta Med. Scand. Suppl.,* **479,** 1
54. Gewurz, H., Pickering, R. J., Mergenhagen, S. E. and Good R. A. (1968). The complement profile in acute glomerulonephritis, systemic lupus erythematosus and hypocomplemententemic chronic glomerulonephritis. Contrasts and experimental correlations. *Int. Arch. Allergy Appl. Immunol.,* **34,** 556
55. Schur, P. H. and Sandson, J. (1968). Immunologic factors and clinical activity in systemic lupus erythematosus. *N. Engl. J. Med.,* **278,** 533
56. Ruddy, S., Britton, M. C., Schur, P. H. and Austen, K. F. (1969). Complement components in synovial fluid: Activation and fixation in seropositive rheumatoid arthritis. *Ann. N. Y. Acad. Sci.,* **168,** 161
57. Ruddy, S. and Austen, K. F. (1970). The complement system in rheumatoid synovitis. I. An analysis of complement component activities in rheumatoid synovial fluids. *Arthr. Rheum.,* **13,** 713
58. Ruddy, S., Everson, L. K., Schur, P. H. and Austen, K. F. (1971). Hemolytic assay of the ninth complement component: Elevation and depletion in the rheumatic diseases. *J. Exp. Med.,* **134,** 259S
59. Ruddy, S. and Austen, K. F. (1973). Activation of the complement system in rheumatoid synovitis. *Fed. Proc.,* **32,** 134
60. De Bracco, M. M. deE. and Manni, J. A. (1974). Serum levels of C1q, C1r and C1s in normal and pathologic sera. *Arthr. Rheum.,* **17,** 121
61. Gwyn-Williams, D., Peters, D. K., Fallows, J., Petrie, A., Kourilsky, O., Morel-Maroger, L. and Cameron, J. S. (1974). Studies of serum complement in the hypocomplementaemic nephritides. *Clin Exp. Immunol.,* **18,** 391
62. Rynes, R. I., Ruddy, S., Schur, P. H., Spragg, J. and Austen, K. F. (1974). Levels of complement components, properdin factors, and kininogen in patients with inflammatory anthritides. *J. Rheumatol.,* **1,** 413
63. Zvaifler, N. J. (1969). Breakdown products of C′3 in human synovial fluids. *J. Clin Invest.,* **48,** 1532
64. Ward, P. A. and Zvaifler, N. J. (1971). Complement-derived leukotactic factors in inflammatory synovial fluids of humans. *J. Clin. Invest.,* **50,** 606

65. Kinsella, T. D., Baum, J. and Ziff, M. (1969). Immunofluorescent demonstration of an IgG-β_{1c} complex in synovial lining cells of rheumatoid synovial membrane. *Clin. Exp. Immunol.*, **4,** 265
66. Koffler, D., Agnello, V., Carr, R. I. and Kunkel, H. G. (1969). Variable patterns of immunoglobulin and complement deposition in the kidneys of patients with systemic lupus erythematosus. *Am. J. Pathol.*, **56,** 305
67. Britton, M. C. and Schur, P. H. (1971). The complement system in rheumatoid synovitis. II. Intracytoplasmic inclusions of immunoglobulins and complement. *Arthr. Rheum.*, **14,** 87
68. Hurd, E. R., Kinsella, T. D. and Ziff, M. (1971). Immunologic studies of synoviocytes and synovial exudate cells. *J. Exp. Med.*, **134,** 296
69. Veroust, P. J., Wilson, C. B., Cooper, N. R., Edgington, T. S. and Dixon, F. J. (1974). Glomerular complement components in human glomerulonephritis. *J. Clin. Invest.*, **53,** 77
70. Alper, C. A. and Rosen, F. S. (1967). Studies of the *in vivo* behaviour of human C3 in normal subjects and patients. *J. Clin. Invest.*, **46,** 2021
71. Hunsicker, L. G., Ruddy, S., Carpenter, C. B., Schur, P. H., Merrill, J. P., Muller-Eberhard, H. J. and Austen, K. F. (1972). Metabolism of third complement component (C3) in nephritis. Involvement of the classic and alternative (properdin) pathways for complement activation. *N. Engl. J. Med.*, **287,** 835
72. Sliwinsky, A. J. and Zvaifler, N. J. (1972). Decreased synthesis of the third component of complement (C3) in hypocomplemententemic systemic lupus erythematosus. *Clin. Exp. Immunol.*, **11,** 21
73. Weinstein, A., Peters, K., Brown, D. and Bluestone, R. (1972). Metabolism of the third component of complement (C3) in patients with rheumatoid arthritis. *Arthr. Rheum.*, **15,** 40
74. Zvaifler, N. J. (1974). Rheumatoid arthritis: An extra-vascular immune complex disease. *Arthr. Rheum.*, **17,** 297
75. Perrin, L. H., Lambert, P. H. and Meischer, P. A. (1975). Complement breakdown products in plasma from patients with systemic lupus erythematosus and patients with membranoproliferative or other glomerulonephritis. *J. Clin. Invest.*, **56,** 165
76. Gewurz, H., Pickering, R. J., Naff, G., Snyderman, R., Mergenhagen, S. E. and Good R. A. (1969). Decreased properdin activity in acute glomerulonephritis. *Int. Arch. Allergy Appl. Immunol.*, **36,** 592
77. McLean, R. H. and Michael, A. F. (1973). Properdin and C3 proactivator; Alternate pathway components in human glomerulonephritis, *J. Clin. Invest.*, **52,** 634
78. Ruddy, S., Fearon, D. T. and Austen, K. F. (1975). Depressed synovial fluid levels of properdin and properdin Factor B in patients with rheumatoid arthritis. *Arthr. Rheum.*, **18,** 289
79. Westberg, N. G., Naff, G. B., Boyer, J. T. and Michael, A. F. (1971). Glomerular deposition of properdin in acute and chronic glomerulonephritis with hypocomplementemia. *J. Clin. Invest.*, **50,** 642
80. Charlesworth, J. A., Gwyn-Williams, D., Sherington, E., Lachmann, P. and Peters, D. K. (1974). Metabolic studies of the third component of complement and the glycine-rich beta-glycoprotein in patients with hypocomplementemia. *J. Clin. Invest.*, **53,** 1578
81. Ruddy, S., Carpenter, C. B., Chin, K. W., Knostman, J. N., Soter, N. A., Gotze, O., Muller-Eberhard, H. J. and Austen, K. F. (1975). Human complement metabolism: An analysis of 144 cases. *Mecidine (Baltimore)*, **54,** 165
82. Ziegler, J. B., Rosen, F. S., Alper, C. A., Grupe, W. and Lepow, I. H. (1975). Metabolism of properdin in normal subjects and patients with renal disease. *J. Clin. Invest.*, **56,** 761
83. Arroyave, C. M., Wilson, M. R. and Tan, E. M., (1976). Serum factors activating the alternative complement pathway in autoimmune disease. Description of two different factors from patients with systemic lupus erythematosus. *J. Immunol.*, **116,** 821
84. Whaley, K., Widener, H. and Ruddy, S. (1977). Modulation of the alternative pathway amplification loop in rheumatic disease. (In press)
85. Frank, M. M., Sergent, J. S., Kane, M. A. and Alling, D. W. (1972). Epsilon aminocaproic acid therapy of hereditary angioneurotic edema. *N. Engl. J. Med.*, **286,** 808

86. Sheffer, A. L., Austen, K. F. and Rosen, F. S. (1972). Tranexamic acid therapy in hereditary angioneurotic edema. *N. Engl. J. Med.*, **287**, 452
87. Lin, T. Y. (1976). Personal communication
88. Fong, J. S. C. and Good, R. A. (1972). Suramin — a potent reversible and competitive inhibitor of complement systems. *Clin. Exp. Immunol.*, **10**, 127
89. Brackertz, D. and Kueppers, F. (1973). A one year's follow up of treatment of hereditary angioneurotic edema with seramin. *Allergol. Immunopathol.*, **2**, 163
90. Naff, G. B. and Ratnoff, O. D. (1968). Conversion of C′1s to C′1 esterase and digestion of amino acid esters by C′1r. *J. Exp. Med.*, **182**, 571
91. Gigli, I. and Austen, K. F. (1969). Fluid phase destruction of $C2^{hu}$ by $C1^{hu}$ II. Unmasking by $C4i^{hu}$ of $C1^{hu}$ specificity for $C2^{hu}$. *J. Exp. Med.*, **130**, 833

Discussion II

Rheumatological Significance of Chemotaxis and Modulation of Complement Activation (Chapters 4 and 5)

K. D. MUIRDEN (Rapporteur): Dr Perper, who presented the first paper, emphasized that multiple factors interacted to cause accumulation of cells in inflammation. With carrageenan induced acute inflammation in rats, neutrophils dominated the lesions at 5 hours and mononuclears at 18 hours. The non-steroidal anti-inflammatory drugs, for example, phenylbutazone and indomethacin, inhibited mononuclear accumulation, it is believed by an effect on cell membranes, and these drugs also suppressed inflammatory oedema. The same agents failed to inhibit and, in certain cases, stimulated the accumulation of neutrophils. Colchicine, which affects the microtubules of cells, inhibited neutrophil accumulation. Corticosteroids inhibited both cell types.

In adjuvant arthritis lymphocytes accumulated at 6 days and mononuclears appeared at 12 days. It was shown that serum factors produced at various times non-specifically stimulated lymphocytes to respond to inflammatory stimuli. Such findings are of obvious importance in considering rheumatoid inflammation, as it appears that cellular events can be modified by drugs and serum factors.

C. M. PEARSON: To the best of my recollection, Dr Whaley, a Dr Jerome Rotstein in the US tried EACA in rheumatoid arthritis many years ago without any significant clinical improvement.

K. WHALEY: I was not aware of that study.

I. F. SKIDMORE: The drugs shown by you, Dr Whaley, all work on the classical pathway for complement activation. What about effects of inhibition of the alternate pathway, especially in view of the suggestions made by Dr A. C. Allison (CRC, Harrow, Middlesex) as to the importance of its role in the maintenance of granulomata.

K. WHALEY: We do not know what they do to the alternative pathway. An important point to stress though is that since the activation of alternative pathway in RA and SLE is in general via recruitment by the C3b feedback, one would prevent alternative pathway activation by blocking the classical pathway.

I. F. SKIDMORE: The last time I heard Dr Allison on this he implied that non-specific or alternate pathway initiation of such a sequence could be obtained. Do we know, or is it possible to determine, the relative importance of classical and alternate pathway activation in a disease such as rheumatoid arthritis?

K. WHALEY: Generally speaking, I believe that patients who have classical pathway activation with recruitment of the alternative pathway have more severe disease. Although it is also reported in the literature that patients with combined classical and alternative pathway activation tend also to be more resistant to conventional therapy, I am not sure how true that is.

J. L. TURK: Surely your remarks on the inter-relationship between types and number of complement pathway activation and severity of disease must be extrapolating a lot from this literature?

K. WHALEY: No, I have done some of the studies myself.

J. L. TURK: Then, tell us about it.

K. WHALEY: I promise to include the data in my manuscript for the proceedings (see p. 59–62).

J. L. TURK: In your studies did you measure complement activation in the actual inflammatory lesion, or in the serum? and how?

K. WHALEY: In the serum, or plasma in SLE; and in the synovial fluid in RA as will be described in the report in the proceedings.

J. L. TURK: People should realize that those who work in industry with the carrageenan model are specifically stimulating the alternative pathway of complement activation. This is a model where the effect of potential anti-complement drugs on an inflammatory situation can be investigated.

S. PROCACCIA: Results of studies we have carried out on complement activation in synovial fluid impress us with the greater importance of classical rather than alternate pathway activation, in RA.

M. B. GOLDLUST: Complement is being discussed today in the sense that it is an inflammatory mediator. But there is now evidence that the activation of C3 may also be involved during the immune response.

K. WHALEY: Absolutely. It is a very good point which I did not have time to mention.

A. J. LEWIS: Dr Whaley, would you know if the inhibitory effects of three compounds upon complement activation was observed *in vitro* only?

K. WHALEY: Not in the case of EACA which we have tested in patients with hereditary angioneurotic oedema.

A. J. LEWIS: Dr Whaley suggests that the pharmacologist might get his hands on these compounds and look at them, I assume, *in vivo*. Has he any ideas on the correct *in vivo* models to use for compounds of this sort?

A. R. MACKENZIE: There is a case reported in the literature of tranexamic acid being used in the treatment of SLE. I believe that it was very successful, but only a single case was recorded.

Section III:
Vasodilation and Increased Vascular Permeability

Chairman: **R. J. PERPER**

6
The Relationship between Increased Vascular Permeability, Hyperaemia, Stasis and Thrombosis in the Microcirculation

H. Z. MOVAT, MARGARET M. KOPANIAK, M. G. JOHNSTON and J. B. HAY

INTRODUCTION

'Inflammation is the reaction of living tissue to injury which comprises the series of changes of the terminal vascular bed, of the blood, and of the connective tissue which tends to eliminate the injurious agent and to repair the damaged tissue'[1].

Of the cardinal signs of inflammation, redness, heat, swelling and pain, the mechanisms underlying swelling have been most thoroughly studied. Quantification of increase in vascular permeability, which leads to exudation and swelling, is relatively simple. It is more difficult to study redness, referred to as erythema when it occurs in the skin. Redness is due to alterations in blood flow. Recently a method has been devised for the quantification of blood flow in the microcirculation[2]. This, together with a method for the quantification of enhancement of vascular permeability[3], enabled us to study the relationship between blood flow and vascular permeability in the microcirculation.

MATERIALS AND METHODS

Measurement of enhanced vascular permeability

The experimental animals were randomly bred albino guinea pigs

(500–600 gm) and rabbits (2.5–3.0 kg). The method of Udaka *et al.*[3] was used, which is based on the fact that intravenously injected ^{125}I-labelled human serum albumin (^{125}I-HSA) and Evans blue (bound to the animals serum albumin) escape into the connective tissue fluid when vessels are hyperpermeable. The HSA was radiolabelled with ^{125}I by the iodine monochloride technique, according to Freeman[4]. The ^{125}I-HSA was adjusted in a γ-spectrometer (Intertechnique, Canatech, Inc., Toronto, Canada) to 20×10^6 counts per minute (CPM) per millilitre. The 2% Evans blue was made up in boiled phosphate buffered saline (PBS) and passed through a Seitz filter. A mixture of Evans blue (1.0 ml/kg) and ^{125}I-HSA (1.0 ml/kg) was given intravenously when only vascular permeability was measured or intra-arterially through a carotid catheter (see below) when both permeability and blood flow were assayed. The blue dye was used to outline the skin lesions and the ^{125}I-HSA to quantify the exudation. At the end of the experiment the skin lesions were punched out with a cork borer (2 cm diameter) and counted in the γ-scaler.

Measurement of blood flow

In order to inject the radiolabelled microspheres hair was removed from the neck region with electric clippers and the animals anaesthetized with 1 gm/kg of urethane (BDH, Toronto, Canada). In addition Lidocaine hydrochloride (1.0% Xylocaine, Astra) was injected into the tissue around the right carotid artery. Polyethylene catheters were positioned in the left ventricle through the exposed right carotid artery[2]. Three types of microspheres were used, ^{85}Sr-labelled (3M Nuclear Products Division, London, Ontario, Canada), ^{57}Co-labelled (New England Nuclear, Montreal, Quebec) and ^{141}Ce (Pharmacia Fine Chemicals, Toronto, Ontario, Canada). They had a diameter of 15 $\mu \pm 5$, and were suspended in 10% dextran. 0.1 mCi was given to rabbits and 0.075 mCi to guinea pigs through the polyethylene catheter. Microspheres were always given at the end of the experiment. If enhanced vascular permeability was measured simultaneously, the Evans blue and ^{125}I-HSA mixture was given 5 minutes before the microspheres. Microsphere trapping was expressed as CPM per lesion. Only the strontium or cobalt labelled microspheres could be used simultaneously with the ^{125}I-HSA. When cerium was used the energy emission interfered with that of iodine.

Elicitation of lesions

Simple transient hyperaemia was induced by injecting prostaglandin E_1 (PGE_1) intradermally[5].

Physical injury was induced by applying heat to the skin. After clipping the hair, the animals were depilated with a paste containing barium sulphide[6]. Heat was applied to the skin of the back by the method of Sevitt[7], using a brass cylinder through which a current of hot water circulated, as described in an earlier publication[8]. One end of the cylinder was held against the skin of guinea pigs for 5, 10 or 15 minutes, the water circulating through the cylinder being 50 °C. The guinea pigs were killed 2½ hours after inducing the lesions. In rabbits the water temperature was 60 °C and the cylinder was applied for 2 minutes at various times before sacrifice (15–120 minutes).

Nitrogen mustard is known to produce inflammatory lesions with serous exudation[9]. Mustargen (Merck, Sharp and Dohme, Montreal, Canada) was injected intradermally into guinea pigs in a dose range of 4.0 to 0.125 mg per injection site (0.2 ml). The animals were killed 4 hours after the intradermal injections.

Immunological injury was produced by eliciting a reversed passive Arthus reaction in rabbits[10]. Arthus lesions are known to be initiated by immune complex deposition in postcapillary venules and PMN-leukocytes play an essential pathogenetic role[11]. Arthus lesions are characterized by aggregation of leukocytes and platelets and formation of thrombin in the microcirculation, which increase as the lesion progresses[12]. To elicit Arthus lesions rabbits were given 3.0 mg bovine serum albumin per kg body weight intravenously. This was followed by 0.2 ml intradermal injections of rabbit anti-bovine serum albumin (0.2 mg antibody N) given between 30 minutes and 24 hours prior to sacrifice. Control sites were injected with normal rabbit serum.

Electron microscopy

For electron microscopy lesions showing stasis were examined in detail. Samples of the Arthus lesions were also examined to confirm earlier observations. The tissue was fixed in paraformaldehyde in sodium cacodylate, postfixed in osmic acid, embedded in Epon and examined as in previous publications[8,10].

RESULTS AND DISCUSSION

Transient hyperaemia is induced by injecting PGE_1 intradermally[5]. The visible erythema disappears when the experimental animal is killed and the circulation stops. When bradykinin was injected simultaneously with the PGE_1 the enhanced vascular permeability induced by bradykinin alone was markedly enhanced. When increasing amounts of PGE_1 were injected with a fixed amount of bradykinin the vascular permeability was enhanced in a dose response fashion, paralleling the enhancement of blood flow through the lesion (Figure 6.1). Further studies showed that the hyperaemia-inducing effect of PGE_1 lasts much longer than the effect of mediators such as histamine and bradykinin[13]. Peak erythema was observed 20–40 minutes after injection of PGE. Furthermore, in contrast with histamine[6], sites injected with PGE_1 did not become refractory to a second or third injection. Accordingly guinea pigs were given 1.0 μg of PGE 3 times at 40 min intervals and the visible

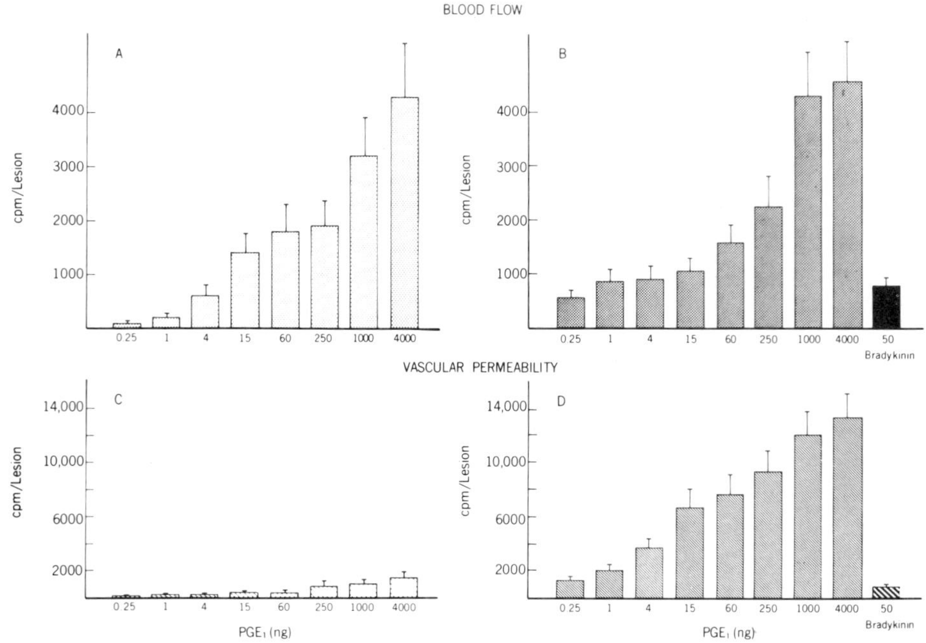

Figure 6.1 Correlation between enhancement of vascular permeability induced by 50 ng of bradykinin and enhancement of blood flow induced by increasing doses of PGE_1 in the rabbit. A = enhancement of blood flow induced by PGE. B = enhancement of blood flow induced by mixtures of bradykinin by PGE_1. C = enhancement of vascular permeability induced by PGE_1. D = enhancement of vascular permeability induced by mixtures of bradykinin and PGE. (From Johnston *et al.* (1976)[5] by permission of *Agents and Actions*.)

hyperaemia persisted throughout the 120 min. At the end of the experiment when the radiolabelled spheres were injected, those lesions showed only slightly more hyperaemia than a single 1.0 μg dose given 40 min before death. A single dose of 3.0 μg of PGE_1, given 90 or 120 mins before death showed no signs of hyperaemia (Figure 6.2).

Ferreira and co-workers[14] postulated that PGE_1 may sensitize blood vessels to the permeability-enhancing effect of other mediators. It is our contention that the enhancing effect of PGE_1 is due to enhanced blood flow. When another mediator, which enhances vascular permeability, was given with PGE_1 more blood flows through the leaky vessels and consequently more plasma and tracer was exuded. If PGE_1 were to sensitize vessels to other mediators, one would assume that the sensitization persists for some time. However, as shown in Figure 6.3 the vascular permeability induced by histamine paralleled the blood flow. The histamine was injected into sites pre-injected 30 or 90 mins before with PGE_1. Only the 30 min lesions, which exhibited enhanced flow, also showed an increase in vascular permeability. Similar observations were made with PGE_1 and bradykinin.

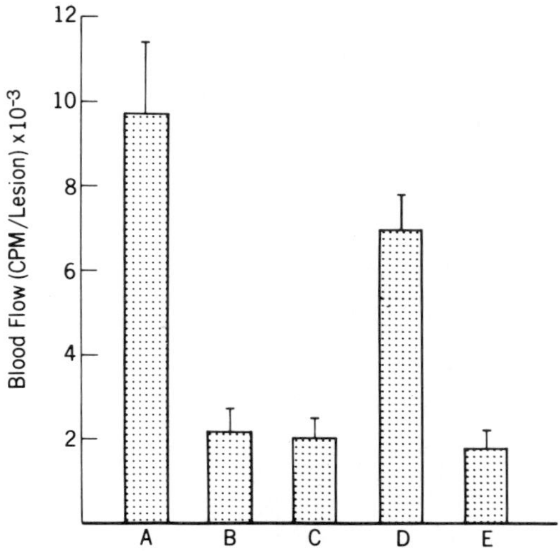

Figure 6.2 Hyperaemia induced by PGE_1. A = three injections of 1.0 μg PGE_1 at 40 min intervals and the animals injected with ^{141}Ce spheres 120 mins after the first injection. B = a single injection of 3.0 μg PGE at the beginning of the experiment. C = three injections of PBS at 40 min intervals. D = one injection of 1.0 μg PGE_1 40 mins before death. E = one injection of PBs 40 mins before death

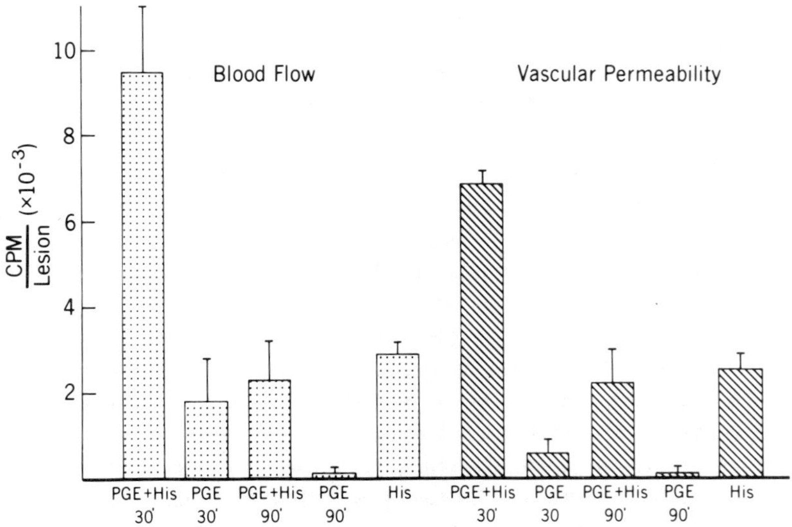

Figure 6.3 Simultaneous measurement of blood flow and vascular permeability in guinea pig skin. After inducing 30 and 90 minute-old lesions with PGE_1 guinea pigs were given Evans blue and ^{125}I-HSA, followed by injections of histamine or buffer into the PGE_1 injected sites. Five minutes later ^{85}Sr-microspheres were injected through a cannula near the left ventricle and the animals killed one minute later. The counts refer to both isotopes. Counts for the buffer were subtracted

Lesions induced with heat show all gradations from mild hyperaemia and enhanced vascular permeability to complete stasis. When 50 °C was applied to the skin of guinea pigs 15 min lesions showed definite stasis, there being less blood flow through the lesions than through normal skin (Figure 6.4). When

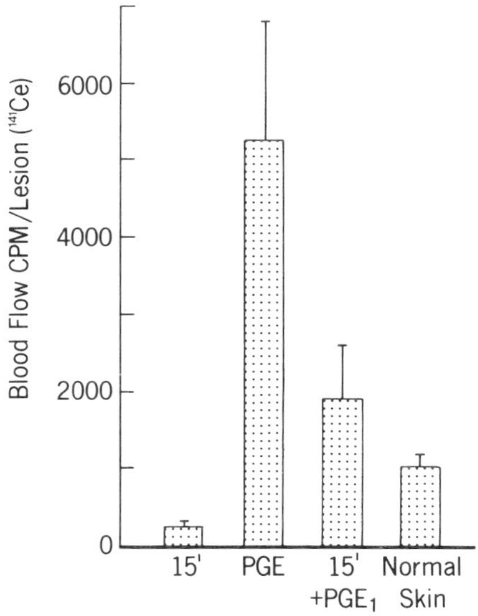

Figure 6.4 Blood flow during stasis. ^{141}Ce-labelled microspheres were injected into guinea pigs which had heat lesions induced by applying 50 °C for 15 mins to the depilated skin. Note that the blood flow is less than in normal skin. The illustration also shows the effect of PGE_1 injected intradermally into normal skin and into skin to which heat had been applied for 15 mins

PGE_1 was injected into such lesions the blood flow increased, but was considerably less than in injected normal skin. It must be remembered however, that the heat has mainly a subepidermal effect whereas an intradermal injection affects deeper lying vessels. With 5, 10 and 15 min lesions the vascular permeability decreased progressively as the lesion and the stasis became more severe (Figures 6.5 and 6.6). Bradykinin was injected in such lesions. The more severe the stasis was, the less effect bradykinin had. The kinetics of the development of heat lesions was studied in rabbits. With 60 °C applied for 2 min a 15-minute lesion showed both enhanced blood flow and increase in vascular permeability. With progressively older lesions the blood flow decreased and the vascular permeability decreased in parallel with it. In the most severe lesions (60 and 90 mins after heat application) the blood flow was below that of normal skin (Figure 6.7). However, the vascular permeability was still slightly above that of normal skin. This is because at the periphery of such lesions the heat has less effect, i.e. insufficient to produce stasis, but sufficient to produce in-

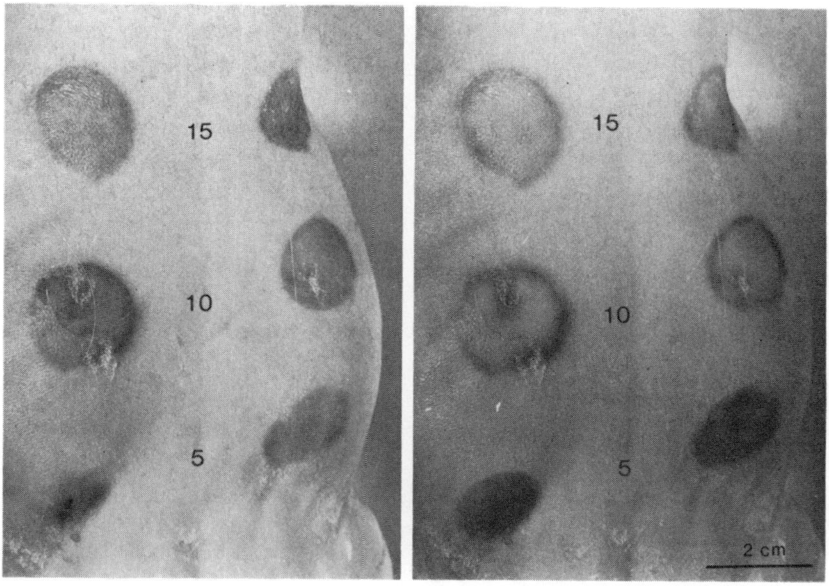

Figure 6.5 Heat lesions of guinea pig skin. Heat (50 °C) was applied as described in Materials and Methods to the depilated backs of guinea pigs for 5, 10 and 15 mins. The animals were killed 2½ hours later. The illustration on the left shows the intense erythema due to stasis (markedly dilated, red blood cell-filled vessels) and was photographed with a green filter to emphasize the red of the erythema. The illustration on the right shows the same lesions after injection of Evans blue, photographed with an orange-yellow filter to emphasize the blue. Note that the 5-minute old lesions show complete bluing, whereas the 10 and 15 min lesions show blue rings at the periphery

crease in vascular permeability. This is illustrated in the right half of Figure 6.5.

With nitrogen mustard an essentially similar effect was obtained, but not as clear cut as with heat. High doses induced stasis and decreased flow in the centre of the lesions and hyperaemia and enhanced vascular permeability at the periphery of the lesions. With lower doses hyperaemia and enhanced permeability was observed.

Arthus reactions were examined ½, 1, 2, 4, 8, 12 and 24 hours after the intradermal injection of antibody. Enhancement of vascular permeability and blood flow were at a peak 4 hours after injection of antibody, followed by a gradual decrease in both parameters. Minimal haemorrhage was first noted in 2 hour-old lesions. In 24 hour-old lesions blood flow was below normal and minimal enhanced permeability was noted at the periphery of the lesions.

With transient hyperaemia no structural abnormality of vessels can be detected. Slowing of the blood and stasis are believed to be associated with a rapid loss of plasma and inspissation, so that individual red cells can no longer be recognized, there seems to be merely a solid red column, when the vessels

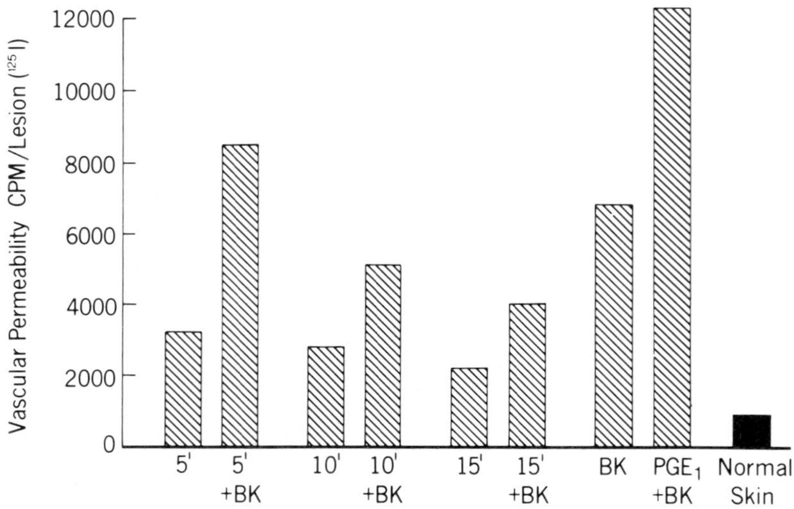

Figure 6.6 Vascular permeability during stasis. Application of 50 °C to the skin of guinea pigs for 5, 10 and 15 mins. Similar sites were injected with 0.1 μg bradykinin. One normal site was injected with bradykinin and one with a mixture of bradykinin and 1.0 μg PGE_1

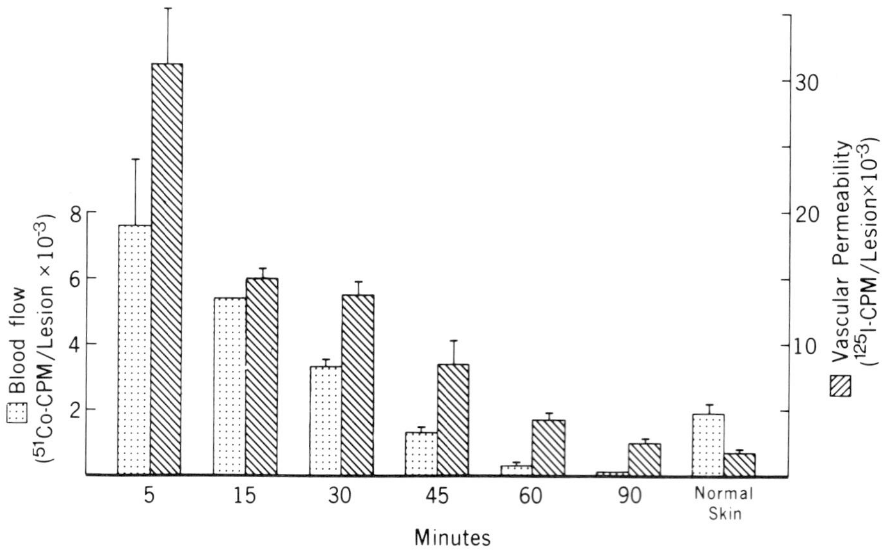

Figure 6.7 Development of stasis induced with 60 °C for 2 mins applied to the rabbit's skin for 5–90 mins

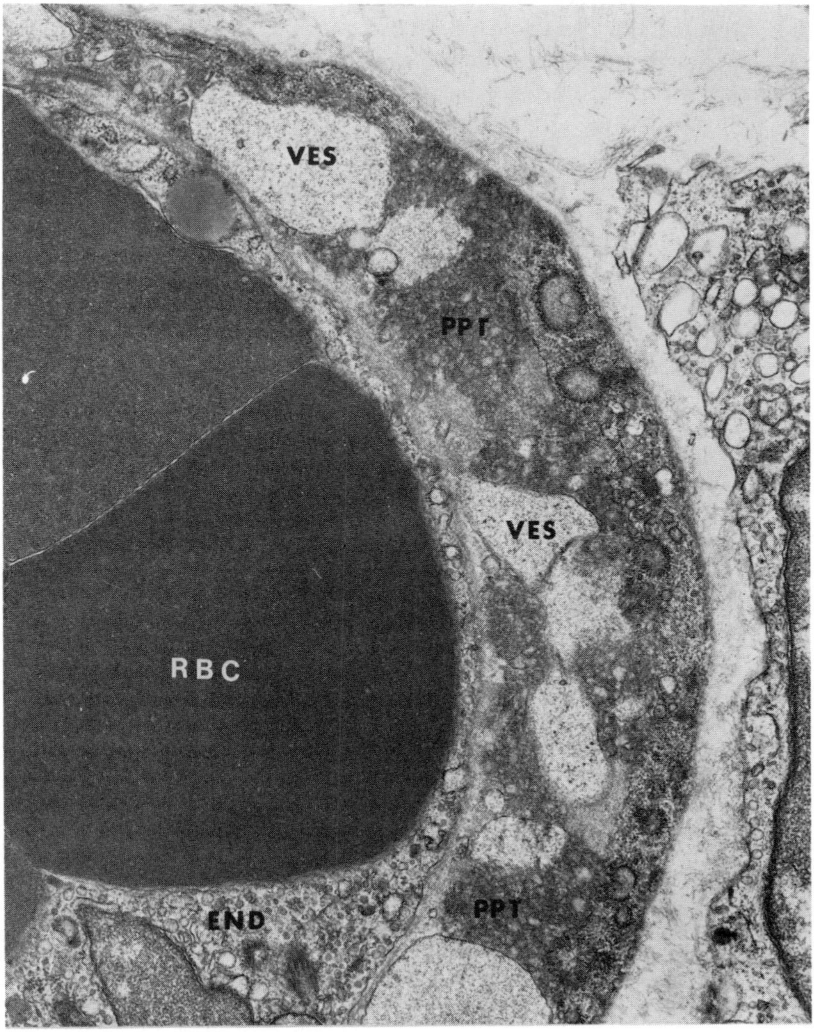

Figure 6.8 Stasis induced with nitrogen mustard. Between the endothelium (END) and a pericite, whose outlines are ill-defined, there are unidentified vesicles (VES) and a dense precipitate (PPT), presumably plasma proteins. RBC = red blood cell: (× 17 700)

are examined *in vivo*. These changes are believed to be due to alteration of the vessel wall[15]. Ultrastructural observations indeed indicate that there is loss of plasma protein which may become entrapped in the vessel wall (Figure 6.8) together with chylomicra (Figure 6.9). Figure 6.9 shows a severely damaged venule, with marked alterations in the endothelium, loss or homogenization of the basement membrane and red cells almost devoid of haemoglobin. This loss of haemoglobin from the red cells is more evident in Figure 6.10, in which

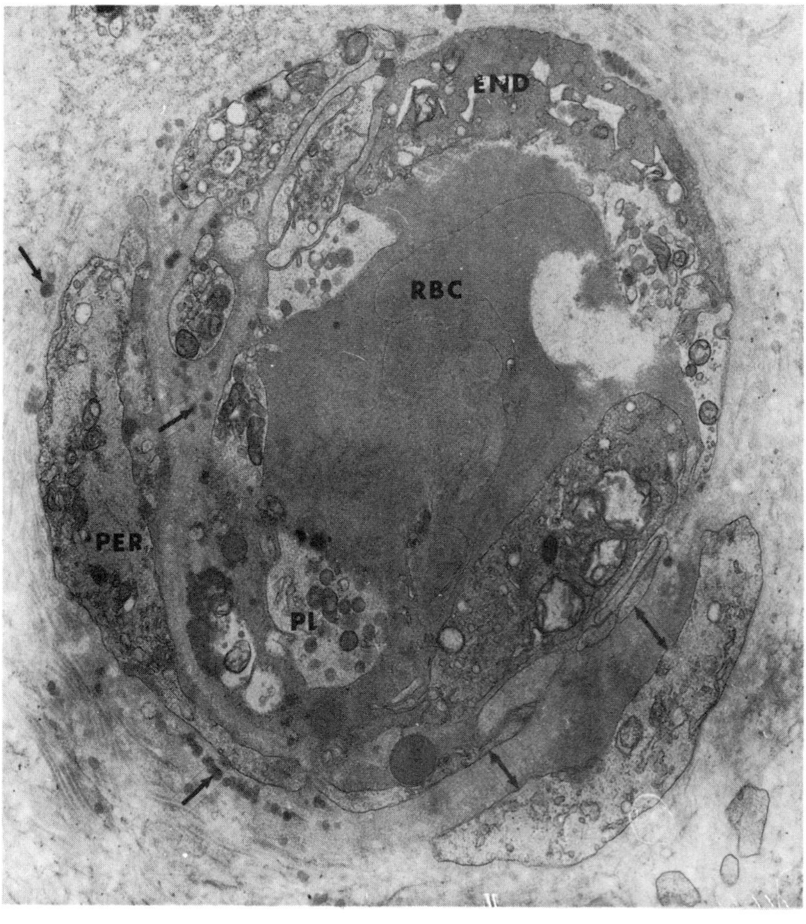

Figure 6.9 Stasis induced by heat. There are regressive changes in the cells of the vessel wall, including vacuolation of mitochondria, and complete absence of endothelium in some areas. The double headed arrows indicate an area occupied by electron dense homogeneous material (? plasma proteins) instead of a basement membrane, which is difficult to recognize in the rest of this venule. The arrows point to chylomicra. END = endothelium, PL = platelet, RBC = red cell ghosts. (× 6800)

several gradations are seen. The Arthus reaction is a more complex lesion and advanced lesions are characterized by platelet aggregation and thrombosis, which impair the blood flow (Figure 6.11).

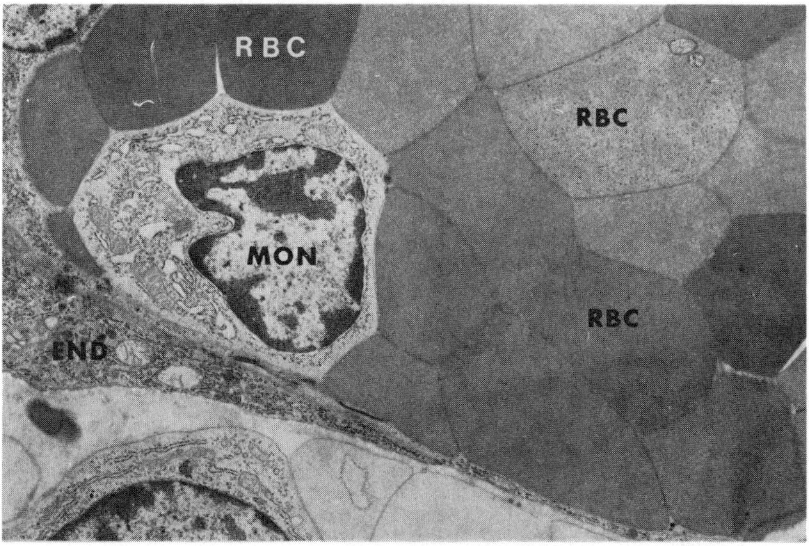

Figure 6.10 Vessel in stasis. Red blood cells (RBC) with varying degrees of electron density due to varying concentrations of haemoglobin. MON = monocyte, END = endothelium. (× 6800)

SUMMARY AND CONCLUSIONS

Enhanced vascular permeability is responsible for one of the cardinal signs of inflammation, swelling. Hyperaemia, another of the cardinal signs of inflammation, is observed in transient lesions such as those induced with prostaglandin E_1. Prostaglandin E_1 augments the vascular permeability induced by mediators such as histamine or bradykinin, by increasing the blood flow and thus providing more plasma to escape through leaky vessels.

In inflammatory lesions induced by physical, chemical or immunological injury there is an early phase in which both increased blood flow and enhanced vascular permeability can be demonstrated. It has been repeatedly observed that the progression of inflammatory lesions is associated with a gradual decrease in vascular permeability. The studies presented demonstrate that these severe lesions are associated with a decrease in blood flow. In very severe lesions the blood flow may be less than in normal skin. The slowing of blood flow is due to either stasis or thrombosis of postcapillary venules.

Ultrastructural studies show that stasis is associated with a loss of plasma from the vessel due to severe injury to the vessel wall. There is also loss of

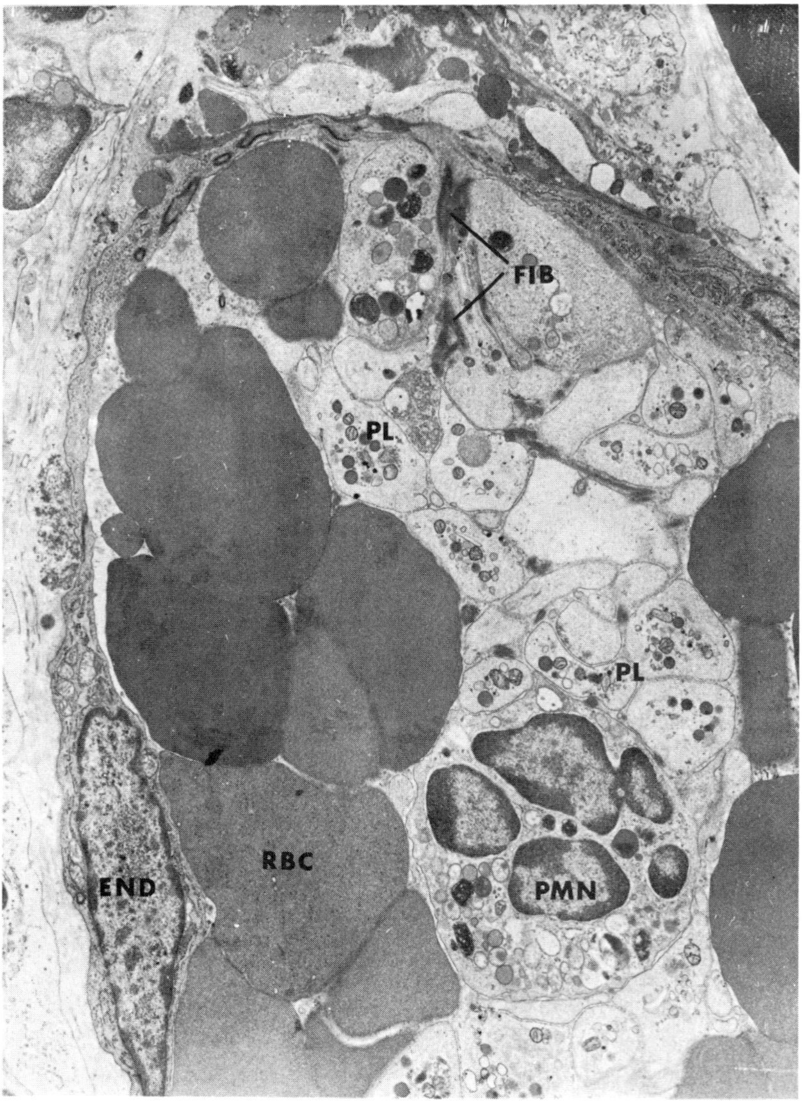

Figure 6.11 Arthus lesion showing aggregation of platelets (PL), a polymorphonuclear leukocyte (PMN), red cells (RBC) and fibrin (FIB) in a thrombus which occludes the vessel. END = endothelium. (× 8000)

haemoglobin from red cells. Impairment of blood flow and of vascular permeability in immunological injury of the Arthus-type is due to gradual occlusion of vessels induced by thrombosis.

Acknowledgements

The authors wish to thank Dr John Pike, Upjohn Co., Kalamazoo, Michigan, for generous supplies of prostaglandins. They also wish to acknowledge the skillful technical and secretarial assistance of Ms Wendy Hunter and Ms Marica Michael.

References

1. Movat, H. Z. (1977). The acute inflammatory reaction. In H. Z. Movat (ed.) *Inflammation, Immunity and Hypersensitivity,* 2nd Edition. (New York: Harper and Row)
2. Hay, J. B., Johnston, M. G., Hobbs, B. B. and Movat, H. Z. (1975). The use of radioactive microspheres to quantitate hyperemia in dermal inflammatory sites. *Proc. Soc. Exp. Biol. Med.,* **150,** 641
3. Udaka, K., Takeuchi, Y. and Movat, H. Z. (1970). Simple method for quantitation of enhanced vascular permeability. *Proc. Soc. Exp. Biol. Med.,* **133,** 1384
4. Freeman, T. (1967). Trace labelling with radioiodine. In D. M. Weir (ed.) *Handbook of Experimental Immunology,* pp. 597–607. (Oxford and Edinburgh: Blackwell Scientific Publications)
5. Johnston, M. G., Hay, J. B. and Movat, H. Z. (1976). The modulation of enhanced vascular permeability by prostaglandins through alterations in blood flow (hyperemia). *Agents and Actions,* **6,** 705
6. Miles, A. A. and Miles, E. M. (1952). Vascular changes due to histamine, histamine liberator and leukotaxine in the skin of guinea pigs. *J. Physiol.,* **118,** 228
7. Sevitt, S. (1958). Early and delayed oedema and increase in capillary permeability after burns of the skin. *J. Path. Bact.,* **75,** 27
8. Uriuhara, T. and Movat, H. Z. (1967). Role of PMN-leukocyte lysosomes in tissue injury, inflammation and hypersensitivity. V. Partial suppression in leukopenic rabbits of vascular hyperpermeability due to thermal injury. *Proc. Soc. Exp. Biol. Med.,* **124,** 279
9. Meyer-Arendt, J. (1953). Über den Ablauf der serösen Entzündung. *Virch. Arch. Pathol. Anat.,* **323,** 351
10. Uriuhara, T. and Movat, H. Z. (1966). The role of PMN-leukocyte lysosomes in tissue injury, inflammation and hypersensitivity. I. The vascular changes and the role of PMN-leukocytes in the reversed passive Arthus reaction. *Exp. Molec. Pathol.,* **5,** 539
11. Cochrane, C. G., Weigle, W. O. and Dixon, F. J. (1959). The role of polymorphonuclear leukocytes in the initiation and cessation of the Arthus vasculitis. *J. Exp. Med.,* **110,** 481
12. Udaka, K. (1971). The Arthus reaction. In H. Z. Movat (ed.) *Inflammation Immunity and Hypersensitivity,* pp. 389–424 (New York: Harper and Row)
13. Kopaniak, M. M., Hay, J. B. and Movat, H. Z. (1978). The effect of hyperemia on vascular permeability. *Microvasc. Res.* (in press)
14. Ferreira, S. H., Moncada, S. and Vane, J. R. (1974). Prostaglandins and signs and symptoms of inflammation. In H. D. Robinson and J. R. Vane (eds.) *Prostaglandin Synthetase Inhibitors — Their Effect on Physiological Functions and Pathological States,* pp. 156–168. (New York: Raven Press)
15. Illig, L. (1955). Experimentelle Untersuchungen über die Entstehung der Stase. *Virch. Arch. Pathol. Anat.,* **326,** 501

7
Evaluation of the Ability of Anti-Rheumatic Drugs to Suppress Hyperaemia and Increased Vascular Permeability

A. J. LEWIS

INTRODUCTION

Ultra-violet (u.v.) irradiation is one of a variety of stimuli known to produce hyperaemia and increased vascular permeability in a number of different species[1]. A biphasic increase in vascular permeabilty consisting of an early transient phase (approximately 20 min after irradiation) and a later prolonged phase for up to 48 hours occurs in both rat and guinea pig[1,2]. The early phase is sensitive to antiserotonin agents, in the case of the rat, and to antihistamines in the guinea pig[3]. The later phases are less sensitive to these amine antagonists but responsive to non-steroidal anti-inflammatory agents such as aspirin[2]. In both species, the concomitant development of hyperaemia, as measured by the production of erythema, appears slightly different from these vascular permeability changes because it is monophasic and maximal between 4 and 6 hours[1,2,4]. The production of erythema in guinea pig skin has been used for the assessment of new anti-inflammatory drugs and a correlation has been demonstrated between the erythema delaying action of systemically applied non-steroidal agents and their anti-rheumatic properties[5]. Recently erythema production in the rat, unlike that of the guinea pig[5,6], has been demonstrated to be sensitive to both the topical and systemic administration of a variety of steroidal as well as non-steroidal anti-inflammatory drugs[4]. Further differences between rat and guinea pig erythema models have also been observed in studies aimed at evaluating the systemic anti-inflammatory activity of copper complexes. More surprisingly, the u.v. erythema model has also been shown responsive to anti-rheumatic drugs such as gold salts and D-penicillamine which are generally considered not to be effective in acute inflammatory responses.

METHODS

Guinea pigs (Dunkin Hartley) and rats (Wistar) were exposed to a u.v. lamp (Hanovia Model 10 Quartz Lamp fitted with a Kodak 18A filter transmitting light above 290 nm wavelength) for 120 sec and 90 sec as previously described[4]. Drugs were administered systemically in 5% mulgofen 1 h prior to u.v. exposure or topically, dissolved in 0.2 ml volumes of absolute ethanol, immediately after irradiation. Changes in erythema intensity after drug administration were expressed as percentage of the erythema intensity at 3 h in vehicle treated animals. All the data were analysed by the randomization test of Siegel[7]. Topically ID_{50} values were calculated after plotting lines of best fit through the data points and expressed as mg drug applied to the skin. After systemic administration the ID_{50}s were calculated for non-steroidal drugs and the ID_{30}s for steroids.

RESULTS AND DISCUSSION

Comparison of topical and systemic application of drugs in the rat

Both non-steroidal and steroidal anti-inflammatory drugs suppressed the erythema produced in the rat when administered topically (Table 7.1). The earliest anti-erythemic activity was detected at 2 h and the drugs were often still effective at 24 h although scab formation at 48 h was unaffected. Several

Table 7.1 Effect of non-steroidal and steroidal drugs administered topically and systemically on u.v. erythema assessed at 4 h in the rat

Type	*Drug*	*Topical* ID_{50} *(mg/rat)*	*Systemic** ID_x *(mg/kg)*
Non-steroidal	Ibuprofen	0.3	22.4
	Indomethacin	1.3	1.3
	Phenylbutazone	5.6	17.2
	Aspirin	9.2	148.0
	Flufenamic acid	10.9	38.5
	Methysergide bimaleate	>15	2.1
Steroidal	Dexamethasone	4.8	0.5
	Prednisolone	7.7	10.5
	Hydrocortisone	9.0	>100

* Systemic ID_{50} values for non-steroidal drugs were calculated after oral administration and systemic ID_{30} values were calculated for steroidal drugs

pharmacological agents, not generally considered to be anti-inflammatory, including cyproheptadine, mepyramine, methysergide, procaine, progesterone and testosterone, were ineffective after topical application. The same anti-inflammatory drugs suppressed the erythema (from 2 to 24 h) after either oral (route used for non-steroidal drugs) or subcutaneous (for steroidal drugs) administration (Table 7.1). Of the variety of non-anti-inflammatory drugs tested systemically on only the serotonin antagonist, methysergide, administered orally, effectively suppressed the erythema.

The effectiveness of the topical and systemic routes of administration often differed for the same drug as might be expected in view of differences in transport mechanisms and the possibility for inactivation. Indeed, none of the steroids tested systemically suppressed the erythema by more than 50% in contrast to their potent topical activity. In comparison, the serotonin antagonist which was very effective after systemic administration was inactive after topical application. It should be noted that neither topical nor systemic administration of any of the the active drugs eliminated the erythema in the rat.

These data extend the observations that non-steroidal anti-inflammatory drugs effectively suppress u.v. induced erythema in the guinea pig both topically [8,9] and systemically[2,5]. The activity of steroidal anti-inflammatory agents in this rat erythema model contrasts with their reported inactivity in the guinea pig after both topical[6] and systemic[4] administration. The observation that topically applied non-steroidal anti-inflammatory agents are effective against local inflammatory responses such as u.v. induced erythema in the rat, guinea pig[8,9] and man[10], and homograft rejection in the rabbit[11] suggests that this route of administration might prove effective in the treatment of joint inflammation. In this way the gastric side effects associated with oral therapy might be circumvented.

Comparison between the effects of different copper salts against u.v. erythema induced in the rat and the guinea pig

The u.v. erythema model has also been used to examine the oral activity of cuprous oxide, cupric chloride and copper aspirinate in both rat and guinea pig. The results expressed in Table 7.2 refer to the effect of each compound on the 4 h erythema response and, in addition, the gastric irritancy of these compounds observable 6 h after administration to starved animals is included. Both cuprous oxide and cupric chloride suppressed the erythema response in the guinea pig but were ineffective in the rat at the same dose. In addition, copper aspirinate was more effective than aspirin in suppressing the erythema in the guinea pig although it was approximately equieffective with aspirin in the rat.

These results would thus appear to support the proposal that copper salts and copper complexes of non-steroidal anti-inflammatory drugs possess marked anti-inflammatory activity[12] at least in the guinea pig. However, examination of the gastric side effects of these compounds demonstrated that the copper salts

Table 7.2 A comparison of the anti-erythemic and gastric irritant effects of orally administered copper salts in the guinea pig and rat

		Guinea pig		*Rat*	
Compound	*Dose (mg/kg)*	*% Inhibition of erythema*	*Gastric* Irritancy*	*% Inhibition of erythema*	*Gastric* Irritancy*
Cu_20	50	62†	++	20	0
$CuCl_2$	50	47†	+++	9	0
Cu	300	N.T.o	N.T.	43†	+
$(Asp.)_2$	100	64†	++	15	0
	30	33†	+	0	0
	10	26	0	N.T.	N.T.
Aspirin	300	51†	+	54†	+
	100	39	+	25	+
	30	2	0	0	+

* Gastric irritation for both species scored as follows: 0, no effect; +minor haemorrhagic lesions: + +moderate haemorrhagic lesions, + + + severe haemorrhagic lesions
† $P < 0.05$
N.T. = not tested

and copper aspirinate are extremely irritant towards the gastric mucosa of the guinea pig. This suggests that it is the gastric irritation which provokes the anti-erythemic response via counter-irritation. The counter-irritant property of copper complexes after subcutaneous or local administration has also been claimed to be associated with their anti-inflammatory action[13]. By contrast, orally administered copper aspirinate is clearly less irritant in the stomach of rats, a finding that confirms previous observations[12].

These data further highlight the difference in sensitivity between rat and guinea pig to the same compound. The results also demonstrate one of the problems in interpreting data obtained from an acute test model aimed at the selection of anti-inflammatory agents, namely the counter-irritation phenomenon.

The effect of gold salts and D-penicillamine on guinea pig u.v. erythema

Both sodium aurothiomalate (intramuscular ID_{50} 30 mg/kg at 3 h) and triethylphosphine gold chloride (oral ID_{30} 30 mg/kg at 3 h) suppressed the u.v. erythema which developed in the guinea pig over the 24 h period of measurement (Figure 7.1). However, orally administered sodium aurothiomalate (3–30 mg/kg; Figure 7.1) and intramuscularly administered thiomalic acid (20 mg/kg) were inactive in this model. Gold serum levels correlated with the anti-erythemic effect in each case[14]. D-Penicillamine (oral ID_{50} 200 mg/kg at 3 h) also suppressed the development of u.v. erythema over the 24 h assessment period.

The relevance of the acute anti-erythemic effects of both sodium aurothiomalate and D-penicillamine, anti-rheumatic agents not normally

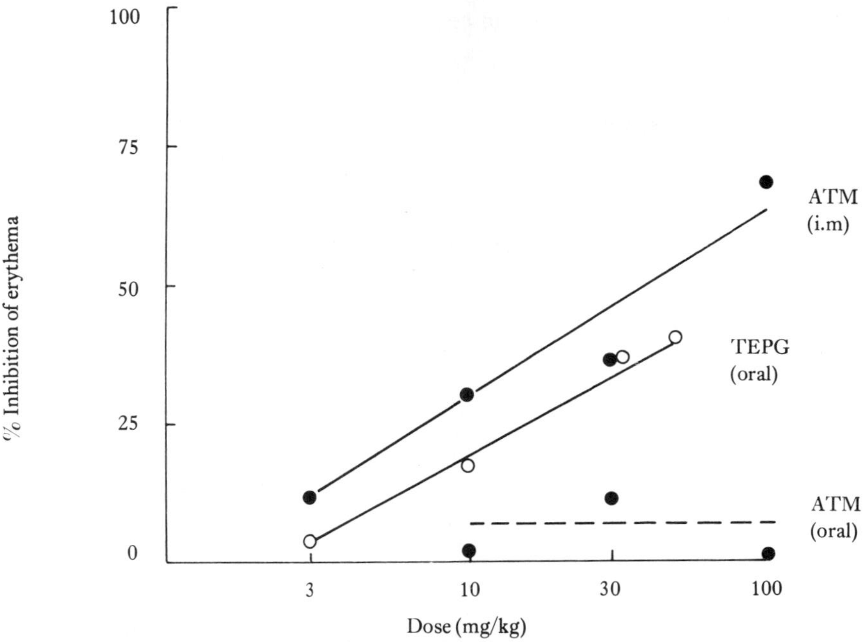

Figure 7.1 Effect of sodium aurothiomalate (ATM: i.m. and oral) and triethylphosphine gold chloride (oral) on the 3h erythema response. Drugs were administered 1h prior to irradiation

associated with acute anti-inflammatory actions[15,16], is uncertain at present. Further studies will be necessary to evaluate the specificity of these responses. However, it is already apparent that neither drug suppresses all erythema responses in guinea pig skin. For instance, they have no effect on the erythema weal produced by intradermally injected histamine.

Possible modes of action for drugs suppressing the development of erythema

In view of the diversity of agents effective against u.v. induced erythema and the qualitative and quantitative differences between species for some of the drugs, a number of theories can be postulated to account for the mechanism(s) of the anti-erythemic actions of the drugs (Figure 7.2). The trigger mechanism for erythema development may involve the formation of highly reactive free radicals which are produced when skin is irradiated with u.v. light[17,18]. Consequently a prime target for drug action might be the mopping up or scavenging of these free radicals. The production of the superoxide free radical (0_2^-) is blocked by a variety of non-steroidal anti-inflammatory drugs in the macrophage[19] although whether free radical production can be influenced by these drugs in u.v. irradiated skin is not yet known. These membrane disruptive species cause lipid peroxidation of polyunsaturated fatty acids with the consequent release of reactive lipid peroxides and aldehydes. The overall result would be severe membrane disturbance should the fatty acid be located in the membrane itself. The peroxidation of the prostaglandin precursor, arachidonic acid, may lead to formation of the highly vasoactive prostaglandin endoperoxides in addition to the prostaglandins themselves. Both the prostaglandin endoperoxides and prostaglandins have been proposed as mediators of inflammatory processes partly on the basis of their ability to cause vasodilatation and to increase vascular permeability. There is mounting evidence that

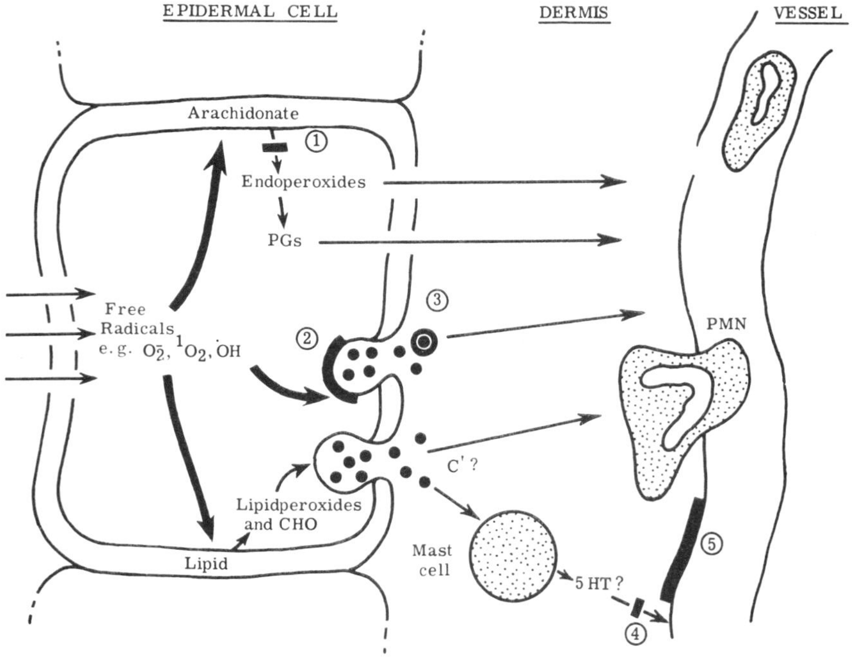

Figure 7.2 Schematic diagram of the possible effect of u.v. irradiation on the skin and some of the major sites of the anti-erythemic effect of drugs

prostaglandins and possibly their endoperoxides may play a role in the mediation of u.v.-induced erythema. After u.v. irradiation prostaglandin formation occurs in rat[20], guinea pig[21] and human[20] skin. Moreover non-steroidal anti-inflammatory drugs are able to inhibit prostaglandin formation in the skin[22] (Site 1: Figure 7.2). Recently, Sekura Snyder [21] has demonstrated that topical application of indomethacin reduces both the erythema and prostaglandin levels present in the u.v. irradiated guinea pig skin. There are also reports that corticosteroids may inhibit the release[23] of these fatty acids. In addition, both gold salts[24,25] and D-penicillamine[25] have been demonstrated to inhibit the formation of prostaglandins.

U.v. light labilizes epidermal lysosomal membranes[26] which may be a further consequence of free radical formation. The concomitant release of hydrolases and neutral proteases may then contribute to the erythema response because these enzymes are known to cause vasodilatation, increases in capillary permeability and chemotaxis[27]. Since steroidal and non-steroidal anti-rheumatic drugs have been shown to stabilize lysosomal membranes[28], this effect may contribute to their anti-erythemic activity (Site 2; Figure 7.2). Gold salts inhibit lysosomal enzyme activity rather than modifying the enzyme release process[29] (Site 3; Figure 7.2) and consequently could also suppress erythema development by this action.

The suppression of erythema in the rat and guinea pig by systemically administered serotonin antagonists, but not anti-histamines, suggests that serotonin may help mediate the erythema (Site 4; Figure 7.2). However, since methysergide has both vasoconstrictor and anti-serotonin activities its use cannot establish if serotonin mediates the u.v.-induced erythema in either species. The cutaneous vasoconstrictor activity of corticosteroids, particularly when they are applied topically, may also contribute to the suppression of the erythema in the rat.

It is evident from this work and other reports[2,5,6] that the erythema produced by u.v. irradiation is affected by a variety of anti-rheumatic drugs. However, not all drugs that demonstrate anti-erythemic activity are of value as anti-rheumatic agents, e.g. the serotonin antagonists. Consequently, the inhibition of erythema cannot be used as a specific predictive model for the evaluation of new anti-rheumatic agents. The comparison of results obtained for the rat and guinea pig erythema studies demonstrates the importance of multi-species testing of a drug before generalization of the drug effect should be made. For example, if steroidal anti-inflammatory agents had been examined in the rat u.v. erythema model a number of years ago the oversimplification that 'steroids are ineffective against u.v. erythema' might not have been made. It would have been qualified by the insertion of the species used to arrive at this statement, in this case the guinea pig. In conclusion, the u.v. models of erythema in the rat and guinea pig provide a quick and simple assessment of newly designed drugs, applied both systemically and topically, prior to more exhaustive evaluation in chronic models of inflammation.

References

1. Logan, G. and Wilhelm, D. L. (1966). The inflammatory reaction in ultraviolet injury. *Br. J. Exp. Pathol.*, **47**, 286
2. Gupta, N. and Levy, L. (1973). Delayed manifestation of ultraviolet reaction in the guinea pig caused by anti-inflammatory drugs. *Br. J. Pharmacol.*, **47**, 240
3. Logan, G. and Wilhelm, D. L. (1966). Vascular permeability changes in inflammation. *Br. J. Exp. Pathol.*, **47**, 300
4. Law, E. and Lewis, A. J. (1977). The effect of systemically and topically applied drugs on ultraviolet induced erythema in the rat. *Br. J. Pharmacol.*, **59**, 591
5. Winder, C. V., Wax, J., Burr, V., Been, M. and Rosiere, C. E. (1958). A study of pharmacological influences on ultraviolet erythema in guinea pigs. *Arch. Int. Pharmacodyn.*, **116**, 261

6. Bonta, I. L. (1969). Microvascular lesions as a target of anti-inflammatory and certain other drugs. *Acta Physiol. Pharmacol. Neerl.*, **15,** 188
7. Siegel, S. (1965). *Non Parametric Statistics.* (New York: McGraw-Hill)
8. Lambelin, G., Vassart-Thys, D. and Roba, J. (1970) Pharmacological studies of bufexamac topically applied on the skin. *Arch. Int. Pharmacodyn. Ther.*, **187,** 401
9. MacDonald-Gibson, W. J. and Schneider, C. (1974). A novel method for evaluating anti-inflammatory drugs in the conscious guinea-pig. *Br. J. Pharmacol.*, **52,** 149
10. Kaidey, K. H. and Kurban, A. K. (1976). The influence of corticosteroids and topical indomethacin on sunburn erythema. *J. Invest. Derm.*, **66,** 153
11. Jasani, M. K., Parsons, R. R., Roberts, J. M. and Tweed, M. F. (1974). The usefulness of homologous pairs of rabbit skin grafts for studying the pharmacology of anti-rheumatic agents. *Br. J. Pharmacol.*, **57,** 152
12. Sorenson, J. R. J. (1976). Copper chelates as possible active forms of the antiarthritic agents. *J. Med. Chem.*, **19,** 135
13. Rainsford, K. D. and Whitehouse, M. W. (1976). Concerning the merits of copper aspirin as a potential anti-inflammatory drug. *J. Pharm. Pharmacol.*, **28,** 83
14. Kamel, H., Brown, D. H., Ottoway, J., Smith, W. E., Cottney, J. and Lewis, A. J. (1977). Serum levels and distribution of gold in guinea pigs after oral administration of different compounds compared to Myocrisin injected intramuscularly. *Arthr. Rheum.* (in press)
15. Walz, D. T., Dimartino, M. J. and Sutton, B. M. (1974). Design and laboratory evaluation of gold compounds as anti-inflammatory drugs. In R. Scherrer and M. W. Whitehouse (eds.) *Anti-inflammatory Agents — Chemistry and Pharmacology*, pp. 209–244. (New York and London: Academic Press)
16. Shen, T. Y. (1974). Non acidic antiarthritic agents and the search for new classes of agents. In R. Scherrer and M. W. Whitehouse (eds.) *Anti-inflammatory Agents — Chemistry and Pharmacology*, pp. 180–207. (New York and London: Academic Press)
17. Norins, A. L. (1962). Free radical formation in the skin following exposure to ultraviolet light. *J. Invest. Derm.*, **39,** 445
18. Pathak, M. A. and Stratton, K. (1968). Free radicals in human skin before and after exposure to light. *Arch. Biochem. Biophys.*, **123,** 468
19. Oyanagui, Y. (1976). Inhibition of superoxide anion production in macrophages by anti-inflammatory drugs. *Biochem. Pharmacol.*, **25,** 1473
20. Mathur, G. P. and Ghandi, V. M. (1972). Prostaglandin in human and albino rat skin. *J. Invest. Derm.*, **58,** 291
21. Sekura Snyder, D. (1976). Effect of topical indomethacin on UVR-induced redness and prostaglandin E levels in sunburned guinea pigs. *Prostaglandins*, **11,** 631
22. Greaves, M. W. and MacDonald-Gibson, W. (1973). Effect of non-steroid anti-inflammatory drugs on prostaglandin biosynthesis by skin. *Br. J. Derm.*, **88,** 47
23. Lewis, G. P. and Piper, P. J. (1975). Inhibition of release of prostaglandins as an explanation of some of the actions of anti-inflammatory corticosteroids. *Nature (London)*, **254,** 308
24. Deby, C., Bacq, Z. M. and Simon, D. (1973). *In vitro* inhibition of the biosynthesis of a prostaglandin by gold and silver. *Biochem. Pharmacol.*, **22,** 3141
25. Newcombe, D. S. and Ishikawa, Y. (1976). The effect of anti-inflammatory agents on human synovial fibroblast prostaglandin synthetase. *Prostaglandins*, **12,** 819
26. Johnson, B. E. (1968). Ultraviolet radiation and lysosomes in skin. *Nature (London)*, **219,** 1258
27. Lazarus, G. S., Hatcher, V. B. and Levine, N. (1975). Lysosomes and the skin. *J. Invest. Derm.*, **65,** 259
28. Ignarro, L. J. (1972). Lysosome membrane stabilization *in vivo*: Effects of steroidal and non-steroidal anti-inflammatory drugs on the integrity of rat liver lysosomes. *J. Pharmacol. Exp. Ther.*, **182,** 179
29. Persellin, R. H. and Ziff, M. (1966). The effect of gold salt on lysosomal enzymes on the peritoneal macrophage. *Arthr. Rheum.*, **9,** 57

8

Role of Hyperaemia and Vascular Permeability in Lymphocyte-mediated Inflammation

CATHERINE S. BACH, M. K. JASANI, K. LOCKWOOD and JEAN M. ROBERTS

INTRODUCTION

Currently available anti-rheumatic drugs, though active against joint pain, fail to arrest the development of rheumatoid joint swelling. Only fresh insight into factors responsible for the initiation and maintenance of such joint swelling can promote improvements in the treatment.

Two types of immunological abnormalities may be responsible for the initiation of rheumatoid inflammation. Firstly, it is believed[1,2] that locally formed immune complexes or circulating immune complexes, which enter the joint, activate the complement sequence. This induces formation of factors chemotactic for polymorphonuclear (PMN) leukocytes. The PMN's then ingest the immune complexes. Such ingestion is accompanied by release of lysosomal enzymes and other mediators[3] the net effect of which is to produce pain, redness, swelling and loss of function in the affected joint.

The second view[4,5] emphasizes a role for locally activated immune lymphocytes or circulating immune lymphocytes which become activated after entering the joint. According to this view, soluble non-antibody mediators, collectively referred to as lymphokines[6,7] initiate the vascular changes characteristic of rheumatoid inflammation. Although much attention has been paid to the role of vascular permeability in inflammation caused by lymphokines[8] and therefore, by implication, by *in vivo* antigenically activated lymphocytes, the contribution of hyperaemia, i.e. increase in blood content of the inflamed tissue, has received less attention.

The present experiments were designed to assess the relative importance of hyperaemia and vascular permeability in the development of swelling caused by antigen-induced activation of immune lymphocytes during rejection of rabbit skin homografts.

MATERIALS AND METHODS

Experiments were made using male albino Norfolk (NFK) rabbits (Morton Commercial Rabbits, Stanstead, Essex) as donors and sex- and weight-matched (2.8 to 3.2 kg) New Zealand White (NZW) rabbits as recipients.

Surgical procedures

Graft-bearing animals

The grafting procedures were as described previously[9]. Full surgical anaesthesia was induced using pentobarbitone sodium (40 mg/kg, i.v.) and maintained by repeated injections (5 mg/kg) via a catheter placed in the marginal ear vein. Four NZW rabbits received grafts.

Homografts, full-thickness (2.5 × 2.5 cm) were dissected from the hind-limb of a NFK rabbit and sutured on to the right hind-limb of a NZW recipient. The donor animal was killed with an overdose of the anaesthetic. Similar sized autografts consisted of skin dissected from the NZW recipient's left hind-limb and sutured on to the sites from which they had been removed. Each rabbit received six grafts per leg, four on the lateral and two on the medial aspect.

After dissection, but before suturing, the grafts were placed in a sterile petri dish on a gauze swab dampened with sterile physiological saline and kept at 4 °C for 15 to 30 min until weighed. Using sterile forceps, each graft was transferred singly to a tared sterile petri dish containing a damp swab, weighed and replaced in the storage petri dish. Once weighed, the grafts were bathed in ice-cold saline for 15 to 60 min. Each graft was held at one corner with dissecting forceps and any blood remaining on its surface removed by gently brushing the convex surface of a pair of tonsil forceps over the graft. The grafts were secured in position with interrupted 5/0 silk sutures, sprayed with Polybactrin powder (Calmic Ltd., Crewe, England) and covered with gauze swabs impregnated with liquid paraffin and Soframycin (Roussel), then dry dressings and finally Elastoplast. The day of grafting is referred to as day 0.

Control animals

Two groups of rabbits not bearing skin grafts were required. In one group, consisting of four NFK and four NZW rabbits, skin (2.5 × 2.5 cm) dissected from each of the six anatomical sites was weighed aseptically, bathed in saline, and the blood lying on the surface removed as described above. All six pieces were then stored at −20 °C until analysis. They were used to determine the amount of blood contained initially in the homo- and autografts. In the second group, also consisting of four NFK and four NZW rabbits, the six pieces of skin (2.5 × 2.5 cm) were dissected 24 h after administration (i.v.) of ^{131}I-HSA. All six pieces were stored at −20 °C, then used to assess the accumulation of ^{131}I-HSA in non-inflamed control skin.

Examination and removal of grafts

The recipient animals were re-anaesthetized daily from day 4 and the grafts inspected. A pair of grafts, consisting of one homograft and one autograft belonging to identical anatomical sites on the opposite legs, was removed daily for quantitative examination. After removal of grafts on day 6, the recipient rabbits were killed with an overdose of the anaesthetic.

After removal, each graft was weighed and a biopsy was taken for histological detection of lymphocytes[10] and fibrin[11]. The remaining tissue was stored at −20 °C.

Substances administered

To minimize uptake of radioiodine by the thyroid, each animal received sterile aqueous iodine solution, B.P., diluted 1:100 (0.1 ml/kg, i.v.) 24 h before administration of the ^{131}I-HSA (Radiochemicals, Amersham) and once daily until the end of the experiment.

^{131}I-HSA (100 μCi; 10 mg protein in 1 ml sterile saline) was injected (i.v.) via the marginal ear vein on day 5.

Blood sampling

A blood specimen was withdrawn on day 6 from the ear artery into a heparinized syringe. A portion 0.10–0.50 ml was used to measure the haemoglobin concentration, $[Hb]_{blood}$, and the remainder (0.3 ml) was placed in a tared counting Bio-vial, weighed and stored at 4 °C until counted.

Measurements

Radioactivity

Tissue and blood radioactivities were measured using a Beckman Biogamma counter. All the specimens belonging to the same experiment were counted on the same day. Counts per minute of all samples were at least 10 times background.

Swelling

This was measured as the increase in weight of each graft, i.e. the difference in weight before suturing and after removal.

Hyperaemia

In this study hyperaemia is regarded as the increase in blood content. It was assessed from the increase in haemoglobin content of the graft.

To measure haemoglobin, the grafts and control skin, which had been stored at −20 °C, were maintained in the frozen state and chopped finely. A portion was homogenized[12] in an aqueous medium to solubilize the blood and tissue proteins, centrifuged and the supernatants (S) removed. Portions of the supernatants (0.5 ml) were mixed with modified Drabkin's reagent (4.0 ml) to convert haemoglobin to stable cyanmethaemoglobin[13]. The reagent contained potassium cyanide (0.774 mM), potassium ferricyanide (0.6 mM) and potassium dihydrogen phosphate (1.03 mM). The mixture was agitated frequently for at least 10 min before determination of E_{542} using a Unicam SP1800 spectrophotometer. Haemoglobin, $[\mathrm{Hb}]_S$, was estimated from a standard curve based on E_{542} of 10 to 200 μg hemiglobin (2 × crystallized, Calbiochem Ltd.) treated as above.

The blood content of each graft was calculated as follows:

$$\text{Blood content (mg)} = \frac{[\mathrm{Hb}]_s\ (\mu\text{g/ml}) \times \text{graft weight (mg)}}{[\mathrm{Hb}]_{\text{blood}}\ (\mu\text{g/ml})}$$

The initial blood content was calculated using the haemoglobin concentration of supernatants of control skin and the graft weight before suturing. The final blood content was calculated from the supernatants of each graft and the weight when removed. The difference between the two values measured hyperaemia, i.e. the increase in blood content.

Vascular permeability

It was measured as the extravascular accumulation of ^{131}I-HSA. ^{131}I-HSA was administered (i.v.) on day 5. Extravascular accumulation of ^{131}I-HSA (cpm/graft) was calculated as follows:

$$\text{Extravascular } ^{131}\text{I-HSA} = (\text{total } ^{131}\text{I-HSA}) - (\text{intravascular } ^{131}\text{I-HSA}).$$

The total ^{131}I-HSA was measured by counting the radioactivity in a weighed portion of finely chopped graft. Intravascular ^{131}I-HSA was calculated by multiplying the increase in blood content by the circulating blood radioactivity at the time of graft removal. Extravascular ^{131}I-HSA in non-inflamed control skin was calculated similarly.

RESULTS

Visual and histological appearance of grafts

Inspection of the grafts *in situ* revealed that on day 6 autografts and homografts showed a similar degree of redness (Table 8.1). Homografts appeared more swollen than autografts and they were also firm, i.e. indurated, on palpation; by contrast, the autografts were as soft as the surrounding skin.

Histological examination revealed the presence of intra- and perivascular accumulation of lymphocytes in homografts but not in autografts (Table 8.1).

Table 8.1 Visual and histological features of rabbit skin grafts. Symbols denote presence (+) or absence (–) of each factor, whereas their frequency reflects degree of severity: +, mild; ++, moderate; +++, severe

Factor	*Autografts*	*Homografts*
Redness	++	++
Swelling	+	+++
Induration	–	++
Lymphocytes	–	++
Congestion	–	++

The blood vessels of autografts were widely dilated but contained only a few cells (Figure 8.1c). Those of the homografts showed congestion, i.e. they were not only more dilated but also plugged full of erythrocytes and leukocytes including lymphocytes (Figure 8.1b). Venules were more congested than arterioles (Figure 8.1b).

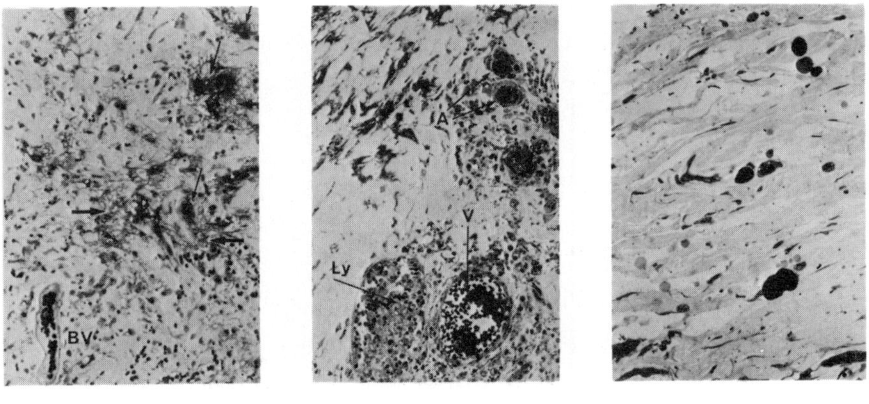

Figure 8.1 Localization of fibrin in the dermis of homograft but not autograft removed from a NZW recipient on day 6, day 0 being the day of transplantation. Light microscope views (×200) of sections (1 μ) of resin-embedded tissue stained with Geimsa 11. Field (a) demonstrates the presence of fibrin meshwork (↓) throughout the dermis. Note that FM is present in the interstitial matrix but not in the congested blood vessel (BV), and is especially prominent around mononuclear lymphoid (↓) cells. Field (b) shows that fibrin was present in distended lymphatics (Ly) but absent from equally dilated venules (V). Note that the fibrin clot has virtually occluded the lymphatic, the venule is grossly congested with leukocytes, and the arterioles (A) are by comparison much less dilated and are plugged instead with erythrocytes. Field (c) shows total absence of fibrin in the interstitial matrix of autograft

The other prominent feature of day 6 homografts was extensive interstitial and intralymphatic filamentous networks (Figure 8.1a and b) which on electron microscopic examination appeared to consist wholly of fibrin. This was confirmed using autoradiography of the grafts 24 h after administration (i.v.) of ^{125}I-human fibrinogen. Light microscopic examination showed large accumulations of radioactivity throughout the dermis of homografts, but only trace amounts in isolated areas in that of autografts. Radioactivity in the homografts was localized predominantly in the interstitial rather than in the intravascular region, and adjacent to mononuclear lymphoid rather than polymorphonuclear leukocytes. Electron microscopic autoradiography showed high silver grain densities associated with filaments and fibrils having a periodicity indentical to that reported for fibrin (200 Å) but not for collagen (640 Å).

Swelling due to hyperaemia

The results in Figure 8.2 show that in autografts almost all of the increase in weight of the grafts was accounted for by an increase in the blood content. In homografts, on the other hand, the increase in blood content accounted for only 50% of the increase in total weight of the grafts.

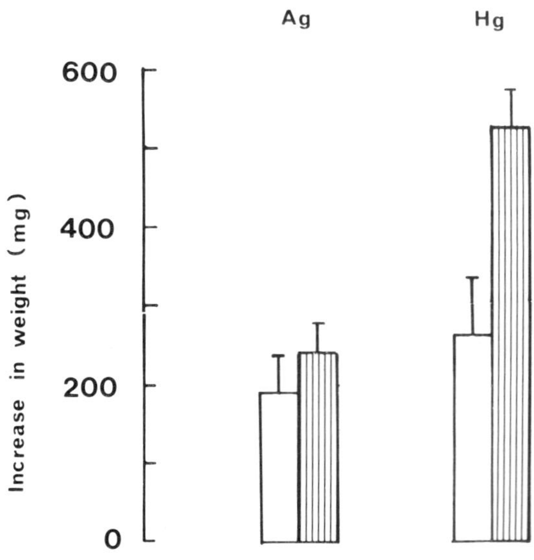

Figure 8.2 Extent to which swelling measured as increase in weight (mg) of rabbit skin grafts is due to hyperaemia, i.e. increase in blood content. Results shown are mean ± s.e. for swelling (▥) and hyperaemia (□) in autografts (Ag) and homografts (Hg) of four NZW recipients on day 6, day 0 being the day of transplantation

Vascular permeability

Figure 8.3 shows that the exudation of protein, measured as extravascular accumulation of ^{131}I-HSA, in homografts was not higher than in comparable autografts. The mean values for both types of graft were, however, significantly higher than the value for control skin, showing that vascular permeability had increased, though to a similar extent in both types of graft.

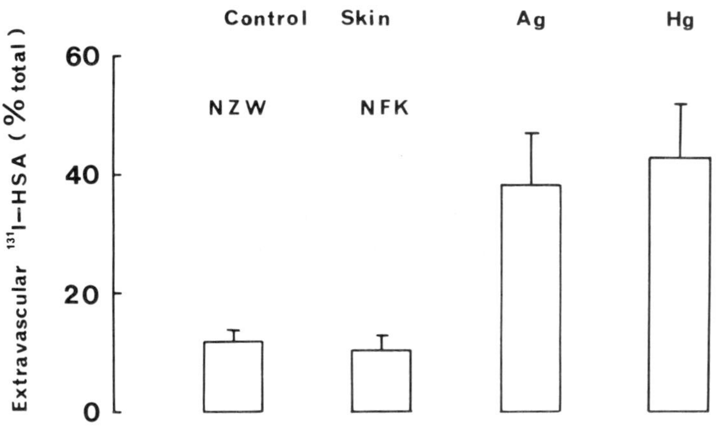

Figure 8.3 Extravasation of intravenously administered ^{131}I-HSA in non-inflamed skin (control) and in rabbit skin grafts. Results are mean ± S.E. for extravascular accumulation of ^{131}I-HSA in control recipient (NZW) and donor (NFK) skin and in day 6 autografts (Ag) and homografts (Hg) in four NZW recipients. Degree of extravasation of ^{131}I-HSA (total–intravascular) is expressed as percentage of total radioactivity per graft

DISCUSSION

The present experiments were designed to define the extent to which vascular permeability and hyperaemia, i.e. increased blood content, account for the swelling associated with lymphocyte-initiated inflammation.

Lymphocytic inflammation was produced using rabbit skin homografts. It is now widely accepted that donor histocompatible antigens in homografts stimulate local activation and transformation of the recipient's immunologically competent lymphocytes[14] and induce intra- and perivascular accumulation of lymphocytic and other inflammatory cells[10,15,16]. Previously[17], it was shown that such accumulation of inflammatory cells not only increases the DNA but also is accompanied by vascular changes that increase the protein and moisture content of skin homografts.

Distinction between lymphocyte-initiated and non-specific swelling in skin homografts

Since homografts also develop a non-specific inflammatory reaction caused by the trauma of surgery, it was essential to recognize the extent to which swelling in homografts was due to lymphocytic as opposed to non-specific inflammation.

Previous investigations[12,17,18] have revealed that when lymphocytic inflammation is prevented, e.g. by treatment with cyclophosphamide, changes in all parameters, which are then due only to the non-specific inflammation in homografts, *equal* those in autografts transplanted simultaneously on to similar sites on the opposite leg of the same recipient. Therefore, differences between comparable homografts and autografts measure the degree of change due to lymphocytic inflammation.

If judged in this manner, the results for swelling, i.e. increase in weight (Figure 8.2), show that only about 50% of the swelling of day 6 homografts is due to lymphocytic inflammation.

Vascular basis for lymphocyte-initiated swelling

Hyperaemia

According to the results illustrated in Figure 8.2, the increase in weight of day 6 homografts due to increased blood content does not differ significantly from that of comparable autografts. Therefore, it is concluded that hyperaemia accounts for only a negligible proportion of the lymphocytic swelling.

Other factors which contribute to the lymphocyte-initiated swelling in homografts include DNA, due to increased cellularity of the homografts, and extravascular accumulation of protein and moisture content, due to increased vascular permeability. Since the increase in DNA accounts for only a negligible increase in the weight of homografts (see Chapter 14, the extra increase in the weight of day 6 homografts, as compared with that of autografts, was due mainly to additional exudation of fluid and protein.

Vascular permeability

Results presented in Figure 8.3 show however, that the extent to which ^{131}I-HSA accumulates extravascularly in day 6 homografts does not differ from that in similar autografts. This being so, how does the additional extravascular accumulation of fluid and protein occur in day 6 homografts in association with the presence of immune lymphocytes?

The fluid content of homografts may increase not only when excessive amounts of fluid leak out of the vessels into the interstitial space but also when the fluid that does exude is not drained adequately by the lymphatics.

Fibrin-induced impairment of lymphatic drainage in homografts

Functional impairment of lymphatic drainage in day 6 rabbit skin homografts, but not in similar autografts, has already been demonstrated using Evan's blue dye injected into the grafts[9]. Additional observations[19,20] have established (a) that the main cause of impaired lymphatic drainage is obstruction of lymph flow by widespread interstitial and intralymphatic deposition of fibrin such as that shown in Figure 8.1; and (b) that immune lymphocytes initiate extravascular accumulation of fibrin.

Thus, presently available evidence indicates that the extra swelling of day 6 homografts as compared with similar autografts (Figure 8.2) is due mainly to extravascular retention of fluid and the accumulation of a water-insoluble protein, namely fibrin, induced by immune lymphocytes.

It is not possible as yet to be certain whether fibrin-induced lymphatic obstruction is solely responsible for the excessive extravascular accumulation of fluid, i.e. oedema, in the homografts. A review of previous literature[21] reveals that oedema occurs in association with lymphatic insufficiency when hyperaemia is passive, i.e. due to venous congestion. In homografts in which venous congestion is recognizable both histologically (Figure 8.1) and as cyanosis[9], is it therefore possible that the lymphocyte-initiated oedema is the combined end-result of venous hyperaemia and fibrin-induced blockage of lymphatics? The suggestion implies that most of the increased blood content of homografts (Figure 8.2) is compartmentalized in the venous rather than the arterial channels, an inference which is supported by results of Figure 8.1 but which requires further investigation.

Relevance to rheumatoid joint swelling

In rheumatoid joint swelling extensive interstitial and intralymphatic deposition of fibrin is a constant feature of the disease process[22]. The fact that fibrin-induced lymphatic insufficiency may be severe enough to result in excessive fluid retention and joint swelling, is indicated by the observations that the osmolality of persistent synovial effusions is that of a plasma transudate rather than that of an exudate[23]. However, it remains to be established whether immune lymphocytes, which have a role in the pathogenesis of rheumatoid inflammation[5], are responsible for the intralymphatic deposition of fibrin in the joint.

Therapeutic implications

For practical purposes, the data presented imply that pharmacological agents which depress the permeability of vessels may prove less effective against the development of swelling associated with clinically-encountered lymphocyte-initiated inflammation than those which can either prevent the intralymphatic formation of fibrin, or promote the removal of such fibrin deposits. In addition, drugs which reduce venous hyperaemia may depress the swelling associated with immune lymphocytes independently of, or in combination with, reduction in the interstitial accumulation of fibrin.

SUMMARY AND CONCLUSIONS

To define the extent to which hyperaemia and vascular permeability account for the swelling associated with lymphocyte-initiated inflammation, the three tissue changes were assessed quantitatively in skin homografts and autografts made simultaneously on to the opposite hind-limbs of rabbits. The appearance and histological changes of the grafts were also examined.

Six days post-operatively the grafts were similarly bright pink but only the homografts showed the presence of intra- and perivascular accumulation of lymphocytes, interstitial and intralymphatic deposition fibrin, and venous congestion.

Swelling measured as increase in weight, was greater in homografts than in autografts. Neither hyperaemia assessed on the basis of hæmoglobin measurements, nor vascular permeability, measured as extravascular accumulation of intravenously administered ^{131}I-human serum albumin (^{131}I-HSA) accounted for the difference. Instead, the extra swelling of homografts was due mainly to retention of fluid occurring in association with venous congestion and lymphatic blockage caused by interstitial and intralymphatic deposition of fibrin. The clinical significance and therapeutic implications for the management of persistent swelling of rheumatoid synovium are discussed.

Acknowledgements

We thank Dr G. R. Bullock for the interpretation of electron micrographs, Mr R. A. Christian and Dr J. R. J. Baker for studies of light and electron microscope autoradiographic localization of intravenously administered ^{125}I-human fibrinogen (results of which are to be published elsewhere), and Mr R. Parsons for the illustrations.

References

1. Zvaifler, N. (1974). Rheumatoid synovitis. An extra-vascular immune complex disesase. *Arthr. Rheum.*, **17,** 297
2. Weissmann, G. (1972). Lysosomal mechanisms of tissue injury in arthritis. *N. Engl. J. Med.*, **286,** 141
3. Henson, P. M. (1971). Interaction of cells with immune complexes: adherence, release of constituents and tissue injury. *J. Exp. Med.*, **134,** 1143
4. Jasani, M. K. (1975). The importance of ACTH and glucocorticoids in rheumatoid arthritis. In Dick, W. C. and Pearson, C. M. (eds.) *Clinics in Rheumatic Disease: Current Management of Rheumatoid Arthritis.* Vol. 1, p. 354. (London and Philadelphia: W. B. Saunders Ltd.)
5. Pearson, C. M., Paulus, H. E. and Machleder, H. I. (1975). The role of lymphocyte and its products in the propagation of joint disease. *Ann. N.Y. Acad. Sci.*, **256,** 150
6. Dumonde, D. C., Wolstencroft, R. A., Panayi, G. S., Mathew, M., Morley, J. and Howson, W. T. (1969). Lymphokines: non-antibody mediators of cellular immunity generated by lymphocyte activation. *Nature (London)*, **224,** 38
7. Stastny, P., Rosenthal, M., Andreis, M., Cooke, D. and Ziff, M. (1975). Lymphokines in rheumatoid synovitis. *Ann. N.Y. Acad. Sci.*, **256,** 117

8. Williams, T. J. and Morley, J. (1974). Measurement of rate of extravasation of plasma protein in inflammation responses in guinea-pig skin using a continuous recording method. *Br. J. Exp. Pathol.*, **55**, 1
9. Jasani, M. K. and Lewis, G. P. (1971). Lymph flow and changes in intracellular enzymes during rejection of rabbit skin homografts. *J. Physiol.*, **219**, 525
10. Bullock, G. R., Jasani, M. K. and Lewis, G. P. (1977). Morphology of immune lymphocytes in homograft lymph. *Cell. Biol. Int. Rep.*, **1**, 123
11. Roberts, J. M. (1977). Detection of fibrin in lymphocyte-initiated inflammation. *Proc. R. Microsc. Soc.*, **12**, 58
12. Jasani, M. K. (1973). The usefulness of enzyme measurement for evaluation of pharmacological agents which modify the homograft reaction. *Biochem. Soc. Trans.*, **1**, 1043
13. Drabkin, D. L. and Austin, J. H. (1935). Spectrophotometric studies. II. Preparations from washed blood cells; nitric oxide haemoglobin and sulfhaemoglobin. *J. Biol. Chem.*, **112**, 51
14. Medawar, P. B. (1963). Introduction: definition of the immunologically competent cell. In Wolstenholme, G. E. W. and Knight, J. (eds.) *The Immunologically Competent Cell*, pp. 1–4. (London: Churchill)
15. Wiener, J., Spiro, D. and Pearl, J. S. (1964). An electron microscopic study of the homograft reaction. *Am. J. Pathol.*, **44**, 319
16. Wiener, J., Lattes, R. G. and Pearl, J. S. (1969). Vascular permeability and leucocyte emigration in allograft rejection. *Am. J. Pathol.*, **55**, 295
17. Bitterli, E. and Jasani, M. K. (1972) A quantitative assessment of tissue changes accompanying homograft reaction; changes in tissue dry weight, DNA and moisture content in rabbit skin homografts. *Br. J. Pharmacol.*, **45**, 138
18. Christian, R. A., Jasani, M. K. and Tweed, M. F. (1977). Role of immune lymphocytes in the development of inflammatory response accompanying the rejection of rabbit skin homografts and its inhibition with the use of cyclophosphamide. (In press)
19. Bullock, G. R., Jasani, M. K. and Roberts, J. M. (1976). Tissue localisation of fibrin in homograft reaction and its relevance to the pathophysiology of rheumatoid synovial swelling. *Proc. R. Microsc. Soc.*, **11**, (Suppl.), 65
20. Bach, C. S. and Jasani, M. K. (1976). Role of lymphocytes in accumulation of fibrin in rabbit skin homografts. *Br. J. Pharmacol.*, **58**, 292
21. Rusznyak, I., Foldi, M. and Szabo, G. (1969). *Lymphatics and Lymph Circulation*, pp. 235–241. (Oxford: Pergamon Press)
22. Caughey, D. E. and Highton, T. C. (1967). Components of the fibrinolytic system in synovial joints. *Ann. Rheum. Dis.*, **26**, 297
23. Lipson, R. L., Baldes, E. J., Anderson, J. A. and Polley, H. F. (1965). Osmotic pressure gradients and joint effusions. *Arthr. Rheum.*, **8**, 29

Discussion III

The Relationship between Increased Vascular Permeability Hyperaemia, Stasis and Thrombosis in the Microcirculation (Chapter 6)

K. D. MUIRDEN (Rapporteur): Dr Movat discussed the relationship between increased vascular permeability, hyperaemia, stasis and thrombosis in the microcirculation using an ^{125}I albumin and Evans blue technique in guinea pigs. PGE_1 was shown to enhance blood flow and vascular permeability with a peak activity 15–40 min after injection. The effects of histamine and bradykinin were potentiated depending on the time interval used. The enhanced vascular permeability was markedly affected by blood flow, for example, stasis induced by heat reduced the swelling caused by PGE_1.

Some elegant electron microscope pictures of blood vessels in the Arthus reaction were shown. Antigen–antibody complexes occurred in walls of vessels and microthrombi developed in small vessels with polymorphs, platelets and fibrin accumulating in the lumen. Stasis lead to necrosis of vessel walls, demonstrated by chylomicrons leaking from the vessels.

T. J. WILLIAMS: When in 1973, Dr John Morley and I observed PGE_1 to agument the accumulation of ^{125}I-HSA at the site of intradermal injection of bradykinin in the guinea-pig (*Nature*, **246**, 215–217), we regarded the effect to represent potentiation of vascular permeability. Since then, however, results of further investigation I have carried out (*Br. J. Pharmacol.*, **56**, 341–342 P; 1976) convince me that the augmented accumulation of ^{125}I-HSA following PGE_1 is due to vasodilatation and the resultant increase in vessel wall area.

I wonder if now we should stop talking about increase in vascular permeability and consider increase in exudation instead. In that event we might understand better not only the chemical basis of inflammation but also the mode of action of non-steroidal anti-inflammatory drugs (NSAIDs).

H. Z. MOVAT: There is a marked difference between the rat which Dr Williams and many others have studied and the rabbit.

T. J. WILLIAMS: We used the guinea pig and the rabbit.

H. Z. MOVAT: The rat has been used in early experiments with PGs in which, in addition to enhanced flow, there was also an actual exudation or enhanced permeability.

Evaluation of the Ability of Anti-rheumatic Drugs to Suppress Hyperaemia and Increased Vascular Permeability (Chapter 7)

K. D. MUIRDEN (Rapporteur): Dr A. J. Lewis noted species differences, and in the rat indomethacin was most effective of five orally administered NSAIDs. Aspirin was the least effective and ibuprofen somewhat mid-way. When topically administered, ibuprofen proved the most, aspirin the least effective and indomethacin intermediate. Systemic steroids curiously enough had less effect, but topically applied steroids were potent inhibitors. An intriguing finding was that both gold and D-penicillamine also possessed anti-erythemic activity in guinea pigs. In considering the mode of action of drugs in the system, it was suggested that release of lipoperoxides and endoperoxides, prostaglandin formation as well as lysosomal enzyme release might be involved.

R. J. PERPER: Did the abstract say that gold and penicillamine worked only in the rat? Did I understand correctly that these two compounds work in the guinea pig?

A. J. LEWIS: I don't think that I wrote that they were effective in the rat. I deal exclusively with these anti-rheumatic agents in the guinea pig.

R. J. PERPER: If that is the case, we use guinea pigs and we must have done penicillamine a thousand times one way and another, and we have also done gold. I could never get any effect on erythema the way we did it. Did I do something wrong, perhaps?

A. J. LEWIS: I do not know. As I said earlier, we were surprised to show these effects. Obviously there are explanations as to why these substances may work in this model. As we know, they tend to take a little time to act in man so that their effect in an acute model of inflammation is rather surprising.

R. J. PERPER: We did exhaustive work on trying to get them to work, and we never could.

G. A. HIGGS: Dr Lewis mentioned the effect of gold salts on prostaglandin biosynthesis, and there was an elevation of PGE production. Was this from *in vitro* work?

A. J. LEWIS: Yes, indeed. Mr Higgs himself has looked at gold *in vivo*, and perhaps that is more relevant to the cases that I have mentioned.

G. A. HIGGS: Yes. In fact, the *in vivo* work that we did with gold salts shows a small but significant reduction in PG production in experimental inflammation, and the PG produced in this type of model is over 80% E_2.

D. C. DUMONDE: I am interested that the vascular response obtained by Dr Lewis is so protracted. I did not quite catch whether he gave ultraviolet light continuously, or whether it was pulsed at the start. If it was pulsed at the start, then the gradual development of erythema and of permeability — with the permeability still rising at 8 hours — looks almost like the beginnings of a delayed-type hypersensitivity reaction.

A. J. LEWIS: It is a pulse of ultraviolet irradiation. I cannot make any useful comment on your other remarks except to recount the fact that the alteration in vascular permeability lasts a considerable period of time; erythema subsides, there being none at 48 hours, and the epidermis undergoes sloughing.

D. C. DUMONDE: I was really asking why?

A. J. LEWIS: I do not know, I am afraid.

J. R. VANE: I wondered whether any of the drugs that were used had any effects on a progression of the erythema into a scab, and then sloughing off.

A. J. LEWIS: So far none of the compounds, including gold, have affected the actual sloughing of the epidermis. This is still a mystery. Ultraviolet light is a very severe insult and it may well be that we shall never ever get a drug which will actually prevent the erythema from appearing.

S. ORLOFF: It is known that several drugs, including the anti-inflammatory drugs, can enhance ultraviolet-erythema. Have any studies been done on spectral absorption of these drugs?

A. J. LEWIS: Not to my knowledge. Enhance the ultraviolet-erythema?

S. ORLOFF: Gold is an example. In man it would enhance the erythema response.

A. J. LEWIS: I do not know of any work that has been done on this.

A. A. J. GOLDBERG: I did not quite catch whether Dr Lewis mentioned the vehicle he used for the administration of his topical drug. Clearly the nature of the vehicle and the thickness of the film that is put on will influence the response to ultraviolet light.

A. J. LEWIS: I did mention it. It was absolute ethanol. We have not looked at any other vehicles. We have stuck with that particular vehicle. Perhaps if we did use a different vehicle we would get a better, or perhaps a different profile of activity. So far we have only used ethanol.

M. K. JASANI: Following on Dr Goldberg's comment I have a brief observation which may make Dr Lewis's work more easily repeatable by others.

There have been reports in the literature (*J. Invest. Dermatol.*, **65**, 238–40; 1975) that the ultraviolet energy imparted to the skin can either induce changes in the vessel which are reversible, or changes which are irreversible. Dr Perper has already referred to his own experience and to his not being able to repeat the type of observations made by Dr Lewis. In the future all such work should perhaps state the type of energy and the type of apparatus employed.

A. J. LEWIS: Dr Perper did not say that he could not reproduce what I have shown. In other models of erythema he has not observed that gold is effective.

R. J. PERPER: In the standard ultraviolet-erythema model we could not get penicillamine or gold to work. I simply asked about the differences in experimental protocol. Dr Jasani is also pointing to that problem. Maybe Dr Lewis has an answer.

A. J. LEWIS: I have one point. We have obviously to find out whether gold is working specifically or non-specifically in this model. We have looked at the erythema induced by histamine to see whether gold has an influence, and gold is inactive against histamine-induced erythema in the guinea pig. It may be something to do with the wave length of light that we use. It might be different in our experiments. Personally I doubt it. The time course of administration may differ.

R. J. PERPER: As Dr Jasani says, the parameters have to be detailed exactly.

M. K. JASANI: Having made an observation which could possibly detract from the work I should point out that overall the effect of the communication that we have just heard would suggest that there is a considerable correlation between the ability to inhibit erythema induced by ultraviolet irradiation and the relief of pain. I am extrapolating from one experimental model to another, but the question which requires to be investigated is whether the correlation reflects similarities between the chemical basis for ultraviolet-induced vascular responses and pain of inflammatory origin.

G. P. LEWIS: Since we know that these anti-rheumatic drugs such as gold and penicillamine have a very long-delayed onset of action where they are effective, would the animals have been pretreated over some period of time? Some of the doses and concentrations that were used looked pretty high. This way they might be brought down.

A. J. LEWIS: They were high. We have not done that experiment — giving gold over an extended period. Obviously it is something that we shall probably try at some stage.

I. F. SKIDMORE: Does the use of this model offer a reasonable chance of developing a new type of drug, and if so, how?

A. J. LEWIS: Personally I do not think that it does. It is interesting from the viewpoint that drugs can be applied topically and systemically. It is also interesting that gold seems to work—in our hands at least—in the model. I would not wish to give the impression that I am advocating that everybody should use a guinea pig ultraviolet-erythema model as a fantastic new screening test. Obviously it is not.

We also have the problem, mentioned already, of false positives, such as methysergide, and, although I do not believe that it is active in rheumatoid arthritis it is a very effective compound here.

So, it has considerable limitations, but at the same time these are interesting observations.

R. J. PERPER: We used to do a bandage on people; putting on tape, taking it off, and getting erythema. Steroids were the only thing that worked, and we always held the opinion that steroids topically had a vasoconstrictive effect, and would work in almost any kind of erythematous model if that was all that we were looking for. The lack of systemic activity of steroids in this model is something that I can confirm. We never could get steroids to work systemically.

Role of Hyperaemia and Vascular Permeability in Lymphocyte-Mediated Inflammation (Chapter 8)

K. D. MUIRDEN (Rapporteur): Dr Catherine Bach described an interesting model for inflammation of an immune type which has not as yet been utilized fully for testing anti-rheumatic drugs (See Chapter 14 by Jasani *et al.*). Experiments involved both homografts and autografts in rabbits, and the role of vascular permeability in lymphocyte-mediated inflammation was studied. In homografts, marked swelling, induration and lymphocyte accumulation occurred and it was found that the swelling was related to venous congestion, lymphatic obstruction and excess extravascular fluid. The minor degree of swelling which occurred in autografts was due to increased vascularity. Evidence was produced that fibrin-induced lymphatic obstruction occurred, but so far fibrinolytic agents have not been assessed as a possible means for modifying the reaction.

K. WHALEY: Would Dr Bach speculate on the mechanism of fibrin deposition and tell us whether fibrinolytic agents prolong survival of homografts.

C. S. BACH: The experiments we carried out using cyclophosphamide revealed (*Br. J. Pharmacol.*, **58,** 292P.; 1976) that when the immunosuppressive agent delays the intra-vascular localization of lymphocytes, it delays also the deposition of fibrin and prevents the development of the lymphocytic component of swelling in the homografts. It is therefore possible that some factor released from the lymphocytes initiates both deposition of fibrin and the development of lymphocytic swelling.

R. J. PERPER: Are there also macrophages in those lesions? I would then speculate that the macrophages might be more responsible for the fibrin.

C. S. BACH: Yes, it is possible.

M. I. V. JAYSON: In a study we undertook several years ago (*Br. Med. J.*, **2,** 555–7; 1963) measuring vascular permeability in rheumatoid patients, we found that in the region between the knee and ankle joints the coefficient of capillary filtration was significantly higher than values observed in the corresponding region of control patients.

Comparison of changes in vascular permeability in rheumatoid patients showing evidence of his oedema with those free of such oedema revealed that the coefficient of capillary filtration was higher in those with oedema. The rate of disappearance of sub-cutaneously injected [^{131}I] human serum albumin (*Ann. Rheum. Dis.*, **30,** 638–9; 1971) was, however, comparable in both the groups, although we would agree that in this sort of problem there does seem to be some obstruction, we did not feel that this particular obstruction of lymphatic clearance contributed towards the oedema problem.

I wanted to draw attention to the fact that there are parallel changes in rheumatoid disease to those that Dr Bach has found in this experimental situation.

H. Z. MOVAT: Dr Perper's remark that fibrin was seen around the mononuclear cells or the macrophages is significant in view of the recent demonstration — over the past several years in fact — of the Rockefeller Group that there is a plasminogen activator in macrophages.

D. C. DUMONDE: The trouble with that argument is that it seems to be the wrong way round. If the lymphocytes were producing lymphokines which activated macrophages to produce a plasminogen activator, one would expect enhanced fibrinolysis rather than impairment, so something else is happening.

R. J. PERPER: Undoubtedly there is an interplay of the several cell types and the mediators.

GENERAL DISCUSSION

J. R. VANE: Could I return to the discussion that started up between Professor Movat and Dr Williams. I believe that Dr Williams said that the increase in permeability was associated with the increase in blood flow. I also thought that Professor Movat said that PGE_1 gave an enormous increase in blood flow without any increase in permeability when it was given by itself. I cannot quite put the two things together.

H. Z. MOVAT: The early findings were all done with the rat and Dr Williams and his colleagues were the first to show that the increase in permeability due to mediators, such as bradykinin and histamine, is enhanced by prostaglandin. It is our view that this is not a 'sensitization' of vessels by prostaglandins, but actually an enhancement of blood flow, so that if there are leaky vessels due to, say, bradykinin, the enhanced flow will allow more plasma to escape into the tissue and increase the swelling.

T. J. WILLIAMS: I was saying that permeability, dilatation and increased blood flow are different events, and I do not believe that the prostaglandins increase the permeability produced by bradykinin. Permeability is the constraint on the passage of the flow of liquid through the vessel wall. We are talking about exudation. We always measure exudation. There is a certain permeability established in the vessel wall produced by bradykinin, and the exudation that is measured can be increased by an increase in dilatation.

We are not increasing permeability *per se*. We are increasing the flow through the holes in the vessel wall that we have established with bradykinin.

R. R. A. COOMBS: I have a question for Dr Perper.

Did the factor in the serum of adjuvant-treated rats adsorb on to the lymphocytes and stay there on these cells when transferred, after a washing? Were the cells and the serum injected without any treatment?

R. J. PERPER: We did wash the cells after each one of those incubations, and so obviously it was adsorbed on there. Perhaps there could be an antibody. We have recently described an anti-lymphocyte antibody developing in adjuvant-arthritic rats.

R. R. A. COOMBS: What about a complex?

R. J. PERPER: It could be complexes. The serum factors also require to be investigated further.

S. MONCADA: Can I ask Professor Movat whether blood platelets play any role in the vascular stasis he observes during the inflammatory process?

H. Z. MOVAT: Platelets do localize intravascularly in severe inflammatory lesions, especially those characterized by rupture of vessels. I think that their role is merely that of haemostasis.

May I ask a question.

Dr Perper tried to defend chemotaxis — I am referring to accumulation in rheumatoid arthritis, and in inflammation in general. It is true that margination, pavementing and extravasation of leukocytes play a role, but surely chemotaxis is the mechanism that leads to all these things.

R. J. PERPER: Obviously something has to trigger the cells to enter the lesion.

R. E. PETTY: To bring ourselves back to rheumatoid arthritis itself, is there any evidence that this inhibition of prostaglandin synthetase does anything to prevent the development of rheumatoid inflammation?

R. J. PERPER: I do not know who best can answer that question. I am sure there are differences of opinion on the question. Maybe we ought to conclude this session on that note of uncertainty.

Section IV:

Immune-complex Mediated Tissue Damage

Chairman: **R. R. A. COOMBS**

9
Localization of Complexes and Rheumatoid-like Joint Lesions in Rabbits*

A. R. POOLE and R. R. A. COOMBS

* As submitted to *International Meeting on Future Trends in Inflammation III* (1977) London.

INTRODUCTION

In man, serum sickness can produce a clinically characterized polyarthritis involving large and medium-sized joints[1,2]. Experimental studies of serum sickness have concentrated mainly on lesions of the kidney, heart and blood vessels: no detailed descriptions of synovial lesions can be traced[3,4] except for a brief mention by Klinge[5] and by Hawn and Janeway[6]. We have recently observed that synovial lesions, closely resembling those seen in early rheumatoid arthritis, can be produced in rabbits which have received intravenous injections of a multiplicity of antigens in the form of bovine serum[7].

New Zealand White rabbits always received a primary intravenous (i.v.) injection of 5 ml of serum per kg body weight: sometimes, additional i.v. injections of 1.0–1.5 ml per kg were given over a period of up to 7 weeks when the knee (stifle) joints were examined. In our earlier work we observed that approximately 20% of all injected rabbits exhibited rheumatoid-like synovial lesions, regardless of the secondary injection schedule employed. These changes were characterized by lining cell hyperplasia, sometimes with villous formation. Hyperplasia was invariably closely associated with the appearance of many lymphocytes and/or plasma cells under the lining cell layer. Lymphocytes appeared first in perivascular sites (around capillaries or venules) and often formed large focal collections. These changes were sometimes accompanied by fibroplasia which spread from under the lining layer into the capsular tissue, with much deposition of collagen. In about one third of animals showing gross lesions, pannus formation was noted. Cartilage proteoglycan was severely depleted in the area close to the invading pannus tissue (as indicated by a marked loss of toluidine blue staining). This pannus was always in continuity with the synovium and was always very vascular. Increased vascularity was frequently a feature of many inflamed synovia. These synovial changes are often associated with an elevated polymorphonuclear leukocyte (PMN) count in the joint fluid[8,9]: the leukocytes were rarely observed in the synovium, as is the case in established rheumatoid synovial lesions in man.

Immunohistochemical examinations of synovia[10] and cartilage[11] in rheumatoid joints in man have revealed the presence of immune complexes. Using fluorescein-labelled antibodies to rabbit IgG, Fab' and C3 we have observed staining in cytoplasmic vacuoles of synovial lining cells and in the superficial cartilage of the patella in joints of animals where lesions have been observed histologically and where PMN counts are elevated. Uninjected rabbits display none of these histological changes or immunohistochemical staining patterns indicative of the presence of immune complexes. It is likely then that immune complexes are lodging in the joints of some rabbits in significant amounts and creating a local allergic response leading to synovial and joint fluid changes that are associated with cartilage destruction.

More recently we have observed that commercial colonies of New Zealand White rabbits produce a variable 'incidence' of gross joint lesions. Whereas in two colonies only 13% of all the rabbits injected in each case developed extensive lesions, 50% of those animals in a third colony displayed marked changes.

This study, which is continuing with other antigens, e.g. bacterial, provides a further animal model for investigating rheumatoid arthritis without any direct injection into the joint. It is hoped that it will be of use in future work concerned with the development and persistence of this disease.

References

1. Boots, R. H. and Swift, H. F. (1923). The arthritis of serum sickness. *J. Am. Med. Ass.*, **80,** 12
2. Shulman, L. S. and Harvey, A. M. (1972). Polyarteritis and other arteritic syndromes. In J. L. Hollander and D. J. McCarty, Jr. (eds.) *Arthritis and Allied Conditions. A Textbook of Rheumatology*. 8th Edition. pp. 918–939. (Philadelphia: Lea and Febiger)
3. Dixon, F. J. (1963). The role of antigen–antibody complexes in disease. *Harvey Lect.*, **58,** 21
4. Cochrane, G. G. and Koffler, D. (1973). Immune complex disease in experimental animals and man. *Adv. Immunol.*, **16,** 185
5. Klinge, F. (1929). Die Eiweissüberempfindlichkeit (Gewebsanaphylaxie) der Gelenke. Experimentelle pathologisch-anatomische Studie zur Pathogenese des Gelenk-Rheumatismus. *Beitr. Path. Anat.*, **83,** 185
6. Hawn, C. V. Z. and Janeway, C. A. (1947). Histological and serological sequences in experimental hypersensitivity. *J. Exp. Med.*, **85,** 571
7. Poole, A. R. and Coombs, R. R. A. (1977). Rheumatoid-like joint lesions in rabbits injected intravenously with bovine serum. *Int. Arch. All.*, **54,** 97
8. Poole, A. R., Oldham, G. and Coombs, R. R. A. (1977). Early rheumatoid-like lesions in rabbits injected with foreign serum: relationship to localization of immune complexes in the living tissues of joints and cellular content of synovial fluid. *Int. Arch. All.* (in press)
9. Coombs, R. R. A. and Poole, A. R. (1977). Rheumatoid-like joint lesions in rabbits injected intravenously with foreign serum: a histopathological and immunopathological study. In J.

L. Gordon and B. L. Hazleman (eds.) *Rheumatoid Arthritis*. pp. 181–191. (Amsterdam: Elsevier/North Holland Biomedical Press)

10. Bonomo, L., Tursi, A., Trizo, D., Gillardi, U. and Dammacco, F. (1970). Immune complexes in rheumatoid synovitis: a mixed staining immunofluorescence study. *Immunology,* **18,** 557
11. Cooke, T. D., Hurd, E. R., Jasin, H. E., Bienenstock, J. and Ziff, M. (1975). Identification of immunoglobulin and complement in rheumatoid articular collagenous tissues. *Arthr. Rheum.,* **18,** 541

10
Evaluation of Anti-Rheumatic Drugs using the Cutaneous Arthus Reaction

M. B. GOLDLUST, T. W. HARRITY and D. M. PALMER

INTRODUCTION

We first became involved with the investigation of new animal models for anti-inflammatory testing about 7 years ago. At that time a meeting sponsored by the Food and Drug Administration was held concerning the pharmacological and clinical evaluation of anti-inflammatory drugs. In discussions held at that meeting, relatively brief mention was made of the effects of anti-inflammatory drugs on Arthus reactions. Generally, the Arthus reaction was considered not good enough to be a primary screen. This conclusion may have been based upon the fact that certain clinically effective anti-inflammatory agents were not effective at reasonable doses in some Arthus tests. As will become apparent, this is exactly the reason we have pursued Arthus models. Being relatively new in the area of non-steroidal anti-inflammatory drug evaluation, we decided to develop a screening programme using non-classical, presumably more mechanistically rational, testing models instead of approaching drug evaluation through established procedures.

The fact that the aetiology of rheumatoid arthritis (RA) is still not known limits pharmacologists to the evaluation of agents in models that mimic the lesions of the rheumatic diseases. By the *in vivo* approach, one can study either models of acute inflammation characterized by marked oedema and polymorphonuclear leukocyte infiltration, or chronic inflammation characterized by mononuclear leukocyte predominance and, in some models, destruction of connective tissues.

Mechanistically, the immune complex-induced Arthus reaction is reasonably well defined[1]. Arthus reactions comprise inflammatory factors that have been implicated in the acute responses in joints of rheumatoid patients[2]. Complement and PMNs are activated via precipitating antigen–antibody complexes leading to an inflammatory focus characterized by oedema, erythema, haemorrhage, and vasculitis. Arthus reactivity becomes maximal between 3 and 24 h after skin challenge depending upon the model.

The discovery and development of new anti-rheumatic drugs involves a number of factors often present in fortuitous combination: appropriate animal screening models, the 'right' chemical structures and low toxicity. The determination of whether Arthus models are useful for screening purposes has involved not only the practical aspects of developing a screening test, for example, the capacity for assaying large numbers of compounds and the ease of assessment of activity, but also the ability to determine just how novel in activity are these Arthus-active compounds. One means by which we have attempted to approach the latter problem is by establishing criteria that include relatively low activity or inactivity in other standard anti-inflammatory tests as a suggestion of specific Arthus activity. Theoretically, agents presently available should not be effective in these Arthus models. A model sensitive to inhibition by currently used agents does not necessarily make it less desirable in terms of specificity. However, since studies of mechanisms of action are not easily extrapolated to *in vivo* situations, it does make interpretation of activity of new compounds in new tests more difficult and necessitates additional testing in secondary procedures.

The various means by which Arthus reactions can be induced are indicated in Table 10.1. Although there may be some differences in these reactions, particularly with respect to factors involved in the initiation of the reactions, the

Table 10.1 Cutaneous Arthus reactions

1.	Active:	actively immunized animal for humoral antibody; intradermal (i.d.) antigen
2.	Direct Passive:	passively administered (intravenous) antibody; i.d. antigen
3.	Reversed Passive:	i.v. antigen; i.d. antibody
4.	Local Passive:	i.d. antigen–antibody complexes

present studies will not take these into consideration. This is not meant to minimize the role of these factors, but in order to implement Arthus testing certain practical considerations have been taken into account. Humoral antibody may be present in the circulation of the recipient, as in the active or direct passive procedures, or antibody may be introduced locally via an intradermal injection such as in the reversed passive or local passive techniques.

Assuming we have a primary model (Arthus) adequately reflecting rheumatoid inflammation, some additional problems involved in a drug screening programme are indicated in Table 10.2. These problems concern such factors as concentrations of inciting agents; animal species — strain, size,

Table 10.2 Potential problems in anti-inflammatory screening tests *in vivo*

1. Specificity of lesion — i.e., pertinent mechanisms
2. Amounts of inflammation-inducing reagents — i.e., sensitivity to inhibition
3. Animal species — strain, size, age, sex
4. Animal health
5. Location of lesion — e.g., skin, joint, paw, pleural cavity
6. Route of administration of compounds
7. Vehicle used for suspending or dissolving compounds
8. Time of evaluation of lesion
9. Method of evaluation

age, sex; animal health; location of lesion; route and vehicle for administration of agents; time of evaluation of lesion; and endpoint and method of evaluation. Differences in any of these factors might contribute to observed activity or lack of it, or to the inability of laboratories to confirm the results of others. As results of our studies are presented, it must be kept in mind that detailed investigations of all the above parameters are difficult to do although some of these factors have been studied.

In Table 10.3 is a list of Arthus models that have been utilized to investigate the inhibitory activities of known anti-inflammatory or other pharmacological agents. It is quite evident that a number of animal species have been studied, and that the location of these lesions may be in the paw, skin, or joint. An Arthus model in the pleural cavity has recently been reported although drug

Table 10.3 Arthus tests used for the evaluation of anti-inflammatory agents

Lesion Location	*Test*	*Species*	*Reference*
Paw	Direct passive	Rat	Megel *et al.*[3]
Skin	Direct passive	Rat	Goldlust *et al.* (present studies)
	Reversed passive	Rat	Chang[4,5]; Malawista *et al.*[6]; Carter and Krause[7]
		Rabbit	Goldlust and Schreiber[8]; Smith and Humphrey[9]; Humphrey[10]
		Guinea pig	Smith and Humphrey[9]
	Antiserum induced Oedema (AIO)	Rat	Yamamoto *et al.*[11]; Komatsu *et al.*[12]; Goldlust *et al.* (present studies)
		Guinea pig	Ungar *et al.*[13]
	Local passive	Rabbit	Humphrey[10]
	Active	Mouse	Goldlust *et al.* (present studies); Kohler and Martinez[14]
		Rabbit	Smith and Humphrey[9]; Butler and Lewis[15]
Joint	Reversed passive	Guinea pig	Blackham *et al.*[16]
	AIO	Guinea pig	Labrid *et al.*[17]; French *et al.*[18]
	Active	Rabbit	Goldlust *et al.*[19]; Blackham *et al.*[20]

evaluations were not performed[21] (also[1], p. 91). Since all classical inflammation models utilize the rat, it is certainly of interest that in some of these investigations other species have also been used.

Data will be presented concerning the evaluation of anti-inflammatory agents using four different cutaneous Arthus models. In addition, some data in a classical acute inflammation model, carrageenan-induced oedema, will also be indicated for comparison. The results demonstrate that Arthus models can be devised that are as easily performed as other standard tests, and that there is the potential advantage of utilizing a model with a more pertinent inflammation mechanism.

MATERIALS AND METHODS

Reference therapeutic agents

The following agents were used in the present studies (the supplier is indicated in parentheses): indomethacin (Merk, Sharp and Dohme); meclofenamic, mefenamic, and flufenamic acids (Parke Davis): niflumic acid (Squibb England); naproxen (Syntex); ibuprofen and ibufenac (Boots Pure Drug); benzydamine (Aziende Chemiche Riunite); phenylbutazone (Ciba-Geigy); acetylsalicylic acid (Monsanto); aurothioglucose (Schering); chloroquine phosphate (Winthrop); sudoxicam (Pfizer); maleopimaric acid (Eastman Organic Chemicals); and colchicine (Calbiochem).

Antisera and other materials

All antisera were obtained from Cappel Laboratories. The following sera were used: rabbit anti-bovine serum albumin (BSA) [lot#6761]; goat anti-rat serum (lot#56732). Pooled normal goat serum was obtained either from Grand Island Biologicals and kept frozen until used, or from Cappel as a lyophilized preparation. Pyrogen-free saline (PFS) was obtained from Abbott Laboratories, and bovine serum albumin (BSA) from ICN.

In vivo assays

Reversed passive Arthus test (RPA) in rabbits

Details of this test have been previously published[8]. Briefly, compounds were tested by intradermal (i.d.) administration after admixing with antibody following i.v. BSA. One or 2 compounds were tested in each animal in replicate sites on the shaved dorsal surface along with replicate, untreated control lesion sites. The effects of compounds were evaluated 6 hours after i.d. challenge by comparing the volumes of treated and untreated lesions as measured by changes in skin thickness and lesion diameters. The activities of systemically administered compounds were determined by first assessing each rabbit's normal 6-hour response in triplicate skin sites followed the next day by treatment of 6 animals per group with compound 1 hour (oral, p.o.) or 0.5 hour (intraperitoneal, i.p.) prior to skin challenge in three additional sites with evaluation 6 hours after the i.d. challenges. Comparisons between pre- and post-compound reaction volumes indicated the extent of inhibition.

Mouse active Arthus test (MAA)

CD® -1 male mice (19–21 g) were obtained from the Charles River Breeding Laboratories. They were sensitized using a procedure modified after Benedict and Tipps[22] by an i.p. injection of 0.5 ml of a 1:1 emulsion of Freund's complete adjuvant (Difco) containing 250 μg of BSA in saline. Five weeks later, the mice were used for testing. Animal reactivity was sufficient for at least two additional weeks. The dorsal skin of the mice was shaved at least one day before testing. Animals were allowed food and water *ad libitum*. At the time of testing mice weighed 35–40 g.

Compounds were suspended using a Polytron® homogenizer (Brinkmann Instruments, Inc.) in sterile 1% sodium carboxymethylcellulose (CMC) in PFS. Each compound was administered in single doses (0.5 ml per mouse) by the i.p. or p.o. route to groups of 6 mice at varying times from 0.5 to 3 hours prior to skin challenge. This i.d. challenge consisted of 0.05 ml of 5 mg BSA/ml PFS. Seven mice were included in vehicle control groups.

Three and one-half hours after skin challenge, the animals were sacrificed by exposure to CO_2 (dry ice vapour) and the lesions were then cut out using the actual perimeter of the oedema as a guide. The average control lesions (not corrected for normal skin) weighed 1.2–1.8 g depending on the batch of mice. The average lesion weight of the group receiving test compound was compared with that of the control group at each time period and the per cent inhibition by the test compound was calculated. Correcting for normal skin weights, about 20 mg of lesion per g of body weight or 700 mg per mouse were produced in these studies.

The reference standard for the MAA was maleopimaric acid[23] administered by the i.p. route at $1\frac{1}{2}$ hours prior to skin challenge. This time was determined to be about optimal. Due to variable responses of maleopimaric acid by the p.o. route, colchicine was used as the p.o. reference agent, administered 1 hour prior to skin challenge.

Antiserum induced oedema test (AIO) in rats

We followed a procedure modified after Yamamoto *et al.*[11]. Charles River CD or Holtzman Sprague-Dawley male rats (100–175 g) were used. Animals were shaved at least one day prior to testing. They were allowed food and water *ad libitum*. Ibuprofen was administered in either saline or 1% aqueous CMC, while other compounds were administered in saline (0.5 ml/100 g body weight) to rats under light CO_2 anaesthesia 1 hour prior to i.d. challenge in two dorsal sites. One site received 0.1 ml of twice concentrated goat anti-rat serum, while the other site was challenged with this amount of normal goat serum. Three hours later, the animals were sacrificed, and the area about each injection site was removed using a 1¼ inch diameter Arch steel punch. The net weights of treated lesions as compared with those of untreated lesions were used to calculate the level of inhibition. In these studies, approximately 4–6 mg of lesion per g of body weight or about 700 mg per rat were produced. No apparent relationship was observed between body weight and size of the lesion.

Direct passive Arthus test (DPA) in rats

A modification of the procedure of Megel *et al.*[3] was employed. Holtzman male rats (85–130 g) were used. The rats were allowed water and feed *ad libitum*. They were shaved at least one day prior to testing. Rats received 0.5 ml of twice concentrated whole rabbit anti-BSA serum i.v. followed within 5 min by an i.d. challenge on the dorsal surface with 0.1 ml of BSA (240 μg in PFS), the rats being maintained under light CO_2 anaesthesia. Compounds were administered in 0.5 ml PFS/100 g body weight 1 hour prior to skin challenge.

Difficulties were encountered in maintaining adequate levels of inflammation; during the course of these studies changes in the amounts of antiserum and BSA were made. We have no obvious indication that these changes affected inhibitory potencies of the agents tested.

Carrageenan-induced paw oedema tests

(i) In rats. The procedure described by Winter *et al.*[24] was modified as indicated. Male Charles River CD Sprague-Dawley rats (150–175 g) were used. They were fasted for 18 hour prior to testing but were allowed water during this period. Test compounds were dissolved or suspended in 1% aqueous CMC and were administered in a volume of 1 ml/rat to groups of seven rats. Two hours after administration of compounds, one hind paw received an intraplantar injection of 0.05 ml of 1% carrageenan (Viscarin®, Marine Colloids) [w/v] in aqueous CMC. Three hours later, the animals were sacrificed and both hind paws cut off at the tibiotarsal junction and weighed. The average increase in paw weights due to carrageenan challenge for treated groups was compared with that in the untreated group receiving vehicle only. Levels of inhibition were then calculated. The approximate average weight of lesion observed in this model was 3–4 mg per g of body weight or 600 mg per rat.

(ii) In mice. A procedure similar to that described by Levy[25] was used. CD-1 mice (25 g) were obtained from Charles River Breeding Laboratories and were utilized up to a weight of 35 g. Animals were allowed food and water *ad libitum*. Compounds were administered orally in 0.5 ml of 1% CMC in PFS to each mouse $1\frac{1}{2}$ or 3 hours prior to paw challenge. Groups of 10 mice were employed. Four hours after paw challenge with 0.025 ml of 1.5% carrageenan (w/v) in PFS, mice were sacrificed and the paws cut off and evaluated as described above for the rat carrageenan model. The approximate weight of lesion in this test was 2–3 mg per g of body weight or 60–80 mg per mouse.

Analgesic writhing test in mice

A modification of the method of Siegmund *et al.*[26] was used. CF-1 or CD-1 male and female mice (20–30 g) were allowed food and water *ad libitum*. Groups of 10 mice received oral doses of compounds (10 ml/kg) in 1% aqueous CMC 1 hour prior to challenge with an i.p. injection of 0.45% acetic acid (1 ml/100 g body weight) to elicit the writhing response. Two to 10 minutes later, the mice were observed for eight minutes and the number of writhing (stretching) responses was determined. The inhibition of these responses was expressed as a percentage of the untreated controls.

Acute toxicity tests (LD_{50})

The acute, single dose toxicity data used in the present studies were based upon average values from two or more published reports except where indicated. The particular agents with references are indicated as follows: colchicine[27]; indomethacin[28]; naproxen[29,30]; sudoxicam[31]; ibuprofen[32]; phenylbutazone[28,33]; acetylsalicylic acid[27,34]; maleopimaric acid (Squibb, p.o., mouse = 1500 mg/kg; i.p., mouse = 70 mg/kg); niflumic acid (Squibb, p.o., rat = 365 mg/kg; p.o., mouse = 500 mg/kg).

These references were selected to indicate approximately the average LD_{50} values, obtained from a larger number of reports, that were used in the calculations indicated in Tables 10.9 and 10.11.

Statistical analysis

The Wilcoxon rank sum test was utilized[35]. Effects were considered to be significant if the P value was less than or equal to 0.05. The minimum level of inhibition giving statistical significance in the procedures in mice was $\leqslant$20%, while in the procedures in rabbits and rats significance was generally observed between 20 and 30% inhibition.

RESULTS

Reversed passive Arthus test (RPA) in rabbits

We utilized the rabbit in our initial studies of Arthus models for two reasons. First, this species was not a classical one for anti-inflammatory testing and therefore might increase the potential of finding more unusual agents. Secondly, it is a larger animal than the normally used rat and the preparation of multiple test sites and drugs on one animal seemed to be an appealing aspect.

Our earliest attempts to design an Arthus screening test culminated in the RPA procedure using i.d. administration of compounds admixed with antibody. Active compounds were then tested by systemic routes. For these systemic tests, the reactivities of individual animals could be controlled as indicated under *Materials and Methods*. Some of these early data and new ones are indicated in the next three tables. Most of the reference anti-inflammatory agents administered by the i.d. route significantly inhibited the lesions; chloroquine and aurothioglucose were ineffective (Table 10.4). Intradermal dose-responses

Table 10.4 Intradermal activity of non-steroidal anti-inflammatory agents in the reversed passive Arthus test (RPA) in rabbits*

Compound†	*% Inhibition of oedema (6hr)*		*Frequency*‡ *%*	
Meclofenamic acid	62	(51–69)§	100	(6)
Niflumic acid	57	(26–76)	98	(132)
Indomethacin	57	(40–77)	100	(15)
Sudoxicam	57	(43–65)	100	(5)
Naproxen	55	(43–70)	100	(7)
Ibuprofen	54	(39–69)	100	(5)
Benzydamine	52	(12–61)	86	(7)
Mefenamic acid	50	(31–62)	100	(5)
Ibufenac	48	(36–67)	100	(5)
Flufenamic acid	46	(31–58)	100	(5)
Phenylbutazone	44	(22–65)	87	(8)
Acetylsalicylic acid	35	(15–50)	71	(7)
Chloroquine**	13	(0–30)	14	(7)
Aurothioglucose	11	(0–23)	0	(5)
Maleopimaric acid**††	18	(3–30)	17	(6)

* The data in this table is presented with permission of the publisher (see reference[8]).
† Compounds were administered at 200 μg/site.
‡ Percentage of tests showing ≥30% inhibition; number of tests (number of rabbits) shown in parentheses.
§ Average percent inhibition; range indicated in parentheses.
** Administered intradermally, 400 μg/site.
†† Reference agent.

have also been obtained (Table 10.5) for three non-steroidal agents, niflumic acid, indomethacin and colchicine, and two steroids. The steroids, halcinonide and triamcinolone acetonide, were the most potent with minimum effective doses of about 0.03 μg/skin site. The minimum effective doses of the non-steroidal agents (0.5–5 μg/site) suggested that our intradermal screening dose of 200μg/site could have been reduced considerably.

A number of reference agents (as well as developmental agents not reported here) were tested by the i.p. and p.o. routes (Table 10.6). Inhibition of Arthus reactivity by these systemic routes was easily observed for the 6 agents indicated. Dose-responses have been obtained for some of these and were

Table 10.5 Intradermal dose–response measurements in the reversed passive Arthus test (RPA) in rabbits*

	% Inhibition†					
	Dose (μg/site):					
Agent	200	50	5	0.5	0.05	
Non-steroids:						
Niflumic acid	60 ± 10 (152)	52 ± 10 (15)	46 ± 13 (8)	9 ± 2 (6)	N.D.	
Indomethacin	57 ± 9 (41)	52 (1)	61 ± 1 (4)	44 ± 17 (7)	12 ± 8 (3)	
Colchicine	68 ± 1 (2)	40 ± 4 (4)	41 ± 6 (4)	15 ± 13 (4)	N.D.	
	Dose (μg/site):					
	300	30	3	0.3	0.03	0.003
Steroids:						
Halcinonide	56 ± 5 (3)	66 (1)	N.D.	52 ± 4 (4)	47 ± 5 (5)	10 ± 5 (3)
Triamcinolone acetonide	43 (1)	N.D.	53 ± 9 (2)	N.D.	43 ± 7 (4)	17 ± 10 (3)

* Two intradermal doses of non-steroidal agents were administered in duplicate sites to each animal; one dose of a steroid was administered in triplicate sites to each animal. Untreated control sites were included on all animals.
† Per cent inhibition ± standard deviation; number of animals is indicated in parentheses.
§ N.D. = Not done.

Table 10.6 Activities of anti-inflammatory agents in the reversed passive Arthus test (RPA) in rabbits *† by systemic routes

Route of administration	*Agent*	*Dose (mg/kg)*	*% Inhibition‡ of oedema (6 hr)*
Intraperitoneal	Niflumic acid	75	50 (33)
	Indomethacin	25	51 (9)
	Ibuprofen	75	43 (11)
	Phenylbutazone	75	52 (7)
	Colchicine	0.5	44§(5)
Oral	Phenylbutazone	75	47 (4)
	Ibufenac	75	46 (4)
		150	53 (4)
	Colchicine	1	67§(6)

* Some of the data in this table is presented with permission of the publisher (see reference[8]).
† 0.2 ml of fractionated antiserum was injected intradermally at each site.
‡ Average percent inhibition; number of animals is indicated in parentheses.
§ Unfractionated antiserum used.

previously published[8]. ID_{50}'s by the i.p. route were obtained for niflumic acid (80–340), indomethacin (16), phenylbutazone (450) and acetylsalicylic acid (480).

Mouse active Arthus test (MAA)

As the rabbit RPA was proceeding, we began investigations of a second Arthus model utilizing a different species, the mouse. This model was suggested, in part, by some limited data that was previously reported[14]. Our objectives at this point were (1) to produce a test in a smaller animal than the rabbit so that systemic dose-response determinations could be more easily obtained with less material than required for the rabbit RPA; (2) to substantiate anti-Arthus activity in another species; and, most importantly, (3) to ascertain the sensitivity of the MAA to some currently available agents.

As indicated in Table 10.7, colchicine was the most potent agent observed in

Table 10.7 Potencies of non-steroidal anti-inflammatory agents in the Mouse Active Arthus Test (MAA)

	$ID_{50}(mg/kg)$†	
Agent†	*Intraperitoneal*	*Oral*
Colchicine	1.1 ± 0.1‡,§	14 ± 3.5‡,§
Indomethacin	40‡	> 30‡(33)**
Naproxen	110	>300 (39)
	>150 (41)	>250 (43)
	170	
Sudoxicam	>150 (48)	~150
		>250 (39)
Niflumic acid	140	>150 (34)
		>200 (38)
Ibuprofen	>150 (30)	>300 (28)
	>150 (36)	>500 (44)
Phenylbutazone	>200 (15)	>150 (34)
	>150 (8)	
Acetylsalicylic acid	120	>200 (16)
	>200 (39)	
Maleopimaric acid††	70 ± 27§	?

* Agents were administered at different times between 0.5 and 3 hours prior to skin challenge with 250 μg of bovine serum albumin. The data indicated are the highest potencies obtained in each test.

† Each value is for an individual dose-response assay. The ID_{50} is that dose that produces a group average of 50% inhibition of the inflammation.

‡ Data for colchicine are the average of 3 assays of intraperitoneal and 27 assays for oral administration. Data for indomethacin are the composite data of 3 assays for intraperitoneal and 16 assays for oral administration.

§ Average ± standard deviation.

** Percent inhibition (in parentheses) is given at the indicated dose if 50% was not attained.

†† Reference agent.

the MAA. Maleopimaric acid, a compound described as an anti-complement agent[23], was used as a reference and has demonstrated an average ID_{50} of 70 by the i.p. route. Accurate oral potency for this agent has not been obtained due to considerable variability in the data. The results with additional reference agents administered systemically are also indicated in Table 10.7. With the exception of colchicine, the i.p. or p.o. potencies of these agents is less in the MAA than by the p.o. route in the rat carrageenan oedema model (Table 10.8). Besides colchicine and indomethacin, none of the anti-inflammatory agents is particularly potent in the MAA.

We next compared the oral potencies of agents tested in the MAA in two

Table 10.8 Potencies of non-steroidal anti-inflammatory agents in Non-Arthus tests *in vivo*

	*Oral ID_{50} (mg/kg)**		
Agent	*Mouse carrageenan*	*Mouse writhing*	*Rat carrageenan*
Colchicine	N.D.	N.D.	16†
Indomethacin	⩾20 (4)‡	0.3	5.3 (102)
Naproxen	740	6§	60 (2)
Sudoxicam	95 (2)	N.D.	3**
Niflumic acid	290 (2)	44	57 (5)
Ibuprofen	>600 (2)	11	62 (2)
Phenylbutazone	>500 (2)	45	94 (3)
Acetylsalicylic acid	664††	53	127 (6)

* The ID_{50} is that dose that produces a group average of 50% inhibition of the inflammation or writhing.
† See reference[5].
‡ Number of determinations are indicated in parentheses; otherwise, results of single assays are presented.
§ Phenylquinone writhing test; calculated from reference[29].
** Estimated from reference[31].
†† See reference[25].
N.D. = Not done.

Table 10.9 Approximate therapeutic ratios (LD_{50}/ID_{50})* for non-steroidal anti-inflammatory agents in various tests *in vivo*

	Mouse Arthus		*Mouse carrageenan*	*Mouse writhing*	*Rat carrageenan*
Agent	IP	PO	PO	PO	PO
Colchicine	3	5	N.D.†	N.D.	4‡,§
Indomethacin	⩽1	⩽1	⩽2	130	3
Naproxen	⩽4	<3	1	180§	7
Sudoxicam	⩽2	⩽2	3	N.D.	52§
Niflumic acid	<4	<3	2	11	6
Ibuprofen	⩽2	<2	<1	73	26
Phenylbutazone	<1	<6	<2	21	7
Acetylsalicylic acid	3	<5	2§	19	10
Maleopimaric acid	1	N.D.	N.D.	N.D.	N.D.

* LD_{50} is that dose that is lethal to 50% of the animals. The ID_{50} is that dose that produces a group average of 50% inhibition of the inflammation or writhing response. At least 2 ID_{50} determinations were made on each compound in each oedema test, except for naproxen (1 assay in mouse carrageenan test). Both the LD_{50} and ID_{50} values used for each ratio were obtained in the same species except as noted. Published LD_{50}'s. See references and comments under *Materials and Methods*.
† Rat LD_{50} not found; used mouse oral LD_{50}.
‡ These calculations utilized additional published data. See footnotes for Table 10.8.
§ Reference agent.
IP = intraperitoneal; PO = oral administration.
N.D. = Not done.

carrageenan models, one in mouse and the other in rat (Table 10.8). Data in the writhing analgesic test in the mouse was also obtained. The results indicated a general order of decreasing potency (based on ID_{50} values) of these agents such that the mouse writhing test was the most sensitive to inhibition followed by the rat carrageenan test which was in turn more sensitive than either the mouse carrageenan or Arthus tests (Tables 10.7 and 10.8).

By using the crude calculation of therapeutic ratios (Table 10.9), we were able to get a better appreciation of both the toxicity and specificity in the MAA. This ratio is simply the acute LD_{50} of a compound divided by the ID_{50} in a particular assay. These ratios have been used as a crude early indication of perhaps a non-toxicity related mechanism of action when the value is high (>10). The ranking of the tests in the order of decreasing ratios was the same as the ranking using potencies indicated in Tables 10.7 and 10.8. These ratios are substantially higher for the carrageenan model in the rat as compared with the comparable test in the mouse. Both the mouse carrageenan testing in the paw and the MAA in the skin, however, gave more comparable but lower ratios than for the rat system. This might suggest that the reference agents were inherently less effective in the mouse. This was not entirely the case, since in another mouse test, the writhing analgesic assay, classical anti-inflammatory agents were quite effective orally with high therapeutic ratios. We therefore concluded that the type of observation and the species were probably contributing to this complex situation. The location of the inflammation might also have been a factor in our observations, but unpublished data we have obtained in the MAA, and in the rat Arthus models to be discussed below, using both skin and paw sites suggested that the skin lesions if anything were more easily inhibited.

Arthus tests in rats

We have more recently extended our studies to two Arthus models in the rat. One of these is the antiserum induced oedema test (AIO)[11]. Our modifications consisted of an i.d. challenge in the dorsal skin with goat anti-rat serum. Basically, this is a reversed passive reaction utilizing serum antigens.

This model has been investigated in an effort to obtain within the same species (rat) more direct evidence that particular compounds possess a greater specificity for the Arthus reaction than for the classical carrageenan model. The results in the AIO with reference agents are indicated in Table 10.10. Colchicine and indomethacin demonstrated some activity. Data from a second rat model, the direct passive Arthus reaction (DPA) in the skin, is also indicated. This DPA appeared to be more sensitive to the agents indicated, but the intragroup variations in inflammatory responses were greater than that observed in the AIO. Once again, the Arthus therapeutic ratios for p.o. or i.p. administration of the anti-inflammatory agents (Table 10.11) tended to compare less favourably with those ratios obtained using the p.o. potencies in the rat carrageenan procedure (Tables 10.8 and 10.9).

The location of the AIO reactions in our studies was the dorsal skin, while carrageenan inflammation was induced in the paw. Data not presented here suggest that the inhibitory effects of 7 of the reference compounds we have been discussing if anything were less when the AIO lesion was induced by subplantar injection as compared with the cutaneous reaction.

Our data support the studies of others in rat Arthus tests in that phenylbutazone[5], acetylsalicylic acid[3,7], and indomethacin[5] are generally weak

Table 10.10 The effects of non-steroidal anti-inflammatory agents in two cutaneous Arthus tests in rats

Agent	Route	ID_{50} (mg/kg)* Antiserum induced oedema (AIO)	Direct passive Arthus (DPA)
Colchicine	IP	3.5 (7)†	1.6‡ (11)
	PO	>20[38]§(2)	4.5‡(2)
Indomethacin	IP	30	13
	PO	20	N.D.
Naproxen	IP	>150 [40]	N.D.
Sudoxicam	IP	> 50 [37]	N.D.
Niflumic acid	IP	>150 [45] (2)	50‡(2)
	PO	300	>150 [47] (3)
Ibuprofen	IP	>150 [0]	>150 [8]
	PO	>150 [35] (8)	N.D.
Phenylbutazone	IP	>200 [9]	>200 [2]
Acetylsalicylic acid	IP	>250 [26] (2)	>250 [45]

* ID_{50} is that dose that produces a group average of 50% inhibition of the inflammation.
† Number of assays (not all dose-responses) are indicated in parentheses. Composite data is presented. Otherwise, the results of single assays are indicated.
‡ Occasional side effects (ruffled fur, sedation, deaths) were observed.
§ Average per cent inhibition is noted in brackets when the level is less than 50% at the dose indicated.
N.D. = Not done.
PO = oral administration; IP = intraperitoneal administration.

Table 10.11 Approximate therapeutic ratios (LD_{50}/ID_{50})* in Arthus and carrageenan tests in rats

Agent	Intraperitoneal Arthus†	Oral Arthus†	Oral Carrageenan‡
Colchicine	3§,**	15§,**	4
Indomethacin	1§	1	3
Naproxen	<3	N.D.	7
Sudoxicam	<3§	N.D.	52
Niflumic acid	7§,**	1	6
Ibuprofen	< 11§	<11	26
Phenylbutazone	< 1	N.D.	7
Acetylsalicylic acid	⩽ 2	N.D.	10

* LD_{50} is that dose that is lethal to 50% of the animals. ID_{50} is that dose that produces a group average of 50% inhibition of the inflammatory response. For LD_{50} data see references and comments under *Materials and Method*.
† The results from the direct passive test were used. When these data were not available, results from the antiserum induced oedema test were used (see Table 10.10).
‡ This data was reproduced from Table 10.9.
§ Oral LD_{50} data used. For colchicine, mouse oral data was used.
** Occasional side effects (sedation, ruffled fur, deaths) were observed.
N.D. = Not done.

or ineffective while colchicine is effective[4,7]. Though our data for indomethacin suggest a somewhat higher potency than previously reported[5], this agent is still effective only at or near toxic doses. Also, colchicine tended to demonstrate better therapeutic ratios than did indomethacin (Table 10.11). We did not demonstrate activity for hydrocortisone or its sodium succinate derivative in the rat AIO (unpublished results) in agreement with the observations of one group[3] but contrasting with oral potency ($ID_{50} = 8$ mg/kg) found by others[7].

DISCUSSION

We have demonstrated that reasonably controlled anti-inflammatory tests can be devised utilizing various Arthus procedures in three animal species. The sensitivity of these tests in terms of the potency of currently available agents seemed to vary, with the rat and mouse models being less sensitive than the rabbit RPA to inhibition. Reasons for different sensitivities of these Arthus models to known drugs may reflect procedural differences as well as species differences with respect to metabolism and quantitative and possibly qualitative differences in inflammatory mediators. We have not done any studies dealing with these important questions.

Utilizing Arthus models, available anti-inflammatory agents generally are less effective when compared with their activities in the classical rat carrageenan model (Tables 10.7, 10.8 and 10.10). Our data and those of others, especially in rat Arthus models[3–5,7,11], suggest that we have achieved one of our goals, that of defining tests with the potential to detect agents differing somehow from current drugs that may be more effective against rheumatoid inflammation. Lacking important information about the aetiology of rheumatoid processes, our alternative is to attack known or presumed pertinent inflammatory mechanisms. A difficulty encountered in detecting mechanistically specific agents *in vivo* concerns the fact that sequences of the inflammatory process probably overlap despite the type of inciting agent utilized. Because of this there is need for secondary tests that may clarify mechanisms of action.

Certain, perhaps relatively minor, discrepancies appeared when our data was compared to those of others[3,5,7]. A number of possible reasons for these have been indicated in Table 10.2. One of these points concerns the methods for quantifying test procedures and is worthy of some further discussion. Because the inflammatory process is a multi-component one, various parameters and methods for evaluating Arthus reactivity have been employed. From the standpoint of drug screening, it is difficult to predict which methodology would be the most profitable. Based on simplicity, we have chosen to measure Arthus reactions either by volume or by weight. The presence of oedema, however, should be reflective of the presence and activation of PMNs in the lesions[1]. Other workers have used a variety of techniques to assess cutaneous Arthus reactivity. These techniques include gross and histological observation and graded scoring[36]; measurement of the area of extravasated dye[7]; quantification of extravasated radiolabelled protein[4]; measurement of increases in water and protein content, histological scoring of PMN infiltration and biochemical analyses[15]. Also, an interesting technique was reported that utilized ^{51}Cr-labelled leukocytes to assess accumulation of cells in paw lesions induced by carrageenan or aggregated gamma globulin[37]. A combination of these techniques may provide valuable secondary information on the mode of action of newer agents, but since a primary screening test usually requires the capacity for evaluating large numbers of compounds, the easiest procedures may be the ones of choice. A compromise between high volume screening and method of measurement may be the best situation we can realistically attain.

Our laboratory studies have concentrated on the acute inflammatory Arthus responses and the effects of current and developmental drugs in these tests with the hope that specific Arthus-active agents may provide greater efficacy than is available with present modes of therapy. A primary test, such as the Arthus, in drug discovery programmes must detect effective agents with some reasonably low frequency. During drug screening, the Arthus models discussed here have demonstrated that between 9 and 12% of the compounds tested were effective by established criteria of dose and potency. Meanwhile, our criteria for pursuing agents in various Arthus and secondary procedures have been subjected to drastic revisions over the 7 years of our involvement in the anti-inflammatory testing programme.

Based on safety and potencies (Tables 10.9 and 10.11), the rat and mouse Arthus models seem not to predict that any one of the currently available agents tested would demonstrate greater anti-rheumatic efficacy than the others. Those Arthus-specific agents with high therapeutic ratios would be valid compounds to determine directly whether Arthus tests predict enhanced clinical efficacy. It will also be of considerable interest to ascertain whether these agents are associated with reduced or peculiar side effects or other activities such as analgesia and anti-pyresis. If these agents have little analgesic activity then clinical anti-inflammatory activity might be more directly observed and measured.

It is not surprising that many laboratories, academic and pharmaceutical, have at one time or another evaluated anti-inflammatory agents in Arthus models (see Table 10.3). What is of some concern is that no reports have been found concerning Arthus-specific agents either in animal or clinical studies. We have some data for developmental agents indicating effectiveness in some Arthus tests but with relatively weak activity in the rat carrageenan model. However, additional problems concerned with demonstrating oral effectiveness and activity in more than one Arthus model, as well as toxicity, indicate that clinical evaluation, unsurprisingly, is not an easily obtainable objective.

The more unusual an agent is with respect to its anti-inflammatory profile, the more difficult may be the problems associated with the development of that agent. However, if we can obtain information from clinical studies of new types of agents, then we can more rationally modify our approach to anti-rheumatic drug discovery and development.

New approaches for the development of anti-rheumatic drugs must be taken. New methods of discovery and development of agents is one approach and should be a major concern of pharmaceutical investigators. These studies should incorporate evaluations not only of acute inflammatory models but also those of chronic inflammation. Investigation of new methods is no guarantee that we will see a breakthrough in anti-rheumatic therapy, but it is likely to enhance this possibility.

SUMMARY

1. Similarities have been noted between the Arthus reaction and acute rheumatoid synovitis, both of which demonstrate the presence of immune complexes, complement activation and polymorphonuclear leukocytes.
2. Non-steroidal anti-inflammatory drugs (NSAIDs) were tested in four Arthus models in the skin: a reversed passive reaction in the rabbit; an active reaction in the mouse; and both direct passive and reversed passive reactions in the rat.
   The eight NSAIDs evaluated in most of these tests were colchicine, indomethacin, naproxen, sudoxicam, niflumic acid, ibuprofen, phenylbutazone and acetylsalicylic acid.
3. Except for colchicine, the NSAIDs tested were more potent by the oral route in the classical rat carrageenan oedema test than in the rat or mouse Arthus procedures, while only limited data is available for the rabbit test. Oral ID_{50}s, the NSAIDs in the carrageenan test ranged from 3 to 127 mg/kg. Colchicine demonstrated high oral potency ($ID_{50} < 20$) in Arthus tests.
4. Seven of the 8 NSAIDs tested demonstrated higher therapeutic ratios (LD_{50}/ID_{50}) by the oral route using the rat carrageenan test potencies (range of ratios, 3–52) than those ratios obtained using rat or mouse Arthus potencies, indicating a lack of Arthus specificity for these agents.
   Only colchicine had apparently equal ratios for the mouse Arthus and carrageenan tests. Although a relatively high ratio was observed in the rat Arthus test for this agent, anti-Arthus activity was accompanied by an exacerbation of drug toxicity.
5. Although Arthus reactions were measured by volume or weight increases in the present studies, other methods or combinations thereof, including histological and biochemical evaluations, may contribute additional information concerning the uniqueness of new, potent Arthus-active agents.

Acknowledgements

The authors thank Mr W. F. Schreiber, Mr A. Plisko and Ms B. Amrein for their technical assistance, and Ms B. Starke of the Squibb Institute's International Research Center for performing the mouse writhing assays.

References

1. Cochrane, C. G. and Janoff, A. (1974). The Arthus reaction: A model of neutrophil and complement-mediated injury. In B. W. Zweifach, L. Grant and R. T. McCluskey (eds.) *The Inflammatory Process*. 2nd Edition, Vol. III, pp. 85–162. (New York: Academic Press)

2. Zvaifler, N. J. (1973). The immunopathology of joint inflammation in rheumatoid arthritis. In F. J. Dixon and H. G. Kunkel (eds.) *Advances in Immunology*. Vol. 16, pp. 265–336. (New York: Academic Press)
3. Megel, H., Raychaudhuri, A., Shemano, I., Beaver, T. H. and Thomas, L. L. (1975). The anti-inflammatory actions of tilorone hydrochloride. *Proc. Soc. Exp. Biol. Med.*, **149**, 89
4. Chang, Y-H. (1975). Mechanism of action of colchicine. I. Effects of colchicine and its analogs on the reversed passive Arthus reaction and the carrageenan-induced hindpaw edema in the rat. *J. Pharmacol. Exp. Ther.*, **194**, 154
5. Chang, Y-H. (1975). Mechanism of action of colchicine. III. Anti-inflammatory effects of colchicine compared with phenylbutazone and indomethacin. *Arthr. Rheum.*, **18**, 493
6. Malawista, S. E., Chang, Y-H. and Wilson, L. (1972). Lumicolchicine: Lack of anti-inflammatory effect. *Arthr. Rheum.*, **15**, 641
7. Carter, G. W. and Krause, R. A. (1976). The reverse passive Arthus reaction in the rat: A potential screen for novel anti-inflammatory agents. *Fed. Proc.*, **35**, 774
8. Goldlust, M. B. and Schreiber, W. F. (1975). Use of the reversed passive Arthus reaction as a test for anti-inflammatory agents. *Agents Actions*, **5**, 39
9. Smith, W. and Humphrey, J. H. (1949). The effect of sodium salicylate upon hypersensitivity reactions. *Br. J. Exp. Pathol.*, **30**, 560
10. Humphrey, J. H. (1951). The effect of cortisone upon some experimental hypersensitivity reactions. *Br. J. Exp. Pathol.*, **32**, 274
11. Yamamoto, H., Saito, C., Okamoto, T., Awata, H., Inukai, T., Hirohashi, A. and Yukawa, Y. (1969). Synthesis and pharmacology of a new potential anti-inflammatory drug, 1-(3′,4′-methylenedioxybenzoyl)-2-methyl-5-methoxy-3-indolylacetic acid (ID-955). *Arzneim.-Forsch.*, **19**, 981
12. Komatsu, T., Saito, C., Awata, H., Sakai, Y., Inukai, T., Kurokawa, H. and Yamamoto, H. (1973). Anti-inflammatory activities of 1-cinnamoyl-2-methyl-5-methoxy-3-indolylacetic acid (cinmetacin). *Arzneim.-Forsch.*, **23**, 1690
13. Ungar, G., Kobrin, S. and Sezesny, B. R. (1959). Measurement of inflammation and evaluation of anti-inflammatory agents. *Arch. Int. Pharmacodyn.*, **123**, 71
14. Kohler, P. F. and Martinez, J. S. (1971). Inactivation of C3 and inhibition of Arthus reactions in mice by flufenamate Na. *Fed. Proc.*, **30**, 472
15. Butler, K. and Lewis, G. P. (1976). The effect of anti-inflammatory compounds on the biochemical changes in the Arthus reaction. *J. Pathol.*, **119**, 175
16. Blackham, A., Radziwonik, H. and Shaw, I. H. (1975). The Arthus reaction in guinea pig knee joints. A test for anti-inflammatory drugs. *Agents Actions*, **5**, 519
17. Labrid, C., Ducher, M., Dureng, G., Moleyre, J., Stevenard, M. and Streichenberger, G. (1973). Etude comparative, chez le cobaye, de quelques inhibiteurs de l'oedème articulaire d'origine immunologique (Comparative study, in the guinea pig, of some inhibitors of immunologically-induced articular oedema). *Therapie*, **28**, 907
18. French, C. E., Allen, J. R. and Davis, K. J. (1955). Bio-assay for anti-inflammatory substances. *Proc. Soc. Exp. Biol. Med.*, **89**, 41
19. Goldlust, M. B., Rich, L. C. and Harrity, T. W. (1977). Effects of anti-inflammatory agents on the acute response of immune synovitis in rabbits. *Arthr. Rheum.*, **20**, 937
20. Blackham, A., Farmer, J. B., Radziwonik, H. and Westwick, J. (1974). The role of prostaglandins in rabbit monoarticular arthritis. *Br. J. Pharmacol.*, **51**, 35
21. Yamamoto, S., Dunn, C. J., Deporter, D. A., Capasso, F., Willoughby, D. A. and Huskisson, E. C. (1975). A model for the quantitative study of Arthus (immunologic) hypersensitivity in rats. *Agents Actions*, **5**, 374
22. Benedict, A. A. and Tipps, R. L. (1954). Actively and passively induced Arthus reactions in the mouse. *Proc. Soc. Exp. Biol. Med.*, **87**, 618
23. Glovsky, M. M., Becker, E. L. and Holbrook, N. J. (1968). Inhibition of guinea pig complement by maleopimaric acid and other derivatives of levopimaric acid. *J. Immunol.*, **100**, 979
24. Winter, C. A., Risley, E. A. and Nuss, G. W. (1962). Carrageenin-induced edema in hind paw

of the rat as an assay for anti-inflammatory drugs. *Proc. Soc. Exp. Biol. Med.*, **111,** 544
25. Levy, L. (1969). Carrageenan paw edema in the mouse. *Life Sciences,* **8,** 601
26. Siegmund, E., Cadmus, R. and Lu, G. (1957). A method for evaluating both non-narcotic and narcotic analgesics. *Proc. Soc. Exp. Biol. Med.*, **95,** 729
27. Spector, W. S. (ed.) (1956). *Handbook of Toxicology.* Acute toxicities of solids, liquids and gases to laboratory animals. Vol. I, pp. 10 and 74. (Philadelphia: W. B. Saunders Co.)
28. Jahn, V. U. and Adrian, R. W. (1969). Pharmakologische und toxikologische Prüfung des neuen Antiphlogisticums Azapropazon = 3-dimethylamino-7-methyl-1,2-(n-propylmalonyl)-1,2-dihydro-1,2,4-benzotriazin. *Arzneim.-Forsch.*, **19,** 36
29. Roszkowski, A. P., Rooks, W. H., II, Tomolonis, A. J. and Miller, L. M. (1971). Anti-inflammatory and analgesic properties of d-2-(6′-methoxy-2′-naphthyl)-propionic acid (naproxen). *J. Pharmacol. Exp. Therap.*, **179,** 114
30. Kuramoto, M., Ishimura, Y., Okubo, T. and Hashimoto, T. (1973). Toxicity of naproxen. Acute and subacute toxicity in mice and rats. *Shikoku Igaku Zasshi,* **29,** 439
31. Wiseman, E. H. and Chiaini, J. (1972). Anti-inflammatory and pharmacokinetic properties of sudoxicam N-(2-thiazolyl)-4-hydroxy-2-methyl-2H-1,2-benzothiazine-3-carboxamide 1,1-dioxide. *Biochem. Pharmacol.*, **21,** 2323
32. Adams, S. S., Bough, R. G., Cliffe, E. E., Lessel, B. and Mills, R. F. N. (1969). Absorption, distribution and toxicity of ibuprofen. *Toxicol. Appl. Pharmacol.*, **15,** 310
33. Hazleton, L. W., Tusing, T. W. and Holland, E. G. (1953). Acute and chronic toxicity of butazolidin. *J. Pharmacol. Exp. Ther.*, **109,** 387
34. Barnes, C. D. and Eltherington, L. G. (eds.) (1973). *Drug Dosage in Laboratory Animals. A Handbook.* p. 30. (Berkeley: Univ. of Calif. Press)
35. Dixon, W. J. and Massey, F. J., Jr. (1969). *Introduction to Statistical Analysis.* 3rd Ed. pp. 545–549. (New York: McGraw-Hill)
36. Ward, P. A. and Cochrane, C. G. (1965). Bound complement and immunologic injury of blood vessels. *J. Exp. Med.*, **121,** 215
37. Perper, R. J., Sanda, M., Stecher, V. J. and Oronsky, A. L. (1975). Physiologic and pharmacologic alterations of rat leukocyte chemotaxis (Cx) *in vivo.* In R. J. Perper (ed.). *Mechanisms of Tissue Injury With Reference to Rheumatoid Arthritis. Ann. N.Y. Acad. Sci.*, **256,** 190

11
Evaluation of Anti-Rheumatic Drugs using Antigen-Induced Arthritis

A. BLACKHAM

INTRODUCTION

Antigen-induced arthritis in rabbit knee joints, first described by Dumonde and Glynn[1], closely resembles rheumatoid arthritis (RA) with regard to histopathology and chronicity. Studies on the immune mechanisms underlying this model of the human disease, implicating both the cellular[2–4] and humoral[5,6] arms of the immune response, have been well documented. Investigation of the activity of anti-inflammatory drugs on the rabbit arthritis have remained largely neglected. A notable exception is the description of the effect of prednisolone on antigen-induced arthritis in the New Zealand White (NZW) rabbit[7]. We have described the production of ovalbumin induced arthritis in NZW, Dutch and Old English (OE) rabbits and showed that the OE rabbits were the best responders[8]. In addition, we tested indomethacin and found that oral administration of 7.5 mg/kg twice daily from day 0–7 reduced the swelling and heat in the inflamed joint without reducing significantly either the joint pathology or the total synovial fluid cell (TSFC) counts. The drug had very little effect on the established arthritis when dosed from day 38–46. Synovial fluid prostaglandin (PG) levels (predominantly E_1) peaked 19 h after challenge in the affected joints of vehicle treated rabbits, while rabbits receiving indomethacin demonstrated very little synovial PG at any time. Since indomethacin reduced the early joint swelling and the increased joint heat, symptoms where PGE_1 was thought to be causally involved, but failed to reduce joint pathology we felt that our results went some way to explaining the clinical activity of indomethacin. The following report describes the effects of a range of anti-inflammatory drugs and agents with claimed anti-rheumatoid activity in man against developing and established antigen-induced arthritis in the rabbit.

METHODS

A monoarticular arthritis was induced in OE rabbits appropriately sensitized to ovalbumin (OA)[8] by injecting OA (5 mg; 5× crystallized, Koch Light Laboratories Ltd.) in sterile saline into one knee joint. The opposite joint was injected with sterile saline (0.5 ml) as control. At this time the rabbits showed delayed hypersensitivity to an intradermal injection of 10 μg OA. The size of the skin induration was later shown to correlate with the severity of the arthritis[9]. The diameters of the knee joints were measured periodically throughout the experiment using either calipers[8] or an electronic device[10]. Joint swelling was calculated as the difference in size between the challenged and control joints expressed in mm. In some experiments joint mobility was measured using a simple goniometer, by recording the angle subtended by the femur and the tibia at the knee, when the hind leg was gently extended. The reduction in mobility of the arthritic joint was calculated as the difference between the challenged and control joints in degrees.

At the end of the experiment the rabbits were killed and the joint space washed out with heparinized saline (1.0 ml) and total and differential cell counts performed. The visual appearance (macroscopy) of the joint tissues was assessed on a 0–3 rating for each of the following 12 parameters; *Synovial fluid* volume, viscosity, discolouration, tissue debris; *Synovium* petechiae, hyperplasia, vascularization, discolouration; *Cartilage and bone* pitting, erosion, new bone formation; *Capsule* fibrosis.

In established arthritis experiments the joints were fixed in formal saline, decalcified, sectioned and stained with haematoxylin and eosin. In the developing arthritis experiments sections were obtained from a piece of infrapatellar synovium. The tissues were evaluated histopathologically using a 0–3 rating for the following parameters: *Joint space* polymorphs, fibrin, mononuclear cells; *Synovial intima* hypertrophy or hyperplasia, villi; *Synovial connective tissue* oedema, polymorphs, lymphocytes, plasma cells, macrophages, giant cells, fibrin, fibrosis, pannus; *Vascular reaction* congestion, haemorrhage, perivascular cuffing, thrombosis; *Cartilage* thinning, irregular chondrocytes, erosion; Macroscopic and histopathological evaluations were carried out blind.

Drugs were given orally once or twice daily (see Table 11.1 and Figures 11.1, 11.2 and 11.3) as a solution or suspension in Tween 80(0.05%; v/v distilled water). Methyl cellulose (1% w/v) was added to aid the suspension of aspirin. Gold sodium thiomalate was injected intramuscularly twice weekly.

The increases in joint diameters of the drug-treated and control animals were compared using Student's *t*-test. Log transformation of the leukocyte counts was necessary to produce a normal distribution upon which Student's *t*-tests were performed. Macroscopy and histopathology scores were analysed using the non-parametric Mann-Whitney U-test. The results were considered significant when $P < 0.05$.

RESULTS

Effect of drugs on established antigen-induced arthritis

Antigen-induced arthritis was induced in a total of 339 rabbits in eleven separate experiments (described in greater detail elsewhere[9]). Just prior to drug dosing 267 rabbits with joint swellings in excess of 2 mm (mean and $SD = 4.31 \pm 1.48$ mm) were considered adequate responders and were used in the drug study. At 4–6 weeks post-challenge the reactor rabbits were divided into groups of 5–10 rabbits each and given increasing doses of drugs for 3 weeks. In the absence of overt signs of toxicity the dose was further increased during the 4th week. The list of drugs and their effects on 4 parameters of the arthritis are shown in Table 11.1. A numerical value for the overall anti-inflammatory activity of each drug is obtained in the final column by adding together the symbols denoting effects on joint swelling, TSFC, joint macroscopy and joint histopathology. The PG synthetase inhibitors aspirin, indomethacin and ketoprofen, in ascending order of potency, reduced one or more parameters of the arthritis. However, increasing anti-inflammatory activity was associated with increasing gastrointestinal toxicity. Gut perforations caused death in 4 rabbits receiving indomethacin or ketoprofen. Sudoxicam was fatal at doses of between 10 and 30 mg/kg, but on retesting at a fixed dose of 10 mg/kg daily for 3 weeks, sudoxicam produced significant inhibition of TSFC. Prednisolone showed good anti-inflammatory activity and was the only drug which significantly reduced the histopathology of the joint. Oral gold (gold triethyl phosphine, SKF 36914), cyclophosphamide and chloroquine produced non-significant inhibitions of TSFC and histopathology, but gold and chloroquine were toxic (the doses of these drugs were not increased during the last week of dosing). Penicillamine, oxisuran and levamisole demonstrated little or no activity. Penicillamine and gold require to be given for prolonged periods in the clinic before they show an effect against RA. These particular drugs were therefore retested at fixed doses of 100 and 3 mg/kg, respectively, for a period of 7 weeks. The beneficial effects of gold on TSFC and histopathology were seen again, but on this occasion the macroscopy was also significantly reduced. Penicillamine was again inactive.

Effect of drugs on developing antigen-induced arthritis

In view of the lack of effect of the so-called anti-rheumatoid drugs on the established disease, interest was directed to the early phase of the arthritis. Cyclophosphamide, procarbazine, prednisolone and intramuscular gold (sodium aurothiomalate) were given to groups of rabbits during the first 4 weeks after

Table 11.1 Effect of sequential oral dosing of drugs on established monoarticular arthritis

Figures in parenthesis refer to the number of rabbits per group where different from starting size.

(From Blackham and Radziwonik[9] (1977) by permission of *Agents and Actions*)

Drug	*Initial No. rabbits per group*	*Total daily dose* (mg/kg)				*Effect on:—*				
		Week 1	*Week 2*	*Week 3*	*Week 4*	*Joint swelling**	*TSFC*	*Macroscopy score*	*Histopathology score*	*Total*
Aspirin	5	10	30	100	200 Div	0	+	0	0	1
Aspirin	8	50	100	200	400 Div	0	0	0	ND	0
Indomethacin	6	3	10	30(5)	60(3) Div	+	+	0	0	2
Naproxen	5	3(4)	10(4)	30(4)	60(4) Div	+	+	+	0	3
Ketoprofen	6	3	10	30	60(5) Div	+	++	++	+	6
Sudoxicam	6	3	10	30(3)	30(0) Div					
Prednisolone sodium phosphate	5	0.3	1	3	6 Div	+	+	+	++	5
D(−)penicillamine hydrochloride	6	10	30	100	200 Div	0	+	0	0	1
SKF 36914	6	1	3	10	10(5)	0	+	0	+	2
Cyclophosphamide	5	1	3	10	20 Div	0	+	0	+	2
Chloroquine diphosphate	5	10	30	100(4)	100(4) Div	0	+	0	+	2
Oxisuran	8	1	10	30	ND	0	+	0	0	1
Levamisole	8	1	3	10	30	0	−	0	0	−1

ND = Not done
TSFC = Total Synovial fluid cells
+ = >20% Inhibition but not significant
++ = >20% Inhibition and significant
− = >20% Increase but not significant
Div = Divided into morning and late afternoon doses
* = Maximum effect occurring at any time during test

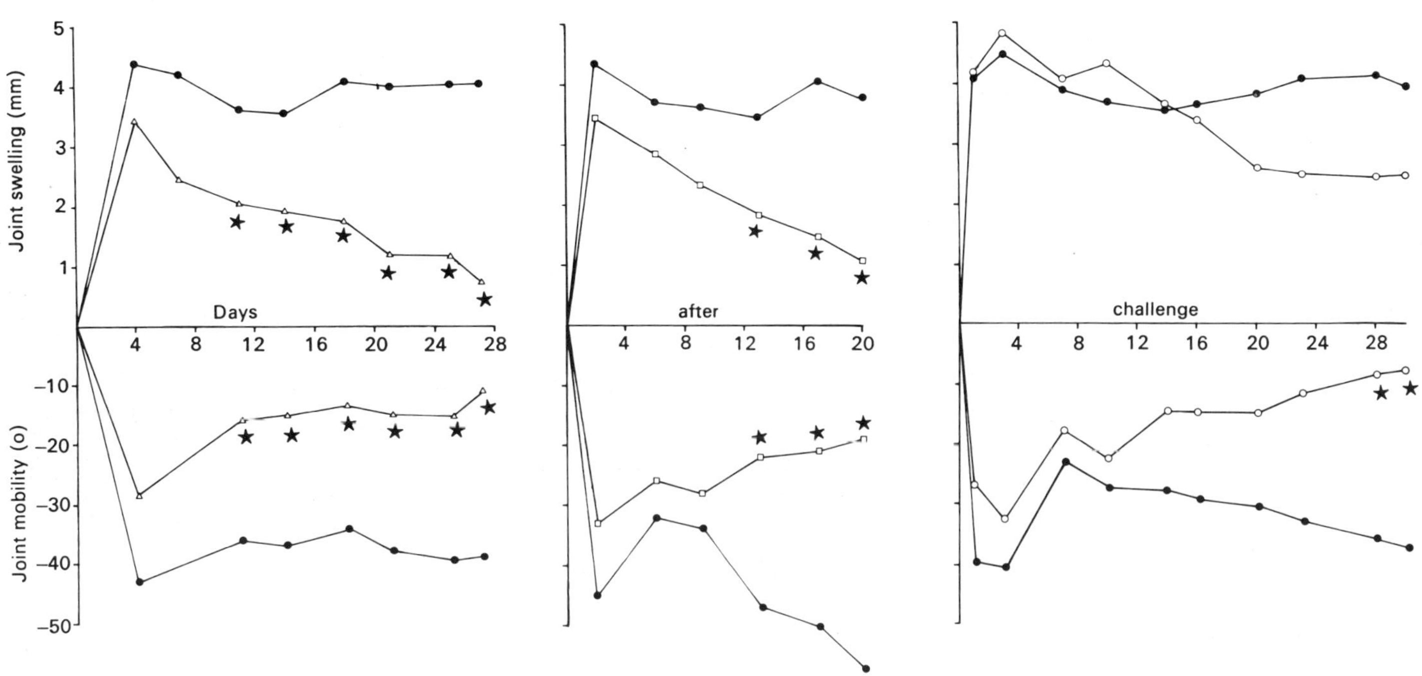

Figure 11.1 Effect of daily oral doses of cyclophosphamide, 20 mg/kg (△), procarbazine HCl, 7.5 mg/kg (□) or twice weekly intramuscular injections of gold sodium thiomalate equivalent to 2.5 mg/kg gold (○), or vehicle (●) on mean joint swelling and mean joint mobility in groups of 5 or 6 rabbits. ★$p < 0.05$ compared with controls

antigen challenge in the joint. The effect of three of these compounds on joint swelling and mobility is shown in Figure 11.1. At the doses chosen all four drugs produced reductions in joint swelling and, with the exception of gold, the inhibitions were significant. Gold, procarbazine and cyclophosphamide also produced a significant increase in the mobility of the inflamed joint (the prednisolone group was not measured). Significant drug-induced inhibitions of joint swelling were reflected by significant inhibitions of TSFC and macroscopy at the end of the experiment (Figure 11.2). Moreover the most active drugs,

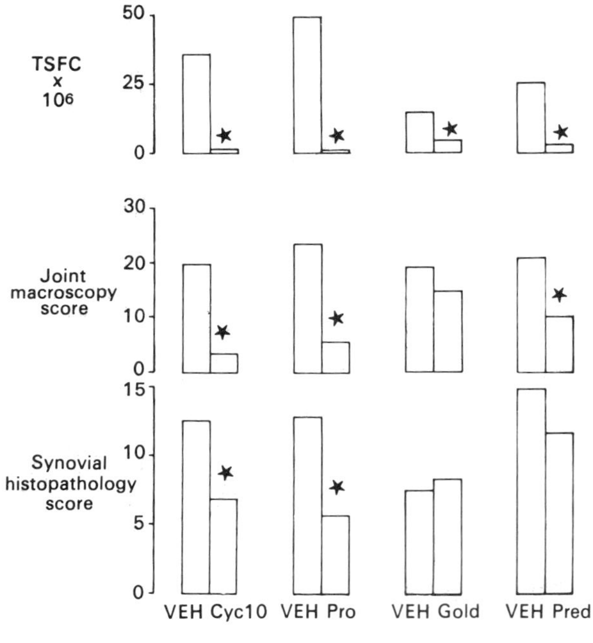

Figure 11.2 Effect of daily oral doses of cyclophosphamide, 20 mg/kg, procarbazine HCl, 7.5 mg/kg, prednisolone sodium phosphate, 1 mg/kg, or twice weekly intramuscular injections of gold sodium thiomalate equivalent to 2.5 mg/kg gold, or vehicle on mean total synovial cell counts (TSFC), mean macroscopy score and mean synovial histopathology score in groups of 5 or 6 rabbits. Dosing was continued during the first 3 or 4 weeks after challenge. *$p < 0.05$ compared with controls

cyclophosphamide and procarbazine, produced significant inhibition of synovial membrane pathology as judged by reduction in synovial hyperplasia and the presence of only a few inflammatory cells in the subsynovium. Gold produced significant inhibition of the mean TSFC and though the macroscopy was reduced by $> 20\%$ the effect was not significant.

The effect of prednisolone and cyclophosphamide on joint swelling appeared to be reversible. In a second series of experiments when dosing was discontinued after 4 weeks the joint swellings increased and at the end of the experiment, 5 weeks later, they were no longer significantly different from arthritic controls (Figure 11.3). In addition, the synovial pathology of the drug-treated rabbits was not significantly reduced as evidenced by villous hyperplasia of the synovial intima and mononuclear cell infiltration of the subsynovium. The effect of procarbazine, however, was more prolonged and although the joint swelling showed signs of returning to nearer control values the difference was still significant at the end of the experiment. This was reflected by significant reductions in macroscopy and TSFC at this time. Nevertheless synovial membrane pathology was not significantly decreased.

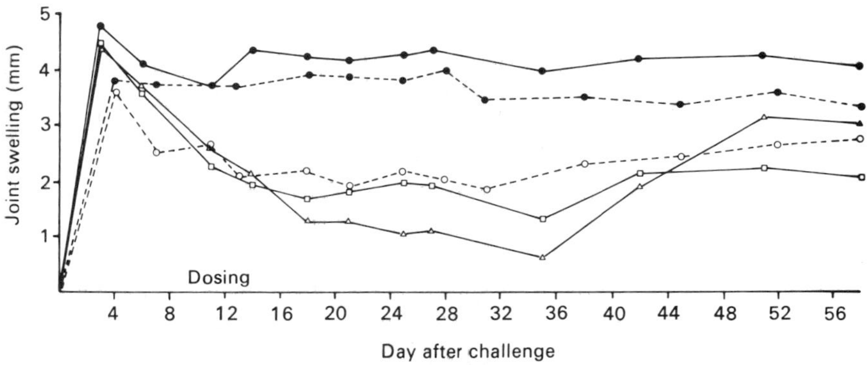

Figure 11.3 Effect of 28 daily oral doses of cyclophosphamide 20 mg/kg (△) and procarbazine HCl, 5 mg/kg (□) or 30 daily oral doses of prednisolone, 1 mg/kg (○), or vehicle (●) on mean joint swelling during the dosing period and for the next 5 weeks (approximately) in groups of 4–7 rabbits. Controls, (—) for cyclophosphamide experiment, (.....) for prednisolone experiment

In other experiments penicillamine failed to reduce any of the parameters of the developing arthritis when given orally at 200 mg/kg daily from the day before sensitization through to the end of the experiment (8 weeks in all), or when injected intravenously as a 5% neutral solution in $NaHCO_3$ at doses of 10 and 20 mg/kg on 5/7 days for 4 weeks beginning on the day of challenge.

DISCUSSION

Measurement of joint swelling provides a very satisfactory means of monitoring the progress of antigen-induced arthritis and correlates very well with the joint pathology. In addition where drugs induced inhibition of joint swelling in developing arthritis inhibitions of at least 2 parameters of joint pathology were also seen. Though joint mobility is a fairly variable parameter and one which is not easy to obtain, it provides another non-intrusive indication of the course of the arthritis. The loss of joint mobility demonstrates the swift, relentless progress of the disease in OE rabbits. Some of the rabbits developed severe flexion deformities (contractures) a few weeks after challenge which restricted the movement of the affected joint by as much as 50%. TSFC and joint pathology parameters have been discussed elsewhere[1,7,8].

Ketoprofen and prednisolone produced moderate inhibition of established arthritis in the rabbit. Although the ascending order of potency of the non-steroidal anti-inflammatory drugs (NSAID) against the arthritis ranked very well with their activities against pig lung PG synthetase (unpublished observations), it is unlikely that their effectiveness is due solely to inhibition of PG synthetase. The dose of indomethacin required to inhibit joint swelling was well in excess of that necessary to severely reduce PG production in the rabbit knee joint[8]. Drug-induced inhibition of inflammatory cell infiltration into the joint, in response to chemotactic factors other than PG, could be a further explanation of NSAID activity. NSAIDs reduce cell infiltration into pleural exudate induced by irritants[11] and antigen-induced joint inflammation (this report) and recently naproxen has been reported to reduce cell counts in rheumatoid synovial fluid[12]. The results obtained with prednisolone agreed with those reported by Davis[7].

Chloroquine, cyclophosphamide, gold and penicillamine, a group of drugs which may do more than control the symptoms of rheumatoid arthritis[13], had little effect on established arthritis in the rabbit. Levamisole which enhances[14] and oxisuran which depresses[15] cell-mediated immune responses also showed disappointing activity. The reasons for the lack of activity shown by these drugs could be manifold; for instance the dosing period may be too short (activity of gold improved when dosing was extended from 4 to 7 weeks), or the dose of drug may be too small or the model, because of the severity of the lesions or the immune status of the rabbits at this time, might be refractory to drugs of this type.

When prednisolone, cyclophosphamide and gold were retested against the developing phase of the disease they all showed greater activity than against established arthritis. Although cyclophosphamide, primarily a B cell suppressant[16], produced a dramatic improvement when given early in the disease, the therapeutic benefit lasted only as long as drug administration continued. On the other hand, procarbazine, a T cell suppressant[17], which caused reduction in thymus weights and depletion of thymocytes in the rabbits, produced an improvement in the arthritis long after dosing was discontinued. This observation suggests a dominant role for T cells in the pathogenesis of antigen-induced arthritis in the rabbit.

Penicillamine had no activity even when tested at high doses during the early phase of the disease. Surprisingly there was no sign of toxicity either when the drug was given intravenously or orally at doses which were far in excess of human toxic doses. This suggests that rabbit handles the drug in a different way to man and may be a reason for the inactivity of penicillamine in this model. At present we have no reliable method of measuring penicillamine levels in biological fluids and therefore this question has not been resolved.

SUMMARY AND CONCLUSIONS

In conclusion, the effects of NSAIDs, steroids, immunosuppressants and gold on the component parts of antigen-induced arthritis in the rabbit fairly accurately reflect their activities in the clinic. It remains uncertain whether drugs like penicillamine, levamisole or oxisuran which may induce subtle changes in the immune response, can be detected by this model. Nevertheless the model may be usefully employed to study the immunopathological events leading to joint destruction and the effect of new therapeutic agents upon these events.

SUMMARY

1. Established antigen-induced arthritis was produced in 264 out of 339 sensitized Old English rabbits 4–6 weeks after a single intra-articular injection of ovalbumin (OA) into one knee joint. In these rabbits the delayed hypersensitivity to OA, in the skin at the time of challenge, correlated very well with the subsequent arthritis at 4–6 weeks. At this time the arthritis was chronic as judged by the presence of villous hyperplasia of the synovial membrane, pannus, lymphocyte and plasma cell infiltration and bone and cartilage erosions.
2. A range of anti-inflammatory drugs and agents with claimed anti-rheumatoid activity in man were tested against four parameters of the arthritis. Drug effects were measured on joint swelling during dosing and on total synovial fluid cell counts, joint macroscopy and joint histopathology at the end of the experiment.
3. Groups of 5–10 rabbits with joint swellings > 2 mm were used in 11 separate experiments. A sequential dosing regimen was used where drugs were given daily by mouth, increasing the dose each week until overt toxicity was seen. Some drugs were retested against established arthritis using a fixed daily dosing regimen.
4. The maximum daily dose of drug, mg/kg, is shown in parenthesis below. In sequential dosing experiments the non-steroidal anti-inflammatory drugs aspirin (200), indomethacin (60), naproxen (60) and ketoprofen (60), in ascending order of activity, produced inhibition of established arthritis. Prednisolone sodium phosphate (6) showed good activity and was the only drug tested which significantly inhibited joint histopathology. Chloroquine diphosphate (100), cyclophosphamide (20) and SKF 36914 (oral gold) (10) had some activity, while levamisole (30), oxisuran (30) and D(–) penicillamine hydrochloride (200) had little or no activity. Sudoxicam (30) was toxic. SKF 36914 showed some improvement when dosed at 3 mg/kg for 7 weeks, but 100 mg/kg D(–) penicillamine hydrochloride was inactive on this schedule.

5. Five drugs were tested against developing arthritis. The compounds were administered daily by mouth for the first 4 weeks after challenge, except gold sodium thiomalate which was injected intramuscularly twice weekly during this period. Drug effects were measured on the 4 parameters outlined above plus a further parameter, joint mobility.
6. Cyclophosphamide (20), prednisolone sodium phosphate (1), procarbazine hydrochloride (5 or 7.5) and gold sodium thiomalate (2.5) produced inhibition of all or most of the parameters of arthritis. The improvement in activity of cyclophosphamide over its effect on established arthritis was dramatic. D(−) penicillamine (100) was inactive.
7. D(−) penicillamine was retested by the intravenous route (20) against developing arthritis, but was again inactive.

Acknowledgements

I thank Miss Audrey M. Woods, Mr H. Radziwonik, Dr J. Mann and Mr R. B. M. Wenham for their help with this work and their valuable comments on the manuscript. I also thank the following companies for generous gifts of drugs: Janssen Pharmaceutica N.V., for levamisole; May and Baker Ltd., for ketoprofen; Merck, Sharp and Dohm Ltd., for indomethacin; Pfizer Ltd., for sudoxicam; Roche Products Ltd., for procarbazine; Smith, Kline and French Laboratories Ltd., for gold triethyl phosphine; Syntex Pharmaceutical Ltd., for naproxen; Ward Blenkinsop and Co., Ltd., for cyclophosphamide; and Warner Lambert Research Institute, for oxisuran.

References

1. Dumonde, D. C. and Glynn, L. E. (1962). The production of arthritis in rabbits by an immunological reaction to fibrin, *Br. J. Exp. Pathol.*, **43**, 373
2. Goldberg, V. M., Lance, E. M. and Davies, P. (1974). Experimental immune synovitis in the rabbit. Relative roles of cell mediated and humoral immunity, *Arthr. Rheum.*, **17**, 993
3. Phillips, J. M., Kaklamanis, P. and Glynn, L. E. (1966). Experimental arthritis associated with autoimmunization to inflammatory exudates. *Ann. Rheum. Dis.*, **25**, 165
4. Andreis, M., Stastny, P. and Ziff, M. (1974). Experimental arthritis produced by injection of mediators of delayed hypersensitivity, *Arthr. Rheum.*, **17**, 537
5. Cooke, T. D. and Jasin, H. E. (1972). The pathogenesis of chronic inflammation in experimental antigen-induced arthritis. 1. The role of antigen on the local immune response, *Arthr. Rheum.*, **15**, 327
6. Jasin, H. E. (1975). Mechanism of trapping of immune complexes in joint collagenous tissues, *Clin. Exp. Immunol.*, **22**, 473
7. Davies, B. (1971). Effects of prednisolone in an experimental model of arthritis in the rabbit, *Ann. Rheum. Dis.*, **30**, 509
8. Blackham, A., Farmer, J. B., Radziwonik, H. and Westwick, J. (1974). The role of prostaglandins in rabbit monoarticular arthritis, *Br. J. Pharmacol.*, **51**, 35
9. Blackham, A. and Radziwonik, H. (1977). The effect of drugs in established monoarticular arthritis. *Agents Actions*, (in press)
10. Blackham, A. and Pugh, I. (1977). Measuring device for recording joint swelling: Possible research and clinical applications. *Agents Actions*, (in press)

11. Blackham, A. and Owen, R. T. (1975). Prostaglandin synthetase inhibitors and leucocytic emigration. *J. Pharm. Pharmacol.*, **27,** 201
12. Katona, G. (1976). Objective methods to assess the anti-inflammatory activity of anti-rheumatic compounds. *Agents Actions,* **6,** 346
13. Constable, T. J., Crockson, R. A., Crockson, A. P. and McConkey, B. (1975). Drug treatment of rheumatoid arthritis, *Lancet,* **i,** 1176
14. Brugmans, J., Schuermans, V., De Cock, W., Thienpont, D., Anssen, P. J., Verhaegen, H., van Nimmen, L., Louwagie, A. C. and Stevens, E. (1973). Restoration of host defense mechanisms in man by levamisole, *Life Sci.*, **13,** 1499
15. Freedman, H. H., Fox, A. E., Shavel, J., Jr. and Morrison, G. C. (1972). Oxisuran: A differential inhibitor of cell-mediated hypersensitivity. *Proc. Soc. Exp. Biol. Med.*, **139,** 909
16. Stockman, G. D., Heim, L. R., South, M. A. and Trentin, J. J. (1973). Differential effects of cyclophosphamide on the B and T cell compartments of adult mice. *J. Immunol.*, **110,** 277
17. Quagliata, F., Phillips-Quagliata, J. M. and Floersheim, G. L. (1972). Immunosuppression by procarbazine. 1. Sites of action of the drug and effect of adjuvant arthritis and circulating antibody responses. *Cell. Immunol.*, **3,** 198

Discussion IV

Localization of Immune Complexes and Rheumatoid-like Lesions in Rabbits (Chapter 9)

G. P. LEWIS: Do we know how the complex gets into the joint? Is it formed in the joint or is it formed in the bloodstream, and then somehow taken into the joint?

R. R. A. COOMBS: We do not know. But our assumption is that it is formed intravascularly, and then carried through.

Z. BENTWICH: Does Professor Coombs have any idea how long the complexes persist in the joints?

R. R. A. COOMBS: We cannot say yet since our main trouble has been getting the arthritic response consistently enough.

Evaluation of Anti-Rheumatic Drugs Using the Cutaneous Arthus Reaction (Chapter 10)

I. F. SKIDMORE: Colchicine, which was the only consistently active compound in the tests, is not — as I understand it — significantly active in rheumatoid arthritis. Could this suggest that the acute Arthus-type reactions that were examined are not an important factor in rheumatoid lesions. If so, Dr Goldlust, is the test a sensible screen for novel anti-inflammatory anti-rheumatic activity?

M. B. GOLDLUST: I suppose that there is an exception to every rule. Therefore, no matter what the model, activity or inactivity of one compound is not a valid basis for acceptance or rejection of a test as a screening procedure.

R. R. A. COOMBS: An equally important question is whether it is not naïve to think that there is just one immunological process operative in the pathogenesis of rheumatoid inflammation.

A. R. MACKENZIE: Is it possible that the high toxic doses of non-steroidal anti-inflammatory drugs that have been used in the tests are working by killing or inactivating cells so that they never arrive at the site of inflammation. Indomethacin at concentrations above 10^{-5} M will start to prove toxic *in vitro*.

M. B. GOLDLUST: It is probably a factor. I was trying to address myself to that particular problem. Where the therapeutic ratios are low, LD_{50}s are easily determined values; especially with single dose experiments. It certainly gives, and early on in the screening programme, some indication that one is looking at a non-specific mechanism, which is what I attempted to demonstrate.

Evaluation of Anti-Rheumatic Drugs using Antigen-Induced Arthritis (Chapter 11).

W. CARSON DICK: It is becoming increasingly obvious that there is a need for combined clinical ward rounds, with pharmacologists and clinicians working together. Some of the statements that have been made today, and in the past weeks, have been unbelievable. Let me remind everyone that rheumatoid joint disease is a symmetrical peripheral chronic polyarthritis associated with extra-articular manifestations and pursuing a relapsing course over perhaps 60 years. It has nothing to do with an acute polyarthritis in an animal, or even a chronic mono-arthritis, and it is ridiculous to extrapolate from animal models. The only model of rheumatoid arthritis is man.

I am particularly concerned over this for two reasons. First, the vast amounts of energy and resources directed to the area, which is an important consideration. Secondly, because we may be selecting variations on a theme of failure to look at ultimately in the clinic whilst throwing out anything that might be useful on the way through.

W. WATSON BUCHANAN: To follow Dr Dick, the doses of indomethacin used would be equivalent to 1–4 g in man which would be toxic to the extreme. The dosage of gold used is enormous if it is related to an average 70 kg man. Is the animal perhaps being stressed to such a degree that it produces hydrocortisone, and that is why an effect of gold can be shown after 1 or 2 days?

A. BLACKHAM: The point is that we did not see very much effect and I had to increase the dose of indomethacin to give it every opportunity to show some effect to evaluate the model. Indomethacin is a very potent drug when it is used in other models of inflammation, including in adjuvant arthritis, but in antigen-induced arthritis it is not at all potent, which therefore reflects its activity in the clinic. That is the point I was trying to put over.

W. W. BUCHANAN: Indomethacin in the dose we use in man is not a potent drug by any stretch of the imagination.

A. BLACKHAM: Exactly. That is what I am saying. In other models of inflammation — adjuvant arthritis — indomethacin shows too much activity for that model to be any use for discovering novel drugs. We are evaluating this model and showing that this is closer to the human situation because the effects of indomethacin cannot be shown.

GENERAL DISCUSSION

J. L. TURK: A question directed at the two clinicians.

I take issue with the point made by Dr Dick that to draw analogy between animal experiments and the human at the dose level is bad science because animals tend to vary a lot between species at the level at which certain drugs will affect various phenomena. This depends a lot on the metabolism of the animal. Animals differ considerably from man. For example, the rabbit is a herbivore and man is an omnivore, and that would have to be taken into account, as would the whole metabolic difference between the different species.

I would come to the defence of our colleagues in the pharmaceutical industry. When they screen compounds they look for maximum effects, and when they get a maximum effect they can try this at a far less toxic dose level in their clinical trials.

W. CARSON DICK: The point that we make is not that the dose alone is not extrapolatable from animal to man, but the activities that they are looking for may be completely wrong.

W. WATSON BUCHANAN: There is the other point that an Arthus phenomenon does not occur spontaneously in man.

J. L. TURK: Professor Coombs has a very nice slide of an Arthus reaction occurring in man. Clinical conditions such as polyarthritis nodosa, allergic cutaneous vasculitis, and erythema nodosum leprosum appear to be fairly good models.

R. R. A. COOMBS: They are usually iatrogenic. But we must stop that there.

H. Z. MOVAT: Did Professor Coombs see immune complexes in neutrophil leukocytes both in the synovium and in the fluid?

R. R. A. COOMBS: Certainly in large macrophage-like cells in the synovium — yes — those were in fact intra-cellular, or so I am told by my experts. But we have not looked at the cells from the joint fluid.

H. Z. MOVAT: I have a number of questions for Dr Goldlust.

First, the pathogenesis of the Arthus reaction consists of an accumulation of antigen–antibody complexes, be it direct or reversed, then fixation of complement, followed by accumulation of neutrophil leukocytes. Either the animal can be de-complemented and there will be no Arthus reaction, or it can be deprived of its leukocytes and there will be no Arthus reaction. With that in mind, it is very difficult to quantify the Arthus reaction because, erythema, oedema, and haemorrhage would all have to be quantified. How did Dr Goldlust go about quantitating this?

M. B. GOLDLUST: We measured the lesions in about the simplest manner possible, by weight, or by volume, in the various models. The other parameters are rather difficult, and depending on the animal species and the type of reaction they occur to significantly different extents. Erythema is not seen too easily in, for example, the mouse. The haemorrhagic response was best seen in the rabbit. According to rough calculations, the intradermal challenge doses of antibody were not all that different. There are a variety of factors. One cannot jump from one model to another and this should not be taken out of context. All the work that has been done in order to devise a testing procedure has indicated that there are some constraints, which is why the easiest way was chosen. I do not necessarily think that we are looking at it in the best way possible, but at least we have been able to generate enough background information with some of these agents that we could be a little more specific in our future approach.

H. Z. MOVAT: But may we have some idea of how, conceivably, these agents act on these parameters.

M. B. GOLDLUST: I can give a very unscientific answer, which may have me banished from the discussion! My feeling is this. There are two approaches. People who take mechanisms from an *in vitro* standpoint and people who hope that the animal will do the job for them. The reason why I describe four models in three animal species is to indicate that they may not all be equivalent even though we can call them all Arthus reactions. The types of antibodies involved in these reactions may be different. I prefer to say let the animal do the job. I cannot begin to say how these agents may be acting.

R. R. A. COOMBS: That is being an empiricist — and there is certainly room for empiricists today!

UNIDENTIFIED SPEAKER: We have investigated the effect of D-penicillamine in the Dumonde–Glynn arthritis using a low-dose long-term regimen, and we have managed to show that it does alleviate the inflammation. But we have found that it is necessary to treat for more than 50 days before any effect can be seen. We did continue treatment for 200 days before we carried out the post-mortem examination on the joints, and we found significant reductions in inflammation by all the criteria that have been mentioned by Dr Blackham.

A. BLACKHAM: Can I add to that. In the New Zealand white rabbit I believe that the erosions occurred 10–15 weeks after the antigen challenge, whereas in our old english rabbit the lesions occur at 4–6 weeks. Our model is far more severe form of inflammation and it may be more difficult to show a drug effect, but we have to use a model like that. Because of lack of time, in the pharmaceutical industry we need to have a model which does not require prolonged administration of drugs.

R. R. A. COOMBS: I shall be very interested in that. We shall go back and use the English rabbits — home produce!

G. P. LEWIS: A small extension of Professor Movat's comments to Dr Goldlust.

If one measures simply erythema, after all the hard work that has been done, might not it be getting just the same effect as if the inhibition of PG synthetase was measured. For example, most of the active drugs in the tables seemed to be synthetase inhibitors.

M. B. GOLDLUST: That is true — but just for the rabbit model. There is a discrepancy. The rabbit model, for some reason, seems to be more sensitive to these agents. That is why we left that model behind some years ago and went into the mouse and the rat. I do not think it a good model for new agents.

M. K. JASANI: The discussion we have had is obviously stimulating but it has to be rounded up. I am not usurping the chairman's role, but I should like to congratulate all the three speakers who have presented their data with great honesty. This is where science begins. Although we may not agree as to their relevance to rheumatoid arthritis, the facts that were presented today have profound implications if we ask the right questions for the future.

R. R. A. COOMBS: On behalf of myself and my colleagues in the dock, thank you.

E. V. BARNETT: In the same vein I would support that Arthus-like reactions are indeed relevant to chronic rheumatoid arthritis because even in the chronic disease synovial fluid has characteristics of ongoing Arthus-reaction as determined by complement activation, immune complexes, anti-immunoglobulins, and polymorphonuclear leukocytes. For an experimental pharmacologist it seems very reasonable to dissect elements of inflammation for drug testing. For the experimental pathologist, however, the goal would be to duplicate as closely as possible all the aspects of rheumatoid arthritis in an experimental model, since in clinical disease it is particularly unlikely that agents are aetiologic by percutaneous injection into the joint of our victims.

Professor Coombs's elucidation of chronic serum sickness with systemic disease targetting the joints seems more relevant, and the use of antigens and the documentation of collagenase anti-immunoglobulins, the use of antigens that contain immunoglobulins, and indeed nucleic acids, may provide a more proximal model to the human situation in other species.

R. R. A. COOMBS: As an immunologist, may I say that if one tries to develop a model for any particular type of immunological reaction, it is extremely difficult to get it absolutely pure. It is always thought to be contaminated by other immunological reactions. This is why it would be appropriate to consider rheumatoid arthritis to comprise of various types of immunological reactions in concert, each one predominating at a particular time. Certainly the serum sickness syndrome has a considerable asset here in that it is a systemic disease, it localizes perhaps in various places and it shows exacerbations and remission. But if one wishes to study the joint, there is no harm in studying one type of immunological response at a time, so long as one does not take it to represent the whole disease.

I think myself that for the model we have just heard described by Dr Blackham there would have to be very powerful therapeutic agents to prevent development of the inflammatory response.

A. BLACKHAM: Rheumatoid arthritis can be as severe as that, Professor Coombs. Severe inflammatory and destructive changes can be seen in a very short length of time in a rheumatoid joint. In that restricted sense at least, the model I have used does not appear to be over severe.

L. E. GLYNN: As one of the two parents of the original model I should like to make some comment, particularly in reply to Dr Dick. If he was willing to provide human patients for the drug tests we would not have to bother with animal models.

I speak as a pathologist interested not only in the treatment of the disease but in its pathogenesis. To have a model which is apparently self-perpetuating almost indefinitely for the rest of the life of the animal provides a unique situation which I do not know of as occurring in any other experimental situation, so that I think it is a model which is well worth considerable attention by the pharmaceutical industry.

The second criticism made by Dr Dick was that it is mono-articular and therefore bears no relation to rheumatoid joint disease. However, I would point out that in many rheumatoid patients the disease starts off as a mono-articular arthritis and remains so for a considerable length of time before becoming poly-articular. For your information, I should also point out that recently Professor Brouilhet of Paris has established that the experimental arthritis also becomes poly-articular, if the immunization schedule is modified so as not to get too strong a response. Professor Brouilhet's experimental rabbits also showed extra-articular manifestations in the form, particularly, of pulmonary lesions; so the antigen-induced arthritis can approximate even closer to RA (work is being published in Kennedy Institute Laboratory Workshop Handbook).

The results of drug treatment as we heard in the paper of Dr Blackham also add to the similarity between the antigen-induced arthritis and rheumatoid arthritis. Both show virtually the same response, or perhaps lack of response, to most drugs which the clinicians are so busy pumping into their patients apparently to no purpose whatsoever.

R. R. A. COOMBS: As a completely impartial chairman I can say that the honours are evenly distributed.

A question to Dr Glynn. Does this model which starts as an Arthus reaction persist as an Arthus reaction or is some other immunological mechanism also becoming involved?

L. E. GLYNN: That is an extremely difficult question. There are — I think — components of the Arthus-reaction probably going on the whole time. The fundamental change is probably not in the nature of the immune reaction, but in the nature of the antigen responsible for it.

DISCUSSION IV

A. G. MOWAT: Could I remind Dr Glynn that the three anti-rheumatic drugs that are currently of any value have actually arisen out of patient studies and have had nothing at all to do with animals, i.e. gold, penicillamine and, levamisole.

With regard to the papers that we have heard in this session, it would be more convincing if so-called non-rheumatic drugs were shown to have absolutely no effect on the systems, e.g. the anti-depressants, the anti-hypertensives, etc. Perhaps those drugs do the same things as the drugs we have heard about.

J. L. TURK: Anti-hypertensives.

M. B. GOLDLUST: So do diuretics.

R. R. A. COOMBS: One of our most distinguished immunologists (Professor Carl Prausnitz Giles) dictated a paper on the influence of hypnosis on the immediate-type hypersensitivity reaction virtually from his death bed (see *Br. med. J.*, **1**, 1291; 1963).

G. P. LEWIS: Are the clinicians really going to stand by and accept that there are only three useful drugs in rheumatoid patients.

From what I heard last week, not much that was good was said about levamisole or D-penicillamine. Surely aspirin is used at least to relieve the signs of the disease, if not to treat it, more than anything else.

P. A. BACON: We are getting confused between the anti-inflammatory effects and the analgesic effects. No one is disputing the analgesic effects of the short-term drugs. They are doubting whether this analgesia does anything to prevent the long-term progress of the disease.

W. WATSON BUCHANAN: I dissociate myself from my other clinical colleagues who have implied that certain drugs have any real effect in rheumatoid arthritis. If we had any drug that had any real effect, we should not have all these patients in wheelchairs.

Section: V
Cell-mediated Immunity and its Suppression

Chairman: J. L. Turk

12

Control Mechanisms in Cell-Mediated Immunity

J. L. TURK and DARIEN PARKER

INTRODUCTION

Anti-rheumatic drugs have in the past been selected for their anti-inflammatory activity. New groups of compounds are now being investigated which increase certain aspects of the immune response. The rationale behind the investigation of these compounds is based primarily upon the observation that rheumatic-like arthropathies can occur following or during the course of a number of acute and chronic infections. It has therefore been suggested that immune complex disease could play a significant role in the pathogensis of these diseases. Moreover, it has been suggested that such immune complexes form under conditions where host resistance is depressed. At the same time as there is increased proliferation of the micro-organisms or release of soluble antigen, there may be normal B-cell function with release of humoral antibody and formation of immune complexes in antigen excess. This will result particularly in arthritis, cutaneous vasculitis and uveitis, well known stigmata of rheumatic disease. As will be discussed later, increased B-cell function may result in a disturbance in the modulating action of B cells on T cells in the immune response and contribute to reduced host resistance which in many cases is T-cell mediated.

Although there is no definitive evidence for the role of infecting organisms in rheumatoid arthritis, there is evidence for the presence of immune complexes in the lesions, especially those containing anti-immunoglobulin antibody, particularly rheumatoid factor. However, the situation is far more complex because there is a further suggestion that the inflammatory reaction could itself be T-cell mediated, as marked improvement has been observed in patients treated by chronic thoracic duct drainage. These two suggestions, that the lesions could be mediated by immune complexes in the face of T-cell depression and that they might be mediated by enhanced T-cell activity resulting in delayed hypersensitivity, have to be reconciled. There is no doubt that a chronic disease such as rheumatoid arthritis is due to a complex system of interactions. It could therefore be that the disease is initiated by an immune complex arthropathy and the chronicity of the lesions is the result of a superimposed specific delayed hypersensitivity.

Two therapeutic approaches have been suggested that would appear to be effective in such a system. The first is to increase cell-mediated immunity by potentiating T-cell function with an immunostimulating drug such as levamisole. The second would be to depress B-cell function independent of T-cell function using a drug such as cyclophosphamide (CY). This would have the added advantage of both reducing the naturally occurring specific modulating effect of B cells on T-cell function and reducing the amount of antibody produced that could react with antigen and form immune complex deposits in the tissues. Both these therapeutic approaches involve a disturbance of the balance caused by normal specific control mechanisms in the immune response.

THE NETWORK OF INTERACTIONS

Early investigators considered that antigen stimulated the central lymphoid tissues to proliferate and differentiate so as to develop specific effector functions. Thus exposure to soluble antigen would result in humoral antibody production and if the antigen was emulsified in Freund's adjuvant, cell-mediated immune mechanisms would be stimulated. The realization that antigenic exposure results in stimulation of a whole network of accelerators and suppressors stems from observations on the effect of simultaneous stimulation of T lymphocytes on humoral antibody production by B lymphocytes. The phenomenon of T-cell–B-cell co-operation in antibody production stems from the observation that there was reduced antibody production to certain antigens in neonatally thymectomized mice and rats. Such co-operation may occur as a result of the action of specific or non-specific mechanisms. Helper T lymphocytes have been envisaged as having specific receptors on their surface that concentrate antigen directly on the B-cell surface. Another mechanism demonstrated by Feldmann[1] was that cell co-operation was mediated by a soluble specific factor derived from specifically sensitized T lymphocytes. This soluble factor was found to be cytophilic for macrophages and it was the macrophages rather than the T cells that focused antigen directly on the B-cell surface. Other workers[2] have described a T-dependent non-specific enhancement of B cells which is also mediated by soluble factors that could be synthesized by macrophages.

T cells can also depress B-cell activation. This is a function of T-suppressor cells that are a different population from T-helper cells. T-suppressor cells have now been demonstrated in a wide range of immunological reactions including the immune response to sheep red cells[3] and account for increased levels of antibodies to polysaccharide and other 'T-independent' antigens following thymectomy.

B-CELL MODULATION OF T-CELL FUNCTION

T-cell reaction can also be modulated by B-cell function. The classical example of this is the phenomenon of immunological enhancement in which humoral antibody blocks tumour immunity dependent on cell-mediated immunity (CMI). This process which allows increased tumour growth, is part of a wider biological process referred to as immunological facilitation[4]. In addition to the modulation of CMI by antibody, B cells can interact directly with T cells, modulating their ability to produce delayed hypersensitivity reactions.

Two forms of delayed hypersensitivity may be observed in guinea pigs sensitive to protein antigens when skin tested by intradermal injection (Figure 12.1). The stronger type of reaction, found in animals immunized with antigens

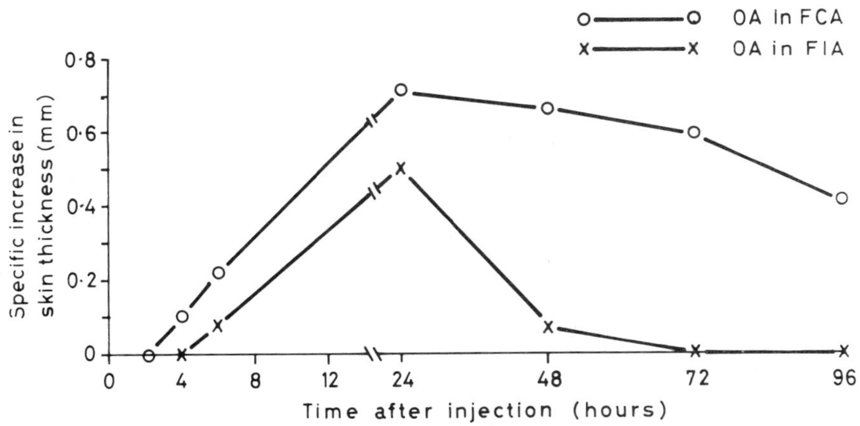

Figure 12.1 Comparison of time course of delayed hypersensitivity reaction (animals immunized with OA in FCA) with Jones–Mote reaction (animals immunized with OA in FIA)

in Freund's complete adjuvant (FCA), bears a close similarity to the classical tuberculin reaction. Erythema and induration appear after 6 h reaching maximum intensity at about 24–30 h and the reactions are still fairly marked after 48–72 h. This type of reactivity is present as early as 7 days after sensitization and persists beyond 14 days. The other form of delayed reaction, found chiefly in animals immunized with antigen in Freund's incomplete adjuvant (FIA) reaches its maximum intensity between 24 and 30 h and is almost imperceptible at 48 h. This form of skin reactivity, which is detected 5–10 days after sensitization and develops into an Arthus or immediate-type skin reaction at 14 days, is frequently referred to as Jones–Mote hypersensitivity. A further form of delayed hypersensitivity in the guinea pig is that which can be elicited by skin contact with a simple chemical sensitizer, such as 2,4-dinitrofluorobenzene (DNFB) or 4-ethoxymethylene2-phenyl oxazolone. The time course of this contact skin reaction is similar to that of a Jones–Mote reaction; however the state of sensitivity persists beyond 14 days.

For many years, it has been known that these reactions are characterized by a mononuclear cell infiltrate consisting of varying proportions of lymphocytes and macrophages. However, more recently the importance of the basophil leukocyte in these reactions, especially in Jones–Mote and contact hypersensitivity, has been emphasized. One of the main features that has always distinguished delayed hypersensitivity and contact sensitivity reactions from antibody-mediated reactions is that the former reactions cannot be passively transferred with serum but can be with cells derived from lymphoid tissues. In a similar manner Jones–Mote hypersensitivity cannot be transferred with serum but can be passively transferred with cells of lymphoid origin.

The effect of cyclophosphamide (CY) on delayed hypersensitivity reactions

A single intraperitoneal injection of 300 mg/kg CY in the mouse and guinea pig was found selectively to deplete lymphocytes from the lymph follicles and cortico-medullary junction in lymph nodes and from the equivalent, non-thymus dependent areas of the spleen. The thymus dependent areas of both the lymph nodes and the spleen appeared to be relatively unaffected. Maximum depletion occurred at 3 days and repopulation could be observed to begin 4 days later. These findings were confirmed quantitatively by the demonstration of a proportional increase in the θ antigen carrying lymphocytes in lymph nodes and spleen of mice treated with CY.

Guinea pigs treated with CY (300 mg/kg i.p.) 3 days prior to sensitization with DNFB or oxazolone were found to develop increased reactivity when skin tested 7 days after sensitization (Figure 12.2). Furthermore these contact sensitive reactions, in CY pretreated animals, were prolonged in that they could still be detected 8 days after skin testing. These findings were not due to increased non-specific reactivity as there was no parallel increase in skin reactions to turpentine. The increased reactivity in CY pretreated animals could be partially reversed by the intraperitoneal transplant of spleen fragments from normally sensitized animals. Also the effect of CY pretreatment was partially reproduced by splenectomy if performed 4 days after sensitization.

However, CY pretreatment was not found to increase delayed hypersensitivity to tuberculin in BCG immunized animals, nor was it found to increase delayed hypersensitivity to ovalbumin (OA) in animals immunized with OA in FCA. In contrast, the effect of CY pretreatment on guinea pigs immunized with OA in FIA was to increase the skin reactions elicited at 7 days (Figure 12.3). These Jones–Mote skin reactions had been converted, by the CY pretreatment,

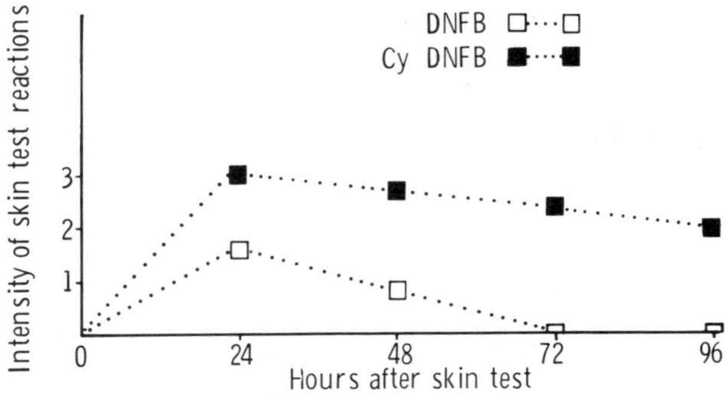

Figure 12.2 Average intensity of contact sensitivity skin reactions after skin test with 0.25% DNFB in CY-treated and control guinea pigs

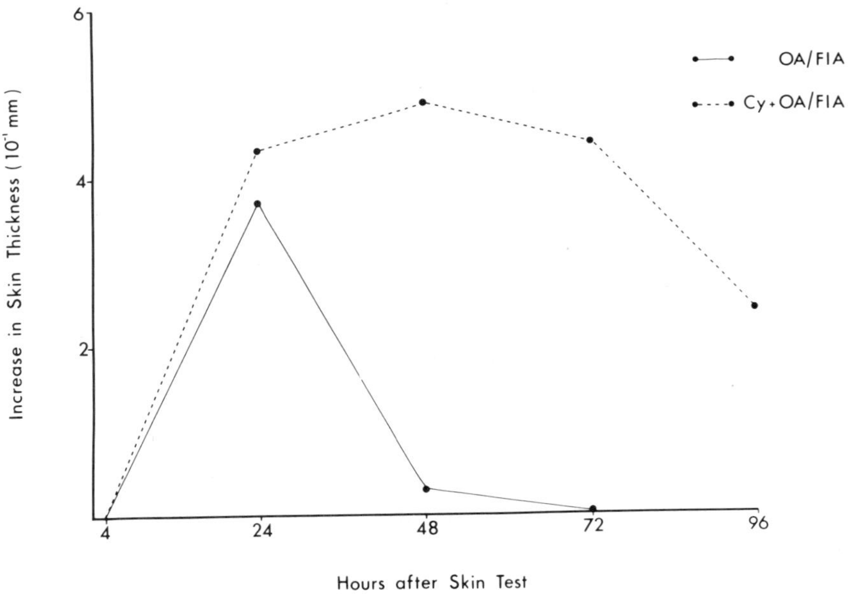

Figure 12.3 Average increase in skin thickness after skin testing with 100 μg OA in animals immunized with OA in FIA. One group of animals was treated with CY 3 days before sensitization

into skin reactions with the intensity and time course of those animals immunized with OA in FCA[5]. The increase in Jones–Mote reactions, following CY pretreatment of OA in FIA immunized animals, was associated with a complete inhibition of IgG_1 homocytotropic antibody production. A partial inhibition of IgG_1 homocytotropic antibody production has also been found in contact sensitized guinea pigs after CY pretreatment.

On the basis of these findings, it might be postulated that CY pretreatment removes a population of cells that modulate the expression of delayed hypersensitivity, as strongly enhanced skin reactions result without this cell population. It would also appear that the cells which are depleted by CY are B lymphocytes. If CY was depleting animals of a population of suppressor cells, normally present at the time of sensitization, the passively transferred cells from these animals should be more reactive than cells from guinea pigs not pretreated with CY. Passive transfer of spleen or PEC from animals, sensitized with OA in FIA 8 days earlier, caused more intense and more indurated reactions in normal recipients when donors had been pretreated with CY 3 days before sensitization, as compared with those reactions transferred from sensitized animals which had not received CY.

In order to demonstrate the presence of suppressor cells, the following model was used. Guinea pigs, treated with CY 3 days before immunization with OA in FIA served as cell recipients 8 days later, as they were potentially susceptible to the effect of suppressor cells which they were lacking. Cells which would reduce the skin test reactions in such animals were found in the spleen and PEC of guinea pigs immunized with OA in FIA, 8 and 14 days previously, and in animals immunized with OA in FCA 8 days previously. This suppression was shown to be antigen specific and to need live cells[6]. In further experiments, the spleen cells from guinea pigs immunized with OA in FIA 8 days previously were passed down plastic bead (Degalan V 26) columns, which had been coated with specifically purified rabbit anti-guinea pig globulin. This process depleted the spleen cells of 90–95% of the immunoglobulin bearing cells (B lymphocytes), as detected by immunofluorescence. These B-cell depleted spleen cells failed to suppress the skin reactions of the animals used for the detection of suppressor cells (i.e. CY–OA in FIA immunized guinea pigs). However, spleen cells passed through normal rabbit serum (NRS) coated columns which were not depleted of B cells suppressed the delayed reactions of the CY treated recipients to a similar degree to the unseparated cells (Figure 12.4). Further, when these B-cell depleted spleen cells were transferred passively into normal guinea pigs, the recipient animals developed increased skin sensitivity similar to that induced by the passive transfer of cells from CY pretreated, OA in FIA donors[7].

The action of CY in reversing certain states of immunological tolerance

The demonstration that CY pretreatment could increase contact reactivity and certain forms of delayed type hypersensitivity by elimination of suppressor cells, led to a study of the action of CY in certain models of immunological unresponsiveness. One of the earliest reports of immunological tolerance in experimental animals was the demonstration, by Chase[8] in 1946, that a state of specific unresponsiveness in contact sensitivity could be induced by feeding 2, 4-dinitrochlorobenzene (DNCB) to non-sensitive guinea pigs. Another model of

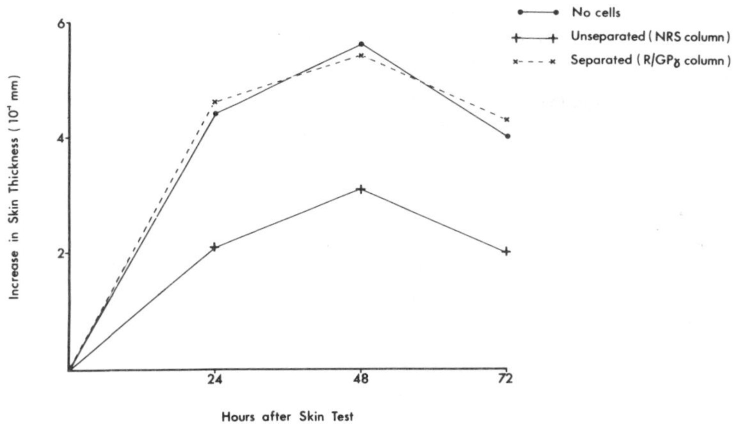

Figure 12.4 Skin reactivity of animals, treated with CY 3 days before immunization with OA in FIA, serving as cell recipients 8 days after sensitization. Donor spleen cells taken 8 days after immunization with OA in FCA

unresponsiveness of this type can be induced by two intravenous injections of dinitrobenzene sulphonic acid sodium salt ($DNBSO_3$) at 14 day intervals before attempting sensitization.

Guinea pigs, treated with 500 mg/kg $DNBSO_3$ twice at 14 day intervals before attempting sensitization with DNCB, were completely unresponsive to DNCB. However if they were treated with CY (250 mg/kg) 3 days before attempting sensitization, they became responsive[9]. In this model, CY pretreatment was effectively able to reverse the tolerant state. Once tolerance had been shown to be broken, the animals remained responsive. However if one allowed a 14 day gap between the CY and attempted sensitization, the animals were subsequently found to remain unresponsive. Thus the effect of the CY was a temporary one and after a limited time the clones of suppressor cells were able to regenerate.

Guinea pigs made tolerant to DNCB with $DNBSO_3$ fail to show T-cell proliferation in lymph nodes draining the site of sensitization. One of the effects of CY pretreatment is to allow T-cell proliferation to develop. It seems therefore, that CY has a preferential action on clones of suppressor cells, releasing effector cells for proliferation in CMI. Animals made tolerant in this way also show a failure of antibody production as well as CMI. CY treatment was able to induce a return of γ_1 homocytotropic antibody production in this system.

Following the demonstration of the reversibility of tolerance induced by intravenous injection of $DNBSO_3$, it was shown (Figure 12.5) that tolerance in-

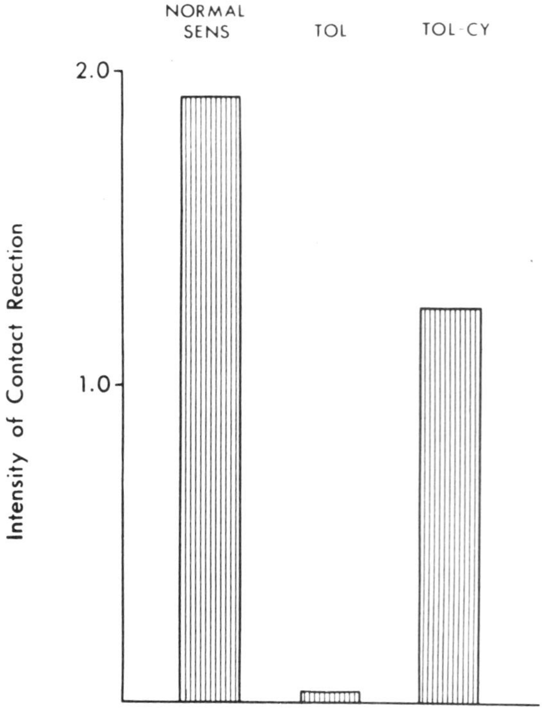

Figure 12.5 Reversal of tolerance to DNCB by cyclophosphamide treatment

duced by feeding DNCB could be reversed by CY in a similar manner[10]. However, the tolerance induced by feeding is not so complete as that induced by intravenous injection. When such partially tolerant animals are treated with CY before attempted sensitization, the resultant sensitivity is far greater than that found after reversal of tolerance in the i.v. $DNBSO_3$ system. The level reached was that found when normal animals were treated with CY before sensitization. This could indicate that the tolerance induced by feeding is completely reversible, whereas that induced by i.v. injection might be a combination of a reversible suppressor cell action with some degree of irreversibility due perhaps to clonal elimination.

The reversibility of tolerance induced by feeding is also accompanied by a return of the ability of lymphocytes to proliferate in the draining lymph nodes following sensitization. In the case of the reversal of tolerance induced by intravenous injection, the number of large pyroninophilic cells in the draining lymph nodes 4 days after sensitization did not return completely to the level found in sensitized controls. The return of sensitivity following treatment with CY in animals made tolerant by feeding was however associated with a complete return of T-cell proliferative activity.

A third model of unresponsiveness in contact sensitivity is one that can be induced by epicutaneous application of a cross reacting compound which is a poor sensitizer in its own right. A partial unresponsiveness to DNFB can be produced by the epicutaneous application of 2% 2,4-dinitrothiocyanate benzene (DNTB), 14 and 7 days before sensitization. This state of partial unresponsiveness can be broken by treatment with 300 mg/kg CY 3 days before sensitization. Suppressor cells, capable of reacting in the periphery, can be demonstrated by passive cell transfer into recipients sensitized to DNFB and depleted of naturally induced suppressor cells by pretreatment with CY. However, the unresponsive state is not associated with a decrease in T-cell proliferation in the draining lymph nodes[11]. This was confirmed in experiments in which $DNBSO_3$ treated animals received lymph nodes from normal syngeneic animals. These animals then behaved like those made unresponsive with DNTB in that they were still unresponsive with respect to their peripheral reactivity, while being able to develop specific proliferation in the draining lymph node[12].

CONCLUSION

Studies taking advantage of the ability of cyclophosphamide to deplete rapidly turning over cells have indicated that there is a balance between suppressor and effector mechanisms in normal immunization schedules. Similar suppressor cells, susceptible to cyclophosphamide, can be demonstrated in reversible models of specific immunological unresponsiveness in chemical contact sensitivity. The reactivity that can eventually be detected in an animal is the resultant of effector and suppressor elements. The Jones–Mote form of delayed hypersensitivity to soluble protein antigens in the guinea pig can now be explained on the basis of such a balance in which the relative proportion of suppressor cells is greater than in the tuberculin type of reaction. These suppressor cells appear to belong to the B population rather than the T population of lymphocytes.

A similar balance can be found in normal contact sensitivity reactions in which depletion of suppressor cells also causes increased reactivity. Moreover when an animal is treated in a number of ways, previously shown to induce specific immunological unresponsiveness, there is preferential stimulation of suppressor cells without activation of effector cells. During tolerance induction in contact sensitivity, suppressor cells have been found which have a central as well as a peripheral action. Data is accumulating to suggest that these actions may depend on two separate populations of cells.

References

1. Feldmann, M. (1972). Cell interaction in the immune response *in vitro*. V. Specific collaboration via complexes of antigen and thymus derived cell immunoglobulin. *J. Exp. Med.*, **136,** 737

2. Waldmann, H. and Munro, A. (1975). The interrelationships of antigenic structure, thymus independence and adjuvanticity. *Immunology,* **28,** 509
3. Gershon, R. K. (1975). A disquisition on suppressor T-cells. *Transpl. Rev.,* **26,** 170
4. Voisin, G. A. (1971). Immunological facilitation, a broadening of the concept of the enhancement phenomenon. *Progr. Allergy,* **15,** 328
5. Turk, J. L. and Parker, D. (1973). Further studies on B-lymphocyte suppression in delayed hypersensitivity indicating a possible mechanism for Jones–Mote hypersensitivity. *Immunology,* **24,** 751
6. Katz, S. I., Parker, D., Sommer, G. and Turk, J. L. (1974). Suppressor cells in normal immunization as a basic homeostatic phenomenon. *Nature* (*London*), **248,** 612
7. Katz, S. I., Parker, D. and Turk, J. L. (1974). B-cell suppression of delayed hypersensitivity reaction. *Nature* (*London*), **251,** 550
8. Chase, M. W. (1946). Inhibition of experimental drug allergy by prior feeding of the sensitizing agent. *Proc. Soc. Exp. Biol. Med.,* **61,** 257
9. Polak, L. and Turk, J. L. (1974). Reversal of immunological tolerance by cyclophosphamide through inhibition of suppressor cell activity. *Nature* (*London*), **249,** 654
10. Polak, L., Geleick, H. and Turk, J. L. (1975). Reversal by cyclophosphamide of tolerance in contact sensitization. Tolerance induced by prior feeding with DNCB. *Immunology,* **28,** 239
11. Sommer, G., Parker, D. and Turk, J. L. (1975). Epicutaneous induction of hyporeactivity in contact sensitization. Demonstration of suppressor cells induced by contact with 2.4.dinitrothiocyanatebenzine. *Immunology,* **29,** 517
12. Polak, L., Frey, J. R. and Turk, J. L. (1973). Dissociation between lymph node and peripheral reactivity in immunological unresponsiveness to DNCB. *Immunology,* **25,** 451

13
The Rheumatological Significance of Lymphokines

D. C. DUMONDE

INTRODUCTION: THE PARADOX OF RHEUMATIC INFLAMMATION

Until quite recently it has been widely held that rheumatic inflammation arises from the development of lymphocyte-mediated specific immunological responses of inappropriate character or duration, following latent exposure to, or established infection with, a variety of extrinsic (microbial) agents: and that this leads somehow to recognizable 'rheumatic' patterns of pathology affecting the lymphoid, vascular and locomotor apparatus[1]. Two principal kinds of derangement have been suggested whereby pathogenetic pathways may operate: (i) an inability to eradicate immunogens or inflammogens from the host and thus from potential sites of rheumatic inflammation; and (ii) failure to stop reactions produced by stimuli that should normally induce only an ephemeral response by a host's immunological or inflammatory mechanisms. Herein lies the paradox of rheumatic inflammation: for to the histopathologist, local tissue lesions often resemble chronic cellular allergic responses; but no extrinsic antigens or other plausible inflammatory agents have been identified with regularity in the rheumatoid synovium or other such inflammatory sites.

Whereas the aetiology of rheumatoid arthritis and related diseases is not yet clear, there is increasing evidence that their pathogenesis involves persistent lymphocyte activation and lymphokine production at sites of inflammation. The identification of lymphokines as effector substances in cell-mediated rheumatic inflammation would have clear implications for the design of test systems by which new therapeutic agents, with more selective actions on the rheumatic process, might be recognized. This chapter examines the evidence that lymphokines are mediators of rheumatic inflammation and identifies current approaches to the recognition of how lymphokine production may be normally controlled in health and inappropriately regulated in diseases such as rheumatoid arthritis.

It is contended that uncontrolled or unbalanced activities of lymphokines may well govern the local accumulation and activation of blood-borne inflammatory cells at 'risk' sites of rheumatic inflammation. The key to further understanding would seem to lie in defining how lymphokine-producing cells may lose responsiveness to physiological mechanisms by which their inappropriate activation is normally restrained; and in defining what kinds of stimuli, immunological or otherwise, can result in such inappropriate lymphocyte activation. Special emphasis is placed upon characterizing mechanisms which may normally control interactions between recirculatory lymphocytes and endothelial cells of the microvasculature and upon finding out how a variety of initiating stimuli might precipitate reactive lymphoendothelial dysfunction in the susceptible subject.

It is concluded that identification of the role of lymphokines and other mediators in lymphocyte:endothelial interactions may lead to a fresh approach to the recognition of pathogenetic processes and of anti-rheumatic agents.

LYMPHOID CELL ACTIVATION IN RHEUMATOID ARTHRITIS AND RELATED DISEASES

Because of the abundance of lymphocytes in the rheumatoid synovium and in other inflammatory rheumatic lesions, it has been natural to assume that rheumatoid arthritis and related diseases represent disorders of the lymphocyte-mediated allergic response. This view is reinforced by the beneficial effects of thoracic duct drainage in severe rheumatoid arthritis; by the recognized efficacy of immunosuppressive and steroid-based drug regimes in severe or relapsing disease; and by additional evidence of a spectrum of immunological aberration and lymphocytic abnormality in association with inflammatory rheumatic syndromatology. The recognition that antigen-activated lymphocytes can generate lymphokines as well as antibodies led quickly to the proposition that lymphokines are important autopharmacological mediators of rheumatic inflammation; that rheumatoid arthritis could be viewed as a disorder of cell-mediated immunity and that once the specific antigen was identified, therapeutic measures might be devised to combat the putative immunopathology[2].

In this section we shall identify two major concepts which arise in pursuing this line of thinking: (a) the concept of 'basic' and 'superimposed' cellular patterns of rheumatic inflammation; and (b) the concept that aberrant lymphocyte function may be an expression of defective cellular control mechanisms, triggered perhaps by specific immunological or infective processes, but mediated by a failure to limit the activation of lymphocytes at potential 'risk' sites of rheumatic inflammation. With this in mind, five areas of discussion would seem to merit consideration: (i) identification of the 'basic' unit of rheumatic inflammation; (ii) identification of the stimulus to lymphocytic accumulation; (iii) identification of the stimulus to lymphocytic activation; (iv) the relationship between lymphocytic accumulation and lymphocytic activation; (v) the identification of lymphokines as mediating the consequences of persistent lymphocytic activation at sites of rheumatic inflammation.

Histopathology of rheumatic inflammation (Figure 13.1)

The most constant histological feature of inflammatory rheumatic disease comprises the perivascular accumulation and activation of lymphocytes, frequently accompanied by enlargement of the endothelial cells of small blood vessels around which the perivascular infiltrate is characteristically observed. This 'basic' histopathological unit is well illustrated in the rheumatoid synovium (Figure 13.1); in the peripheral regions of rheumatoid granulomata[3], in the classical histopathology of skin and muscle in dermato/polymyositis[4]; in the dermal and visceral lesions of systemic sclerosis[5]; and even in the synovium in osteoarthritis[6]. 'Superimposed' upon this basic lymphoendothelial pathology

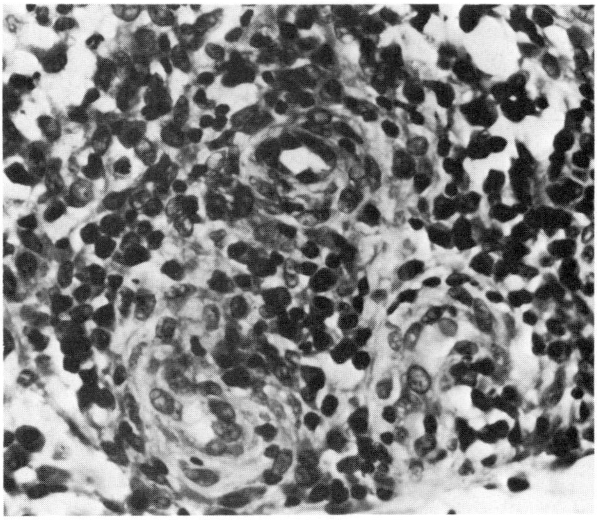

Figure 13.1 The 'basic' unit of 'lymphoendothelial' pathology in a synovial biopsy from a patient with rheumatoid arthritis. The figure shows three small blood vessels surrounded by lymphocytes which can also be seen emigrating through the microvasculature. Endothelial cells of the small blood vessels have taken on a plump appearance and resemble endothelium of post-capillary venules in the paracortex of lymph nodes. Emigrated lymphocytes appear to be in various stages of activation. (H & E × 250)

there is a tendency for other patterns of inflammatory response to become established. Thus in systemic sclerosis and systemic lupus erythematosus, there is frequently endothelial hyperplasia and fibrosis, especially in long-term lesions; in the rheumatoid nodule there is accumulation of activated macrophages and fibroblasts which often assume geographical 'palisading' patterns; in the rheumatoid synovium there is frequently extensive infiltration by activated macrophages, follicular aggregation of lymphocytes, cytodifferentiation of plasma cells and lymphoblasts, intimal cell hyperplasia, fibroblast proliferation and fibrosis[4]. In rheumatoid disease, it is the erosion of cartilage and bone by synovial pannus which provides the most striking superimposed pattern of chronic inflammation and which has given rise to so much research directed at elucidating the role of mononuclear phagocytes in the hope of finding ways and means of suppressing the processes and consequences of macrophage activation at such sites[7].

It may be argued that these 'superimposed' patterns of inflammation, whilst of clear importance in mechanisms of tissue damage and functional impairment, have tended to obscure the more fundamental unit of lymphoendothelial pathology whose recognition and investigation may lead to an understanding of why early rheumatic inflammation may develop in the first place.

The stimulus to lymphocytic accumulation

The key to this problem seems to lie in considering why lymphocytes should accumulate at sites outside the lymphoid system shortly after their passage across microvascular endothelium: and it is this very problem which gives rise to a 'paradox' of lymphocytic accumulation in rheumatic disease. The paradox may be stated in terms of two major difficulties. First, to the pathologist, the articular and extra-articular lesions of rheumatoid and allied diseases resemble chronic local reactions of hypersensitivity brought about by interaction between an antigen and a host's immunological apparatus; yet there is no microbiological or immunological evidence which would implicate the presence of specific microbial antigens or other specific allergens at such sites in amounts sufficient to initiate or maintain a state of chronic allergic inflammation[1].

Having identified this first or 'immunological' difficulty we then encounter a second, more general problem in the field of chronic inflammation: the search for a local stimulus. Again, to the pathologist, a second easily understood cause of persistent inflammation is the local persistence of an aetiological agent either because of failure of host defence, or the undegradable nature of an inflammatory agent, or inadequate removal of necrotic material from a local site[8]. In rheumatoid disease there is at present no evidence for a specific immunological deficiency state against identifiable classes of bacteria, viruses or other microorganisms; no evidence which suggests that inadequate clearance of substances from the joint space is responsible for the *initiation* of perivascular lymphocytic accumulation; nor is there evidence to implicate the presence of nonbiodegradable microbial residues or other such substances in the rheumatoid joint. In the development of ideas on the nature of inflammatory processes, it has been rewarding to investigate the consequences of applying an inflammatory agent to a site under consideration. Because no such acceptable inflammogens have been identified in sites of rheumatic inflammation, other pathogenetic explanations have continued to be based on primary (systemic) disorders of collagen (more generally, 'connective tissue') metabolism[9], or of vascular endothelium[10] or of the lymphoid system itself[11]; and it is appropriate to consider how far these have provided an explanation of perivascular lymphocytic accumulation in rheumatic disease.

Although recirculatory lymphocytes must course through the ground substance of connective tissue on their way to the smallest 'initial' lymphatic channels[12], no evidence has yet emerged that primary biochemical abnormalities of collagen or proteoglycan metabolism underly perivascular lymphocytic accumulation in rheumatoid arthritis. In recognition of microvascular abnormalities, the generic term 'collagen disease' was replaced by the term 'collagen-vascular disease', both of which are probably now obsolete; and this focused attention on the more severe pathology of blood vessels, particularly in advanced lesions of rheumatoid vasculitis, scleroderma and systemic lupus: again, without contributing to an understanding of perivascular lymphocytic positioning. The view that rheumatic inflammation arose primarily through tissue-directed autoimmunity[13] was not really substantiated by subsequent work; and has itself been modulated by 'immune-complex' theories in which the (genetically) susceptible host is viewed as depositing soluble immune complexes from the circulation into sites of inflammation. In idiopathic rheumatic disease, neither of these 'immunological' mechanisms would seem to account for the widespread distribution of lymphocytic perivasculitis. Accordingly it would seem more acceptable to view the development of autoimmunity, circulating immune complexes, or both, as contributing to patterns of superimposed inflammation rather than as initiating causes of widespread 'basic' lymphoendothelial pathology.

The stimulus to lymphocytic activation

If we view rheumatoid inflammation as arising from the activation of locally accumulated lymphocytes, it is logical to enquire into the nature of the stimulus to lymphocyte activation. Two approaches are possible, according to which of two kinds of derangement we might consider.

Firstly, if we think that chronic rheumatic inflammation arises because of the host's failure to eliminate a persistent stimulus, we will ask what is its class (e.g. microbial or non-microbial immunogen), where is its primary location (e.g. inside or outside the joint), how is it delivered (e.g. a single insult, or a series of repeated insults), and does the 'stimulus' act directly or indirectly (e.g. does it require 'processing' by the susceptible host). In fields of inflammation and immunology this may be called a 'classical' approach; and it led predictably to an enormous amount of work which has aimed to ascribe rheumatoid disease and allied syndromes to the operation of an unusual stimulus or the untoward persistence of known classes of environmental immunogenic or inflammatory stimuli which in the normal host would be expected to give rise to self-limiting episodes of lymphocyte activation.

Secondly, we may take an 'alternative' view by suggesting that these processes result from a failure in switching off what would otherwise be self-limiting responses, initiated by lymphocyte activation due to either immunogenic or non-immunogenic stimuli, wherever they may arise. If we take this alternative view we are then led to enquire how antigen-mediated lymphocyte activation is normally controlled *in vivo*; how the production of lymphokines and the response to lymphokines is regulated during physiological immune reactions; what stimuli other than immunological may initiate lymphocyte activation and lymphokine production and what kinds of defects in host response systems could permit the persistence of lymphocyte activation and lymphokine production at anatomical sites that we know to be preferential sites of rheumatic inflammation. On this basis we could return to the chronic 'rheumatic' host and search for the occurrence of behavioural defects in the control of lymphocyte activation, as judged by lymphokine production and by other criteria, in comparison with the behaviour of lymphocytes of healthy subjects or from subjects with self-limiting 'post-infective' rheumatic syndromes complicating known microbial infection[14].

Relationship between lymphocytic accumulation and lymphocytic activation

Given that lymphocytes accumulate and become activated in sites of chronic rheumatic inflammation we may now ask whether these phenomena should be regarded as inseparable or separable features of the behaviour of lymphocyte populations *in vivo*. Again, there are two approaches to the discussion.

Firstly, we recognize that persistent activation of T cells, B cells and accessory cells (e.g. macrophages) in the rheumatoid joint results in the generation of lymphokines, Ig:anti-Ig complexes, complement activation products, proteolytic enzymes, and doubtless other agents, any or all of which may recruit further haematogenous lymphocytes into the site of inflammation by damaging vascular endothelium or by acting as chemotactic agents[1]. On this basis we may accept that lymphocyte accumulation will necessarily follow local lymphocyte activation, however this is initiated; and that lymphokine-mediated mechanisms will be found to provide positive feedback systems to ensure continued arrival and consequent activation of fresh lymphocytes and other leukocytes into the local environment, to increase its resemblance to ectopic lymphoid tissue, or merely to balance local cell loss by cell recruitment and exudation.

However, there is a second area of enquiry which seems to be crucial to the genesis of lymphocyte-mediated chronic rheumatic inflammation: that of whether the first 'inflammatory' lymphocytes accumulate in an activated or non-activated state. If we think that the rheumatic lesion starts by the emigration of already activated lymphocytes, then local lymphokine production may well take place inevitably as soon as these cells have migrated across the microvasculature. The therapeutic problem would then be to devise ways of arresting lymphocyte activation before 'arrival'. If however we think that a rheumatic lesion might start by the local accumulation of lymphocytes emigrating in a previously quiescent state, we are led to enquire into whether mechanisms normally exist for ensuring that recirculatory lymphocytes migrate away from sites of transmural passage; and whether lymphocyte activation may follow lymphocyte accumulation if these mechanisms become defective.

The consequences of persistent lymphocyte activation

Whether local lymphocyte activation is caused by the local presence of some elusive agent, or by the arrival of already activated lymphocytes, or by a failure to maintain the quiescence of locally recirculating lymphocytes, its consequences as viewed histopathologically are explicable to a large measure on the basis of persistent lymphokine production. We shall 'accommodate' the role of antiglobulin and antinuclear responses by accepting that the consequences of untoward lymphocyte activation in such subjects will then include superimposed phenomena of immune complex disease whose pharmacological implications are discussed elsewhere in this symposium.

In building 'models' for the recognition of anti-rheumatic agents we shall single out the lymphokine system as a principal means whereby lymphocytes take action at sites of rheumatic inflammation. Any such model should accommodate the architectural similarities between advanced rheumatoid synovitis and immunologically stimulated lymphoid tissue which support the concept of the rheumatoid synovium as a site of ectopic lymphoid tissue formation. In the paracortex of normal lymph nodes the 'basic' architectural unit is itself a lymphoendothelial element comprised of a segment of the microvasculature surrounded by a cuff of recirculatory lymphocytes and other features of lymph node architecture are 'superimposed' upon a three-dimensional array of such units[15]. In the rheumatoid synovium we appear to have this lymphoendothelial element as the 'basic' structural unit, superimposed upon which are patterns of cellular accumulation and proliferation together with disorganization of adjacent articular structures. In the next section we shall summarize the current concepts of lymphokine function and the nature of evidence which implicates lymphokines as mediators of rheumatic inflammation.

Table 13.1 Illustrative activities of lymphokines which may be relevant to the pathogenesis of tissue damage in rheumatic inflammation

*Cell type affected and designation of lymphokine activity ('soluble factor')**	*Feature of the normal cellular immune response in which lymphokine activity is inferred*	*Feature of rheumatic inflammation in which lymphokine activity may be implicated*
Affecting macrophages		
Macrophage migration-inhibition factor	Encourages retention of emigrated macrophages at effector site	Continued macrophage activation results in secretion of proteolytic enzymes (e.g. depolymerizing proteoglycans), of E-type prostaglandins (promoting bone resorption) and of plasminogen activator (with local activation of coagulation, fibrinolytic and complement pathways)
Macrophage chemotactic factor	Encourages emigration of macrophages into local site	
Macrophate-activating factor	Activates metabolic, phagocytic, microbicidal capacities of emigrated macrophages	
Macrophage-aggregating factor	Promotes aggregation of emigrated macrophages	
Macrophage-arming factor	Promotes extracellular cytotoxicity of recruited macrophages	
Macrophage spreading-inhibition factor; and macrophage slowing factor	Acute changes at the cell surface might facilitate passage of mononuclear phagocytes through inflamed microvasculature	Continued recruitment of macrophages into granuloma and positive feedback in potentiating lymphokine production (if lymphocytes unresponsive to PGE suppression)
Macrophage-disappearance factor	Promotes adherence of macrophages to endothelial surfaces	

Affecting lymphocytes		
Lymphocyte-mitogenic (blastogenic) factors	Recruits non-committed lymphocytes into metabolic activity at local effector site	Perivascular lymphocyte positioning in 'basic' inflammatory pattern; LK-mediated recruitment of cells in superimposed pleomorphic inflammation
Lymphocyte transforming factor and potentiating factors	Augments lymphocyte activation by specific antigen	
Suppressing factors (DNA synthesis)	Limits or modulates extent of lymphocyte response at effector site	
Co-operating or helper factors	Facilitates B-cell response to T-dependent antigens	Over-production of non-specific Ig and of Ig: anti-Ig complexes with 'by-pass' of T-cell suppression
Affecting fibroblasts		
Cytotoxic factors ('lymphotoxin')	Illustrates indirect mechanism of restricting the growth or metabolism of aberrant (tumour) cells	Impairment or stimulation of fibroblast metabolism with cell destruction or cell mitosis, collagen deposition and fibrosis; ? mediates synovial intimal hyperplasia
Cloning-inhibitory factor		
Fibroblast-stimulating factor	'Repair' of chronic allergic inflammatory lesions	
Interferon-like factor	Protects host cells against virus infection	
Affecting vascular endothelium		
Erythrogenic factor	Vasodilatation to encourage arrival of sensitized cells	Contributory stimuli to microvascular proliferation and endothelial activation
Permeability-increasing factor	Increased vascular permeability in delayed hypersensitivity	
Inflammatory factors	Encourages emigration of leukocytes into sites of allergic inflammation	
Lymph-node activating factor	Facilitates lymphocyte emigration into paracortex during immune response	Inappropriate LK production may selectively damage vascular endothelium
Affecting polymorphs		
Granulocyte migration-inhibition and chemotactic factors	Contributes to pleomorphic character of delayed hypersensitivity responses	Provides mechanism to encourage polymorph emigration into synovial fluid

* For further details see Refs. 21, 25, 28, 73

LYMPHOKINES AND RHEUMATIC INFLAMMATION

Nature and biological activities of lymphokines (Table 13.1)

The possibility that activated lymphocytes produce a special class of macromolecules other than immunoglobulins arose from the discovery some 10 years ago that soluble products generated during antigen activation of guinea pig lymphocytes would inhibit the centrifugal migration of cultured guinea pig macrophages[16–18]. It soon became evident that guinea pig lymphocyte activation products possessed a number of other biological activites which appeared relevant to the expression of cellular immune responses *in vitro* and *in vivo*, such as the production of a pleomorphic inflammatory cell response on intradermal injection[19]; an ability to enhance DNA metabolism of cultured lymphocytes[20]; and a cytotoxic effect on cultured fibroblasts[21]. The action of lymphocytes in effecting cellular immune responses became viewed in terms of two principal mechanisms; (i) a 'direct' pathway involving interaction of (T-) cell populations with antigen sequestered in a local biological environment; and (ii) an 'indirect' pathway involving amplification of lymphocyte activities by means of soluble non-antibody mediators appearing as a local result of antigen:lymphocyte interaction[22].

In 1969 we proposed the generic term 'lymphokines' to denote the existence of a group of autopharmacological substances, generated by antigen-activated lymphocyte populations, which differed from immunoglobulins in their physicochemical characteristics and to which an increasing number of biological activities would become attributed[23]. The term 'lymphokine' was introduced to indicate the 'usual' sources of these materials (i.e. derived by lymphocyte activation); their putative distinction from immunoglobulin; their putative physiological significance ('lymphokinesis'); and the proposition that they may function physiologically both as mediators and regulators of cellular immune responses to specific antigen[23, 24]. It now seems[25] that there may be 30 or more recognizable activities of lymphokines and recently-developed methods of parallel bioassay and physicochemical separation now indicate that some of the lymphokine activities must be ascribable to different molecular species of protein or glycoprotein generated by activated lymphocytes[21,25,26].

Table 13.1 illustrates a partial list of soluble lymphocyte factors whose circumstances of production and action would fit their inclusion under the generic term 'lymphokines'; and the table also illustrates those features of the cellular immune response in which it seems likely that the particular lymphokine is involved. Current evidence suggests that lymphokines may act physiologically upon at least the four major cell families found in connective tissue (mononuclear phagocytes; lymphocytes; fibroblasts; microvascular endothelial cells) as well as upon polymorphonuclear leukocytes and other formed elements of the blood (with the possible exception of red cells). Physicochemical studies indicate that lymphokines derived from antigen-activated lymphocytes may range in molecular weight from 12 000–120 000 although it is not yet known how far the many lymphokine activities may be ascribed to different and distinct molecular entities.

In addition to being generated by 'classical' means (i.e. lymphocyte activation by specific antigen) it has become clear that lymphocyte populations activated by 'alternative' pathways may also generate products with lymphokine activity. Two such phenomena seem particularly relevant: (a) the generation of lymphokines by activation of non-neoplastic lymphocytes with the aid of phytomitogens, microbial endotoxins or membrane-active chemical reagents[25,27,28] and (b) the 'spontaneous' generation of lymphokines by transformed or neoplastic lymphocyte lines or by lymphocyte populations in long-term culture[29,30,31]. The activation of lymphocytes to release lymphokines is therefore not invariably a phenomenon confined to antigenic stimulation and the sequence of biochemical events in the lymphocyte or its surface components, which precede lymphokine production, have yet to be defined[25].

Future trends in lymphokine research

When we coined the term 'lymphokines' we suggested that they might act not only as 'cell cooperators' but also as 'traffic regulators' in the sense of controlling the trapping of lymphoid cells at sites of allergic inflammation or immune induction and in controlling the physiological passage of recirculatory lymphocytes through microvasculature of blood and lymphatic vessels[24,32]. Support for such a role of lymphokines in immunologically activated lymphoid tissue was obtained by studying patterns of lymphocyte retention and mitotic activation within guinea pig lymph nodes following injection of small quantities of lymphokines into afferent lymphatics[33,34]. More recently Anderson *et al.* have suggested that the ultrastructural features of transmural migration of recirculatory lymphocytes in the unstimulated lymph node are compatible with a chemotactic stimulus directing lymphocyte emigration which might itself be a lymphokine[35]. If the 'physiological' migration of lymphocytes involves a directional chemotactic response by lymphocytes to small quantities of lymphokines released in the extravascular microenvironment, then some physiological mechanism must clearly exist for ensuring that lymphokine production does not get 'out of hand'. One of the important areas of future research, relevant to the physiology of the lymphokine system, will be to study the mechanisms by which lymphokine production is modulated or 'switched off' during self-limiting reactions of Type IV hypersensitivity[36].

A second inter-dependent area of research will be to exploit methods of quantitative biological assay, including the use of reference standards, in the physicochemical and biological characterization of lymphokines[37]. Interest is now developing in the use of biological standards of lymphokine activities for research purposes: to aid the purification and measurement of lymphokines in different laboratories, to provide a biological basis for the development of immuno-assays of different lymphokines and to advance understanding of the role of the various lymphokine activities in surveillance, immunoregulatory and inflammatory functions of specific cell-mediated immunity.

A third area of anticipated research relates to the clinical significance of lymphokines; for measurement of lymphokine production may well be viewed as examining the integrity of an important component of immunological homeostasis[11]. It seems likely that selective abnormalities of cellular immune function in neoplastic, inflammatory, and infective disease may involve an imbalance of 'physiological' lymphokine production and action, in all its heterogeneity. On this basis the clinical expression of cellular immunological disorders may depend upon which features of lymphocyte or lymphokine function are abnormally reactive or under-represented. In addition to providing a pharmacological approach to the study of specific cellular immune responses, the lymphokine concept provides an approach to the investigation and classification of abnormal cellular immune responses in human disease, in which human lymphokine standards have an important part to play. Such work should form the basis for research into antagonists and promoters of lymphokine activity, some of which may find application in controlling the cellular immune response. As part of the more general field of clinical immunopharmacology, the study of human lymphokines has obvious relevance to inflammatory disease; future research will seek to simplify what seems at the present time (1977) to be a problem of investigative complexity[25]. Development of this field will be much assisted by parallel studies of lymphokine function in both animals and man and with some optimism, may yield a predictive basis for control of the cellular immune response.

Lymphokines in experimental models of rheumatic inflammation

Experimental models of the rheumatoid process, in synovium, subcutis, lymph nodes and peripheral microvasculature, can be brought about by intense or persistent immunopharmacological stimulation to lymphocyte emigration, accumulation and activation at various sites in (genetically) normal laboratory animals. Analysis of the circumstances under which these experimental models are generated provides strong circumstantial evidence for a similar role of lymphokines in the pathogenesis of inflammatory rheumatic lesions.

The direct injection of sufficient foreign antigen into a synovial joint of a specifically sensitized rabbit, guinea pig or chicken results in a sequence of synovial and articular pathology mimicking faithfully the histopathological spectrum in rheumatoid arthritis[38–40]. Analysis of these arthritis models reveals the importance of specific T-cell mediated immunity[39]; and the generation of lymphokines by explants of inflammatory synovium[41]. Repeated injection of homologous lymphokine into rabbit[42] or guinea pig[43] knee joints results in a mononuclear synovitis; and a single injection of lymphokine mixed with non-immune but inflammatory lymphocytes and macrophages into the guinea pig knee joint produces a protracted response which mimics the time course of a delayed hypersensitivity reaction in the joint[40]. We can therefore say that antigen-induced arthritis becomes chronic because of local persistence of antigen:lymphocyte interactions with persistent lymphocyte emigration, accumulation, and activation to lymphokine production. The role of lymphokines is viewed as coordinating and recruiting the overall chronic inflammatory response, which is driven by persistent antigen. A similar explanation accounts for persistent subcutaneous granulomata as models of the rheumatoid nodule[44].

The direct injection of a single small quantity of guinea pig lymphokine into the afferent lymphatic of a guinea pig lymph node results in a sequence of changes in lymph node architecture which resemble the histopathology of lymph nodes in rheumatoid disease[33,34]. An early phase of paracortical distension with acute retention of lymphocytes[34] is rapidly followed by follicular hyperplasia and mitotic activation of cells within the follicles[33]. If an antigen is given intralymphatically in relation to the injection of lymphokine there is accelerated cytodifferentiation of antibody-forming cells in the node[45] with an even more enhanced resemblance to the rheumatoid lymph node. Analysis of the model suggests that lymphokines, released within lymphoid tissue, may act on lymphocytes, macrophages and microvascular endothelium to promote lymphocyte recruitment, retention and activation within different compartments of the node[33,34,45].

At this descriptive level it therefore seems that extravascular generation of lymphokines can provide the local stimulus to lymphocytic emigration, perivascular positioning, lymphocytic activation and the recruitment of accessory macrophages in experimental animals at sites chosen for their predilection to involvement in human rheumatic inflammation. Studies of the effects of known anti-rheumatic drugs on lymphokine-induced histopathology have yet to be undertaken; but from the experimental point of view it can be said that certain of the 'Dale criteria'[37] would seem to be satisfied to implicate lymphokines as mediators of rheumatic inflammation.

Identification of aberrant lymphokine production in rheumatic disease

Circumstantial evidence that the rheumatoid synovium is busy generating lymphokines has been provided by the predominance of T cells in areas of rheumatoid synovitis[46] and in cell populations recovered by elution from rheumatoid synovia[47]. Ziff's group have evidence that lymphokine-like substances with migration-inhibition activity can be generated by short-term culture of rheumatoid synovial explants[31] and various workers have reported cytotoxic and mitogenic factors in rheumatoid synovial fluid, although the identity of these lymphokine-like substances with an antigen-induced lymphokine remains to be demonstrated. We agree that rheumatoid synovial explants can generate lymphokine-like substances in short-term culture[48] but we have two principal qualifications: (a) that the migration inhibition activity seems more polydisperse on Sephadex chromatography and molecular sieve ultrafiltration than antigen-induced lymphokines from normal peripheral blood; and (b) that a more limited spectrum of lymphokine activity seems to be generated than expected from antigen-activated lymphocytes[49].

The findings raise the possibility that the lymphokine-generating cell populations in the rheumatoid synovium may be 'different' in character or function to those of normal antigen-activatible cell populations; and that in sites of rheumatic inflammation, alternative pathways of lymphocyte activation may be operating. Could this be due to persistence of an unusual stimulus at sites of inflammation, or could it be due to defective control of lymphocyte activation mechanisms at such sites?

Identification of aberrant lymphocyte function in rheumatic disease

Many features combine to reinforce the growing view that regulation of lymphocyte activation and migration may both be defective in several ways in rheumatic disease. *First*, there are the phenomena of autoimmunity[11] which now include the demonstration of anti-lymphocytic antibodies[50]. *Second*, surface-marker studies and lymphocyte function studies on peripheral blood reveal a number of abnormalities including the unexplained presence of circulating immunoblasts[51,52], the occurrence of subpopulations of unclassifiable cells[53], and deviations from normality in respect of lymphocyte activation responses to phytomitogen and to 'recall' antigens[47,48]. *Third*, there are associations between inflammatory rheumatic disease and states of lymphoid malignancy and of frank immunodeficiency. *Fourth*, lymphoid cells in rheumatoid synovium can take on a Sezary-like appearance[47]; synovial fluid lymphocytes are less responsive than peripheral blood lymphocytes to stimulation by phytomitogen[47] or to suppression by E-type prostaglandin[54]; and such lymphocytes have a high mitotic index[47]. *Fifth*, although no specific immunogenic stimulus has been incriminated in the rheumatoid process, there is microscopic evidence of immunoblasts leaving rheumatoid lymph nodes[40].

Taken together, these features contribute to give a picture of the 'rheumatic' lymphoid system as having lost some degree of responsiveness to factors which may normally control lymphocyte activation, positioning and compartmentation: with a resulting propensity of recirculatory lymphocytes to become inappropriately activated in circumstances where lymphocyte quiescence would appear to be physiological. This recalls the problem of identifying the elusive stimulus to lymphocyte activation (see above) or the site at which such defective control mechanisms would seem to be operative.

RHEUMATOID ARTHRITIS VIEWED AS A DISORDER OF LYMPHOCYTE POSITIONING

The hypothesis of lymphoendothelial dysfunction (Figure 13.2)

There are many indications for considering regulatory disturbances of microvascular function in inflammatory rheumatic diseases (see Refs.[14] and [40] for reviews). The hypothesis that a primary abnormality of vascular endothelium was involved in inflammatory rheumatic disease[10] has been somewhat over-shadowed by the prominence of immunological abnormalities in these syndromes. Microvascular endothelium responds to many injuries by increased passage of protein and leukocytes; yet the inflammatory response that characterizes the lesions of rheumatoid disease appears to involve the selective accumulation and local activation of lymphocytes as in sustained local reactions of Type IV hypersensitivity[39]. In the absence of evidence for a sufficient (immunogenic) stimulus at sites of rheumatoid inflammation, comparable to what is needed in the experimental models, it seems that non-immunological alterations in the migratory behaviour of lymphocytes, at sites of transmural passage, may play an important part in the persistence and distribution of inflammatory rheumatic lesions. The histopathology of rheumatoid disease, with prominent 'lymphoendothelial' inflammatory elements in lymph nodes, subcutis, synovium, muscle, nerve and sometimes viscera, suggests that the 'risk' sites at which such defective control mechanisms would seem to operate are those where lymphocyte:endothelial interaction may play an important part in controlling lymphocyte recirculation and hence lymphocyte positioning.

The hypothesis of 'lymphoendothelial' dysfunction in inflammatory rheumatic disease is illustrated in Figure 13.2 which proposes the existence of a body 'system' concerned with regulating the traffic and activation of recirculatory lymphocytes in connection with their passage through microvascular endothelium. This lymphoendothelial system will clearly involve close physiological interactions between lymphocytes and endothelial cells, a situation which could be so easily disturbed by abnormalities of the lymphocyte, abnormalities of the endothelial cell, or abnormalities affecting the plasma milieu in which these interactions take place (Figure 13.2). The passage of lymphocytes for example through the complex structure of a post-capillary venule must be associated with considerable physical deformation of the membranes of the lymphocyte as well as the endothelial cell; and in view of the variety of ways in which peturbation of the lymphocyte surface may lead to lymphocyte activation and lymphokine production, some homeostatic mechanism presumably exists to control this. The 'rheumatoid' response suggests the failure of feedback control of the activation of such recirculatory lymphocytes to stimuli which would otherwise elicit only a self-limiting or subclinical lymphocyte activation episode, at or shortly after the transmural passage of cells through postcapillary venular endothelium. At such sites, the multiple actions of lymphokines on all major cell types in connective tissue

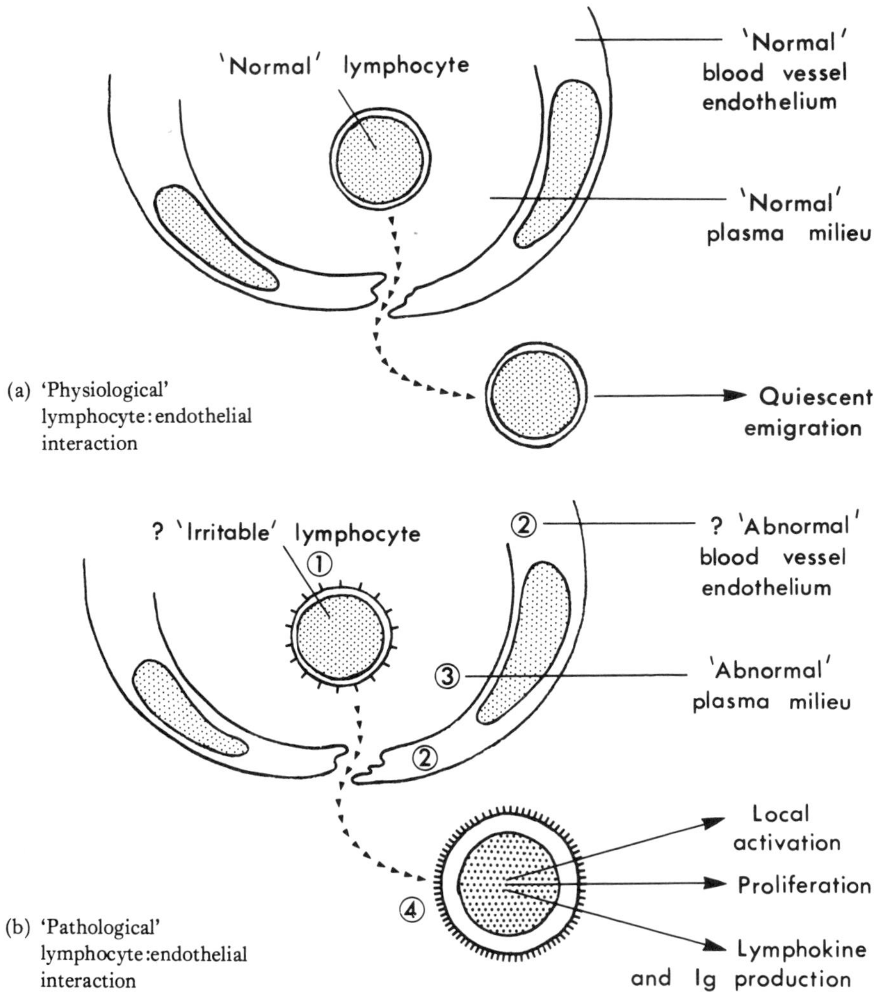

Figure 13.2 Hypothesis of lymphoendothelial dysfunction in rheumatic disease
Diagrammatic representation of a proposed body system (the 'lymphoendothelial system') which is envisaged as regulating the traffic and activation of recirculatory lymphocytes through microvascular endothelium within lymphoid tissue and at widely distributed sites outside the lymphon itself (e.g. subcutis; synovium). The 'system' is viewed as ensuring that when lymphocytes are entering extravascular connective tissue they will normally remain quiescent and migrate away from the site of transmural passage. The diagrams depict the essential differences envisaged between lymphocyte behaviour when the lymphoendothelial system is 'normal' and when it is 'disturbed' by regulatory defects.

Regulatory disturbances in lymphocyte:endothelial interaction could arise by virtue of: (1) primary 'disease' of the lymphocyte (e.g. aberrant C-type virus expression; hormonal disturbance); or (2) primary 'disease' of vascular endothelial cells (e.g. paramyxovirus or other infections; bacterial toxins; vasomotor or pharmacological abnormalities . . .); or (3) primary 'disease' of the milieu or environment in which these cellular interactions take place (e.g. presence of could offer many opportunities for abnormally activated lymphocytes to set in motion the mechanism which could lead to chronic inflammation at these 'risk' sites of reactive pathology (Figure 13.2).

Implications of the 'lymphoendothelial' model (Figures 13.3, 13.4)

A first implication is that a feed-back system for controlling lymphocyte activation and lymphokine production may be identifiable. It is known that prostaglandins of the E series will inhibit lymphokine production in guinea pigs[55,72], direct cytolysis and haemolytic plaque formation by murine lymphocytes[56,57], and mitogen-induced stimulation of murine lymphocytes[58]. Likewise, normal human lymphocytes are responsive to the suppressive effects of E-type prostaglandin, which will suppress phytomitogen-induced DNA synthesis and lymphokine production[59–62].

The second implication is that prostaglandins of the E series might act as physiological modulators of lymphocyte-mediated responses[63]; for vascular endothelial cells, at least in culture, can generate very large quantities of E-type prostaglandin[64]. Thus we find that supernatants from cultured porcine endothelial cells will suppress the transformation of pig peripheral blood lymphocytes in partial concordance with their content of E-type prostaglandin[65].

The third implication concerns the way in which such a feedback mechanism might operate. Figure 13.3 suggests a hypothesis by which normal lymphocytes are thought of as being kept in a quiescent state by E-type prostaglandins from contiguous vascular endothelial cells during transmural migration; and that the passage of activated lymphocytes through vascular endothelium is viewed as stimulating the production of feedback inhibitor, either by cell contact or by means of the short-range activity of small quantities of lymphokines generated by the 'irritable' lymphocytes.

The hypothesis presented in Figure 13.3 is based on the remarkable ability of activated lymphocytes to penetrate between contiguous vascular endothelial cells in confluent co-cultures where within 24 hours a model 'lymphoendothelial' tissue is established *in vitro* (Figure 13.4). Experiments are in progress to determine whether integration of activated lymphocytes into endothelial monolayers results in the potentiation of prostaglandin E_2 production

---

vasoactive mediators, immune complexes, etc. in the plasma):- leading to (4) failure to keep lymphocytes 'quiet' during emigration.

Rheumatoid arthritis and allied rheumatic diseases are then viewed, not as 'primary' diseases of the connective tissue, but as disorders of the lymphocyte traffic which connective tissue carries. For example, the multiple actions of lymphokines on all major cell types in connective tissue could offer many opportunities for abnormally activated lymphocytes to set in motion the mechanisms which could lead to chronic inflammation at certain 'risk' sites of reactive pathology (see Figure 13.3).

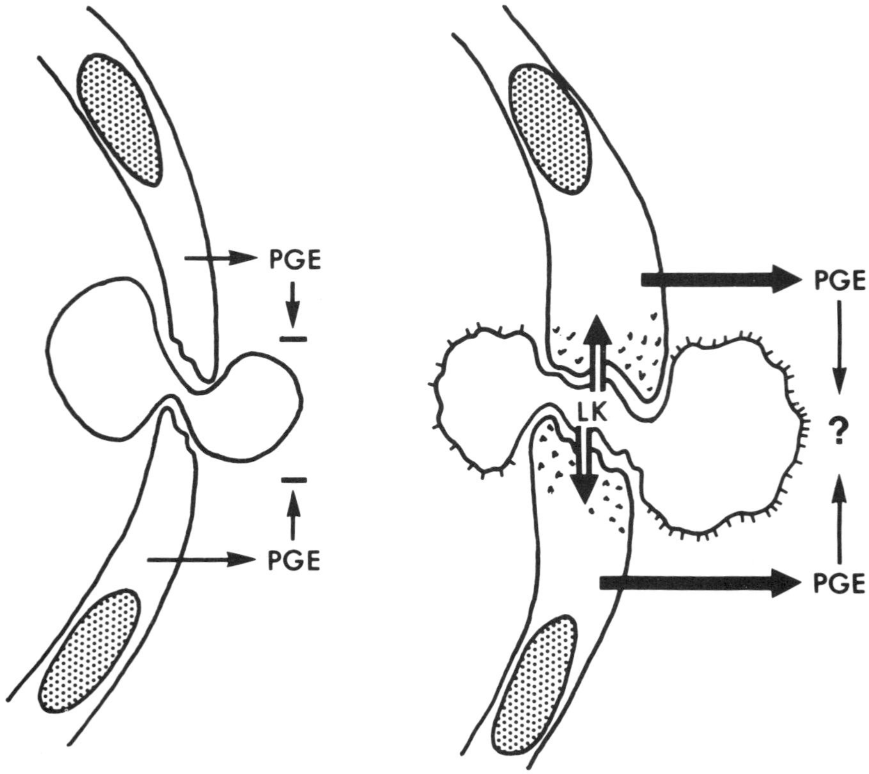

(a) 'Physiological' (b) 'Pathological'

Figure 13.3 Proposed role of lymphokines and prostaglandins in lymphocyte: endothelial interaction.

In Figure 13.3a a normal recirculatory lymphocyte is depicted as migrating between microvascular endothelial cells whose production of (E-type) prostaglandin is viewed as being sufficient to maintain the lymphocyte in a quiescent state during transmural migration, or to wind down lymphocyte activation in self-limiting reactions of type IV hypersensitivity.

In Figure 13.3b an activated lymphocyte is stimulating (E-type) prostaglandin production (PGE) of contiguous vascular endothelial cells by the local action of lymphokines. Lymphoendothelial pathology is illustrated as arising from defective response of vascular endothelium to metabolic stimulation by activated lymphocytes (or by their locally-secreted lymphokines); or by defective suppression of lymphokine secretion by (E-type) prostaglandins generated by contiguous vascular endothelial cells.

The hypothesis presented in these figures leads to the corollary that a variety of stimuli, acting *via* the lymphocyte, the endothelial cell or the (plasma) milieu, could precipitate reactive lymphoendothelial dysfunction at a distance from the primary site of action of the initiating stimulus on the susceptible host (see also Figure 13.2).

by endothelial cells; and if so, whether this may be ascribed to the local secretion of lymphokines by the integrating lymphocytes.

The fourth implication is simply that if lymphocytes 'escape' this control process, for example if they lose their sensitivity to modulatory prostaglandins[36], a basic unit of lymphoendothelial pathology could well become established. The possibility that activated rheumatoid lymphocytes can lose their sensitivity to modulatory prostaglandins[66] arises from the substantial production of both lymphokines and E-type prostaglandins by rheumatoid synovia[67,68], where hypertrophied vascular endothelial cells have been shown to contain considerable amounts of PGE_2 as judged by immunofluorescence[69]. This high degree of lymphokine and prostaglandin production suggests that such a feedback mechanism is no longer operating properly and that attempts to suppress PGE production (by inhibiting prostaglandin synthetase) may only make matters worse by encouraging even further lymphokine secretion.

Lymphokines in 'superimposed' inflammation

The reasoning illustrated in the previous section points to lymphokine release during normal lymphocyte migration as a mechanism which might activate or potentiate E-type prostaglandin production by vascular endothelial cells. In addition to this physiological situation, potentiation of PGE production might serve to wind down self-limiting reactions of Type IV hypersensitivity when lymphocytes are the dominant emigrating cell population[55] and when endothelial activation, including microvascular proliferation, is known to occur[70]. On this basis, lymphokine production would be regarded as a 'good' thing; and 'blanket' attempts to suppress lymphokine function might interfere with the physiology of lymphocyte recirculation and with the control of antigen-mediated type IV hypersensitivity responses. However, in rheumatic inflammation, continued lymphokine production at sites of transmural migration will be expected to recruit and activate mononuclear phagocytes as part of the processes of 'superimposed' cell accumulation and activation. As lymphokine-activated macrophages can produce E-type prostaglandin, a second opportunity arises for feedback inhibition of lymphocyte activation, both in pleomorphic reactions of Type IV hypersensitivity and in less-understood sites of rheumatic inflammation[36]. Perhaps at this stage a therapeutic approach to the selective suppression of lymphokine production is warranted in the knowledge that a 'first line of defence' has already been broken.

Implications of lymphokine heterogeneity (Table 13.2)

When we first implicated lymphokines in the pathogenesis of rheumatic lesions[2] we pointed to their potential heterogeneity, later confirmed by bioassay[26]; and suggested that future approaches to the recognition of anti-rheumatic drugs, with actions on the lymphokine system, would seek to affect

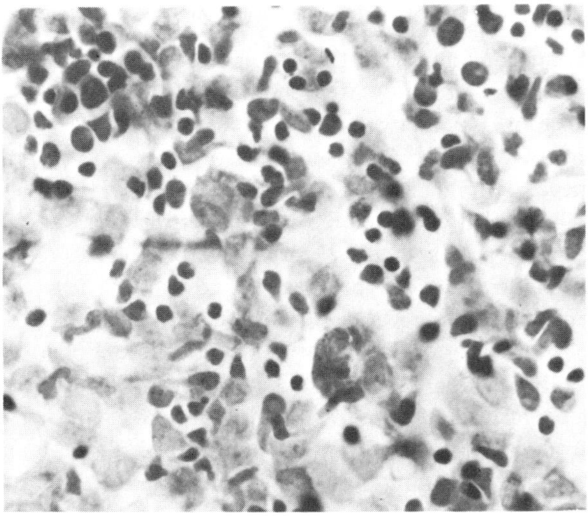
Figure 13.4a

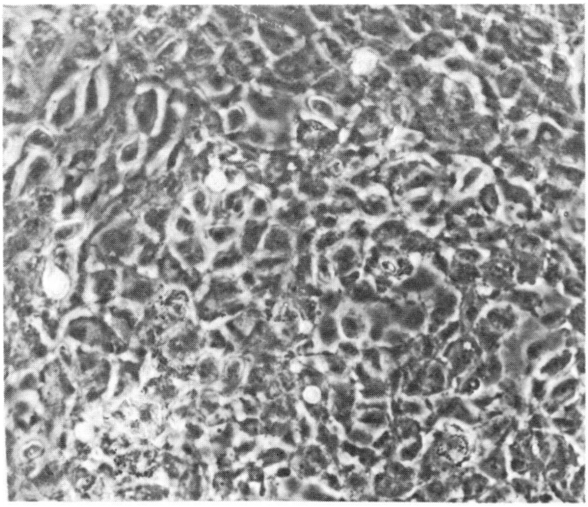
Figure 13.4b

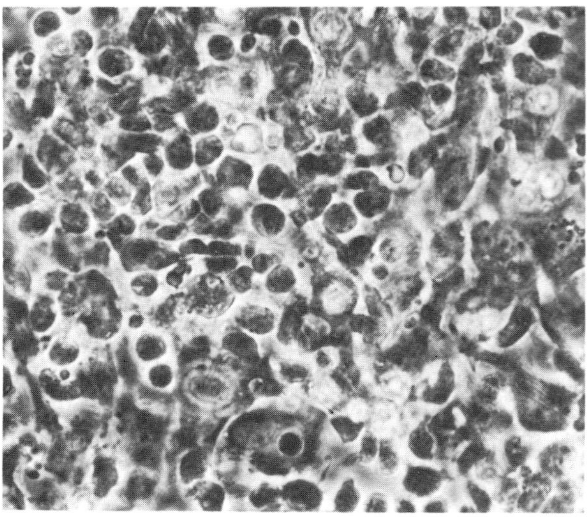
Figure 13.4c

lymphokines selectively rather than globally. If the concepts of lymphoendothelial dysfunction, inappropriate lymphocyte activation and loss of sensitivity to controlling mediators can be investigated in model systems (see Figure 13.3), we may obtain some clues as to which of the many lymphokine activities could be operating at sites of rheumatic inflammation and how to develop a selective approach to manipulation of the lymphokine system (see Table 13.2).

In recalling the concept of lymphokines as 'cell cooperators' and 'traffic regulators'[24], we must appreciate that research in this field is still only 10 years 'old'; nevertheless, the rheumatological significance of lymphokines is now becoming accepted with increasing enthusiasm. More work is needed on the characterization of lymphokines produced by antigen-specific and by other methods of lymphocyte activation. In particular, the extent of heterogeneity needs to be defined; the macromolecules which carry lymphokine activity need to be purified and isolated; agonists and antagonists of lymphokine production and activity need to be developed; and it is to be expected that this research will lead to the recognition and classification of abnormalities in lymphokine production or responsiveness in human disease. When one considers the growth of knowledge in other fields of inflammation, it is clear that the characterization of a mediator system involves the study of cell receptors and cell interactions as well as the synergistic and antagonistic effects of one mediator system upon another. In going deeper into the rheumatological significance of lymphokines, these enquiries will prove to be at least as complex as in other areas of mediator pharmacology; but it is hoped that the development of simplified systems as 'models' of certain aspects of cell behaviour in rheumatic inflammation will be of predictive value in the design of new therapeutic approaches to the enigmatic behaviour of lymphocytes in rheumatic disease.

Acknowledgements

I thank my colleagues in the laboratory for their enthusiasm and continued collaboration; and the Medical Research Council and Arthritis and Rheumatism Council for continued support.

Figure 13.4 Stages in the formation of 'lymphoendothelial' aggregates during co-culture of porcine vascular endothelial cells with pig peripheral blood lymphocytes previously activated by $NaIO_4$ to be in a state of lymphokine production.

Figure 13.4a shows the adherence of lymphocytes to vascular endothelium 2 hours after the addition of a lymphocyte suspension to an endothelial monolayer. (H & E: × 600). Figures 13.4b (× 250) and 13.4c (× 600) shows phase-contrast appearances of the co-cultures at 24 hours where the activated lymphocytes have penetrated between previously confluent endothelial cells so that the nuclei of both cell types come to lie in the same optical plane.

The photomicrographs illustrate lymphocyte integration into endothelial monolayers and the apparent development of 'lymphoendothelial tissue' *in vitro*.

Table 13.2 Rheumatological significance of lymphokine heterogeneity

Illustrative features of the normal cellular immune response		*Rheumatological consequences of inappropriate lymphokine production or of inappropriate response to lymphokines*
Quality of response	*Putative combinations of lymphokine activity*	
Allergic inflammation Delayed hypersensitivity; granuloma formation; allograft rejection; graft-*v*-host reactions . . .	Inflammatory (complex); chemotactic; macrophage-aggregating; macrophage-arming; lymphocyte mitogenic . . .	Inappropriate control of lymphocyte activation leads to both 'basic' and 'superimposed' patterns of chronic cell-mediated inflammation
Protective cellular immunity Restriction of tumour growth and parasite multiplication; destruction of parasitized cells; activation of host macrophages; restriction of (parasitized) macrophage metastasis . . .	Cytotoxic; proliferation-inhibitory; macrophage-activating; macrophage-arming; migration-inhibition; interferon-like . . .	Inappropriate lymphocyte responses in peripheral blood or tissues may mimic states of immunodepression or states of cellular hypersensitivity
Immunoregulation Control of cell traffic through microvasculature and lymphoid system; cooperation between lymphoid cells in immune induction; termination of antigen-mediated cellular responses	Lymphokinetic, migration-inhibitory, lymphocyte-mitogenic, macrophage-activating, chemotactic, permeability-increasing; vasodilatory . . .	Inappropriate stimulation of lymphocytes within lymphoid tissue may generate immunoblasts into peripheral blood with enhanced potential for emigration into tissues (e.g. synovium)

References

1. Dumonde, D. C. (1976). (ed.) *Infection and Immunology in the Rheumatic Diseases.* (London: Blackwell Scientific Publications)
2. Dumonde, D. C. (1971). Rheumatoid arthritis as a disorder of cell-mediated immunity. p. 447. In *Rheumatoid Arthritis, Geigy Colloquium, Basle* (W. Muller, H–G Harwerth and K. Fehr eds.).(London: Academic Press)
3. Sokoloff, L. (1963) The pathophysiology of peripheral blood vessels in collagen diseases p. 120. In *The Peripheral Blood Vessels* (J. H. Orbison and D. E. Smith eds.).(Baltimore: Williams and Wilkins)
4. Gardner, D. L (1978), Pathology of rheumatoid arthritis. p. 273. In *Copeman's Textbook of the Rheumatic Diseases.* 5th Edn. (J. T. Scott ed.).(Edinburgh: Churchill Livingstone) Livingstone)
5. D'Angelo, W. A., Fries, J. F., Masi, A. T. and Shulman, L. E. (1969). Pathologic observations in systemic sclerosis (scleroderma). A study of fifty-eight autopsy cases and fifty-eight matched controls. *Am. J. Med.*, **46,** 428
6. Fassbender, H. G. (1975). *The Pathology of Rheumatic Diseases* (G. Loewi ed.). (New York: Springer-Verlag)
7. Allison, A. C. and Davies, P. (1974). Mechanisms underlying chronic inflammation. p. 449. In *Future Trends in Inflammation* (D. A. Willoughby and J. P. Giroud eds.). (London: Piccin Medical Books)
8. Glynn, L. E. (1977). Discussion of 'future trends'. p. 259. In *Perspectives in Inflammation* (D. A. Willoughby, J. P. Giroud and G. P. Velo eds.) (Lancaster, MTP Press)
9. Klemperer, P., Pollack, A. D. and Baehr, G. (1942). Diffuse collagen disease: acute disseminated lupus erythematosus and diffuse scleroderma. *J. Am. Med. Assoc.*, **119,** 331
10. Gross, L. (1940). The cardiac lesions in Libman-Sacks disease. With a consideration of its relationship to acute diffuse lupus erythematosus. *Am. J. Pathol.*, **16,** 375
11. Burnet, F. M. (1972). *Auto-immunity and Auto-immune Disease.* (Lancaster: MTP Press)
12. Casley-Smith, J. R. (1973). The lymphatic system in inflammation.p. 161. In *The Inflammatory Process*, Vol. 2 B. W. Zweifach (L. Grant and R. T. McCluskey eds.).(New York: Academic Press)
13. Burnet, F. M. (1959). *The Clonal Selection Theory of Acquired Immunity.* (Cambridge: Cambridge University Press)
14. Dumonde, D. C. and Steward, M. W. (1977). The role of microbial infection in rheumatic disease.p. 222. In *Copeman's Textbook of the Rheumatic Diseases.* 5th Edn. (J. T. Scott ed.). (Edinburgh: Churchill Livingstone)
15. Kelly, R. H. (1975). Functional anatomy of lymph nodes. I. The paracortical cords. *Int. Arch. Allergy*, **48,** 836
16. Bloom, B. R. and Bennett, B. (1966). Mechanisms of a reaction *in vitro* associated with delayed-type hypersensitivity. *Science*, **153,** 80
17. David, J. R. (1966). Delayed hypersensitivity *in vitro* and its mediation by cell-free substances formed by lymphoid cell-antigen interaction. *Proc. Nat. Acad. Sci.*, **56,** 72
18. Dumonde, D. C. (1967). Role of the macrophage in delayed hypersensitivity. *Br. Med. Bull.*, **23,** 9
19. Dumonde, D. C., Howson, W. T. and Wolstencroft, R. A. (1968). The role of macrophages and lymphocytes in reactions of delayed hypersensitivity. p. 263. In *Immunopathology: Vth International Symposium* (P. A. Miescher and P. Grabar, eds.).(Basel: Schwabe)
20. Wolstencroft, R. A. and Dumonde, D. C. (1970). *In vitro* studies of cell-mediated immunity: Induction of lymphocyte transformation by a soluble 'mitogenic' factor derived from interaction of sensitized guinea pig lymphoid cells with specific antigen. *Immunology*, **18,** 599
21. David, J. R. and David, R. (1972). Cellular hypersensitivity and cellular immunity. *Progr. Allergy.*, **16,** 300
22. Cerottini, J. C. and Dumonde, D. C. (1971). *In vitro* models of cell-mediated immunity. p.

141. *Proc. 1st. Internat. Congr. Immunol.*, 1971; In *Progress in Immunology* (D. B. Amos ed.) (New York: Academic Press)

23. Dumonde, D. C., Wolstencroft, R. A., Panayi, G. S., Mathew, M., Morley, J. and Howson, W. T. (1969). Lymphokines: non-antibody mediators of cellular immunity generated by lymphocyte activation. *Nature* (London), **224,** 38
24. Dumonde, D. C. (1971). 'Lymphokines': mediators and regulators of cellular immunity. p. 289. In *Immunopathology, VIth International Symposium,* (Grindelwald, 1970) (P. A. Miescher ed.). (Basel: Schwabe)
25. Cohen, S. *et al* (1977). Current state of studies of mediators of cellular immunity: a progress report. *Cell. Immunol.*, **33,** 233
26. Bray, M. A., Dumonde, D. C., Hanson, J., Morley, J., Wolstencroft, R. A. and Smart, J. V. (1976). Heterogeneity of guinea pig lymphokines revealed by parallel bioassay. *Clin. Exp. Immunol.*, **23,** 333
27. Bressler, J., Krzych, V. and Thurman, G. (1976). Release of lymphokines from periodate-treated lymphocytes. *Fed. Proc.*, **42,** 389
28. Dumonde, D. C., Kelly, R. H., Preston, P. M. and Wolstencroft, R. A. (1975). Lymphokines and macrophage function in the immunological response. p. 375. In *Mononuclear Phagocytes* (R. van Furth ed.).(London: Blackwell Scientific Publications)
29. McDaniel, M. C., Laudico, R. and Papermaster, B. W. (1976). Association of macrophage activation factor from a human cultured lymphoid cell line with albumin and α_2 macroglobulin. *Clin. Immunol. Immunopathol.*, **5,** 91
30. Papageorgiou, P. S., Sorokin, C. K. and Glade, P. R. (1974). Similarity of migration-inhibitory factors produced by human lymphoid cell line and phytohaemagglutinin and tuberculin-stimulated human peripheral blood lymphocytes. *J. Immunol.*, **112,** 675
31. Yoshida, T., Kuratsuji, T., Takada, A., Takada, Y., Minowada, J. and Cohen, S. (1976). Lymphokine-like factors produced by human lymphoid cell lines with B or T-cell surface markers. *J. Immunol.*, **117,** 548
32. Dumonde, D. C., Kelly, R. H. and Wolstencroft, R. A. (1972). Molecular pharmacology of cell-mediated immunity. p. 705. In *Microenvironmental Aspects of Immunity* (B. D. Jankovic ed.).(New York: Plenum Press)
33. Kelly, R. H. and Wolstencroft, R. A. (1974). Germinal centre proliferation in response to mitogenic lymphokines. *Clin. Exp. Immunol.*, **18,** 170
34. Kelly, R. H., Wolstencroft, R. A., Dumonde, D. C. and Balfour, B. M. (1972). Role of lymphocyte activation products (LAP) in cell-mediated immunity. II. Effects of lymphocyte activation products on lymph node architecture and evidence for peripheral release of LAP following antigenic stimulation. *Clin. Exp. Immunol.*, **10,** 49
35. Anderson, A. O. and Anderson, N. D. (1976). Lymphocytic emigration from high endothelial venules in rat lymph nodes. *Immunology*, **31,** 731
36. Morley, J. (1976). Prostaglandins as regulators of lymphoid cell function in allergic inflammation: a basis for chronicity in rheumatoid arthritis. p. 511. In *Infection and Immunology in the Rheumatic Diseases* (D. C. Dumonde ed.).(London: Blackwell Scientific Publications)
37. Morley, J., Wolstencroft, R. A. and Dumonde, D. C. (1973). The measurement of lymphokines. Ch. 28. In *Handbook of Experimental Immunology,* 2nd Edn. (D. M. Weir ed.). (Edinburgh: Blackwell Scientific Publications)
38. Dumonde, D. C. and Glynn, L. E. (1962). The production of arthritis in rabbits by an immunological reaction to fibrin. *Br. J. Exp. Pathol.*, **43,** 373
39. Dumonde, D. C., Jones, E. H., Kelly, R. H. and Oates, C. M. (1977). Experimental models of rheumatoid inflammation. p. 4. In *Experimental Models of Chronic Inflammatory Diseases* (L. E. Glynn and H. D. Schlumberger, eds.).(Heidelberg: Springer-Verlag)
40. Dumonde, D. C., Kelly, R. H. and Morley, J. (1976). Lymphoid and microvascular dysfunction in experimental models of rheumatoid inflammation. p. 375. In *Infection and Immunology in the Rheumatic Diseases* (D. C. Dumonde, ed.). (London: Blackwell Scientific Publications)

41. Stastny, P., Cooke, T. D. and Ziff, M. (1973). Production of macrophage migration inhibitory factor in rabbits with experimental arthritis. *Clin. Exp. Immunol.*, **14,** 141
42. Andreis, M., Stastny, P. and Ziff, M. (1974). Experimental arthritis produced by injection of mediators of delayed hypersensitivity. *Arthritis Rheum.*, **17,** 537
43. Franco, M. de F. and Dumonde, D. C. (1975). Unpublished observations
44. Dumonde, D. C. and Glynn, L. E. (1965). The reaction of guinea pigs to autologous and heterologous fibrin implants. *J. Path. Bact.*, **90,** 649
45. Kelly, R. H., Harvey, V. S., Sadler, T. E. and Dumonde, D. C. (1975). Accelerated cytodifferentiation of antibody-secreting cells in guinea pig lymph nodes stimulated by sheep erythrocytes and lymphokines. *Clin. Exp. Immunol.*, **21,** 141
46. Williams, R. C. (1977). Lymphocyte abnormalities in rheumatoid arthritis. *Arthritis Rheum.*, **20,** (6): suppl. p. 34
47. Van de Putte, L. B. A., De Vries, E., van Leewen, A. W. F. M. and Meijer, C. J. L. M. (1977). T-lymphocytes and rheumatoid inflammation. p. 103. In *Non-articular forms of Rheumatoid Arthritis* (T. E. W. Feltkamp, ed.).(Leyden: Stafleu's Scientific Publishing Co.)
48. Maini, R. N., Roffe, L. M. and Horsfall, A. C. (1977). Lymphocytes, lymphokines and rheumatoid arthritis. p. 111. In *Non-articular forms of Rheumatoid Arthritis* (T. E. W. Feltkamp, ed.). (Leyden: Stafleu's Scientific Publishing Co.)
49. Horsfall, A. C., Roffe, L. M., Maini, R. N., Hanson, J., Wolstencroft, R. A. and Dumonde, D. C. (1978). Lymphokine production by explanted rheumatoid synovia (in preparation)
50. Bresnihan, B., Oliver, M. and Hughes, G. R. V. (1977). Lymphocytotoxic antibodies in systemic lupus erythematosus: association with cerebral manifestations. *Ann. Rheum. Dis.*, **36**, 481P
51. Bacon, P. A., Sewell, R. L. and Crowther, D. (1975). Reactive lymphoid cells ('immunoblasts') in autoimmune and haematological disorders. *Clin. Exp. Immunol.*, **19,** 201
52. Eghtedari, A. A., Esselinckx, W. and Bacon, P. A. (1976). Circulating immunoblasts in polymyalgia rheumatica. *Ann. Rheum. Dis.*, **35,** 158
53. Greaves, M. F. and Williams, R. C. (1978) Standardization of lymphocyte surface marker tests. In *Laboratory Tests in the Rheumatic Diseases* (D. C. Dumonde and M. W. Steward eds.). (Lancaster: MTP Press)
54. Zurier, R. B., Doty, J. and Goldenberg, A. (1977). Cyclic AMP response to prostaglandin E_1 in mononuclear cells from peripheral blood and synovial fluid of patients with rheumatoid arthritis. *Prostaglandins*, **13,** (1), 25
55. Gordon, D., Bray, M. A. and Morley, J. (1976). Control of lymphokine secretion by prostaglandins. *Nature*, **262,** 401
56. Henney, C. S., Bourne, H. R. and Lichtenstein, L. M. (1972). The role of cyclic 3′, 5′ adenosine monophosphate in specific cytolytic activity of lymphocytes. *J. Immunol.*, **108,** 1526
57. Melmon, K. L., Blurne, H. R., Weinstein, Y., Shearer, G. M., Kram, J. and Bauminger, S. (1974). Haemolytic plaque formation by leukocytes *in vitro*. *J. Clin. Invest.*, **53,** 13
58. Webb, D. R. and Jamieson, A. T. (1976). Control of mitogen-induced transformation: characterization of a splenic suppressor cell and its mode of action. *Cell. Immunol.*, **24,** 45
59. Goodwin, J. S., Bankhurst, A. D. and Messner, R. P. (1977). Suppression of human T-cell mitogenesis by prostaglandin. *J. Exp. Med.*, **146,** 1719
60. Lomnitzer, R., Rabson, A. R. and Koornhoe, H. J. (1976). The effects of cyclic AMP on leukocyte inhibitory factor production and on the inhibition of leukocyte migration. *Clin. Exp. Immunol.*, **24,** 42
61. Quagliata, F., Lawrence, V. J. W. and Phillips-Quagliata, J. M. (1973). Prostaglandin E_1 as a regulator of lymphocyte function. *Cell. Immunol.*, **6,** 457
62. Smith, J. W., Steiner, A. L. and Parker, C. W. (1971). Human lymphocyte metabolism: effects of cyclic and non-cyclic nucleotides on stimulation by phytohaemagglutinin. *J. Clin. Invest.*, **50,** 442
63. Bourne, H. R., Lichtenstein, L. M., Melmon, K. L., Henney, C. S., Weinstein, Y. and

Shearer, G. M. (1974). Modulation of inflammation and immunity by cyclic AMP. *Science*, **184,** 19

64. Dumonde, D. C., Jose, P. J., Page, D. A. and Williams, T. J. (1977). Production of prostaglandins by porcine endothelial cells in culture. *Br. J. Pharmacol.*, **61,** (3) 504
65. Kasp-Grochowska, E., Page, D. A., Jose, P., Williams, T. J. and Dumonde, D. C. (1978). Suppression of lymphocyte transformation by products of cultured vascular endothelial cells (in preparation)
66. Morley, J. (1974). Prostaglandins and lymphokines in arthritis. *Prostaglandins*, **8,** 315
67. Dayer, J. M., Robinson, D. R. and Krane, S. M. (1977). Prostaglandin production by rheumatoid synovial cells: stimulation by a factor from human mononuclear cells. *J. Exp. Med.*, **145,** 1399
68. Robinson, D. R., Smith, H., McGuire, M. B. and Levine, L. (1975). Prostaglandin synthesis by rheumatoid synovium and its stimulation by colchicine. *Prostaglandins*, **10,** 67
69. Husby, G. Bankhurst, A. D. and Williams, R. C. (1977). Immunohistochemical localization of prostaglandin E (PGE) in rheumatoid synovial tissues. *Arthritis Rheum.*, **20,** 785
70. Polverini, P. J., Cotran, R. S. and Sholley, M. M. (1977). Endothelial proliferation in delayed hypersensitivity: an autoradiographic study. J. *Immunol.*, **118,** 529
71. Dumonde, D. C. and Maini, R. N. (1971). The clinical significance of mediators of cellular immunity. *Clin. Allergy*, **1,** 111
72. Koopman, W. J., Gillis, M. H. and David, J. R. (1973). Prevention of MIF activity by agents known to increase cyclic AMP. *J. Immunol.*, **110,** 1609
73. Editorial (1978). Lymphokines: an increasing repertoire. *Br. Med. J.*, (i) 62
74. Stastny, P., Rosenthal, M., Andreis, M. and Ziff, M. (1975). Lymphokines in the rheumatoid joint. *Arthritis Rheum.*, **18,** 237

14
Recognition of Anti-Rheumatic Drugs using the Homograft Reaction

M. K. JASANI, JEAN M. ROBERTS, M. D. TALBOT and M. F. TWEED

INTRODUCTION

Although between six and ten potential anti-inflammatory (AIF) compounds are patented every month there is still much scope for an innovative approach to their pharmacological evaluation. This is because the currently employed predictive tests involving for example stabilization of lysosomes, inhibition of the biosynthesis of prostaglandins, suppression of experimental foot-pad oedema, cotton pellet granuloma test, u.v.-induced erythema test and adjuvant arthritis, have failed so far to recognize compounds which could reverse joint swelling, arrest synovial hypertrophy and prevent erosive articular damage in rheumatoid arthritis (RA).

An important reason why such tests might not select desirable anti-rheumatic drugs is that, apart from adjuvant arthritis, none of them involves a role for immunological factors, e.g. immune complexes and immune lymphocytes, known to be important in the development of rheumatoid synovial inflammation.

It is possible that maximally-tolerated doses of presently available anti-rheumatic drugs, while relieving joint pain, fail to inhibit rheumatoid synovitis and erosive articular damage because they cannot suppress inflammation caused by immune lymphocytes. To test this hypothesis, the pharmacological action of several compounds was characterized using rabbit skin homografts. The present report reviews these observations and discusses why the homograft reaction may provide a better means for the recognition of more efficacious anti-rheumatic drugs.

BACKGROUND TO LYMPHOCYTE HYPOTHESIS

Phagocytosis of immune complexes by polymorphonuclear leukocytes or macrophages results in the release of lysosomal enzymes (Figure 14.1) which, according to the antibody hypothesis[1,2], are chiefly responsible for the initiation of rheumatoid inflammation and erosion of bone and cartilage. If this were the only explanation for the development of rheumatoid inflammation, drugs capable of inhibiting the release of lysosomal enzymes should prevent all the consequences of the disease process.

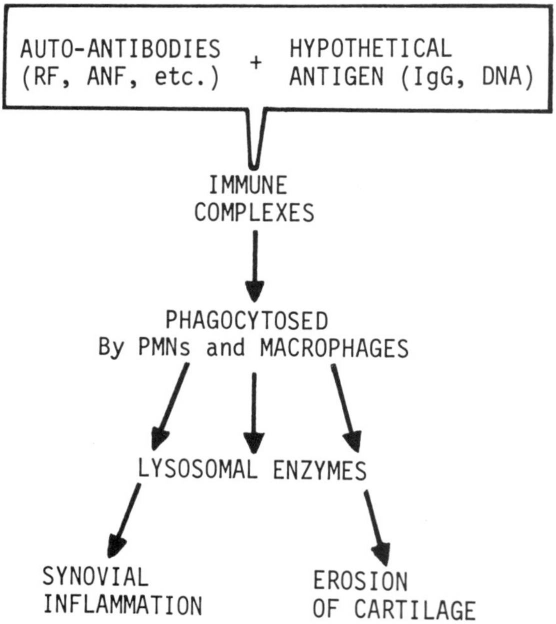

Figure 14.1 The antibody hypothesis (1968) to explain the pathogenesis of rheumatoid joint inflammation

However, as is the common clinical experience, in many patients the inflamed joints and tendon sheaths remain swollen despite adequate relief of pain with maximally-tolerated doses of drugs such as indomethacin and corticosteroids which are known to inhibit the release of lysosomal enzymes[3,4]. In time, the joints which remain swollen become grossly deformed owing to erosive destruction of bone and cartilage.

To account for the therapeutic failure, it was proposed[5], as outlined in Figure 14.2, that the immunological disorder underlying RA involves not only a role for immune complexes but also for immune lymphocytes of the type which initiate the rejection of kidney homografts; and that the failure of drugs such as indomethacin and corticosteroids to arrest rheumatoid inflammation reflected

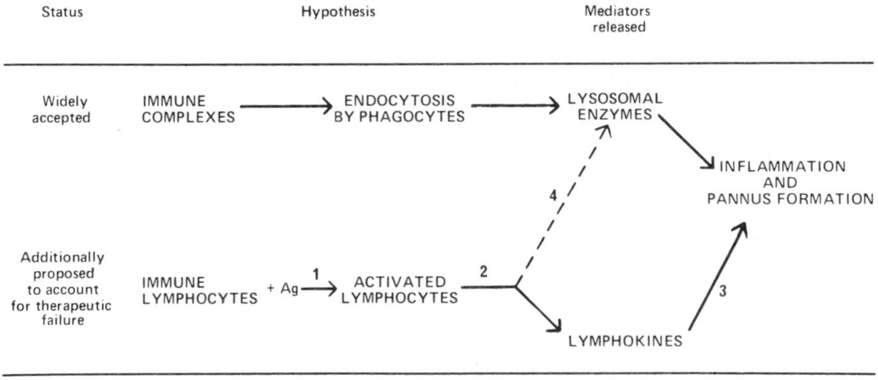

Figure 14.2 A revised view of the pathogenesis of rheumatoid joint inflammation incorporating a role for immune lymphocytes in addition to that widely accepted for the immune complexes. Inability of currently available anti-rheumatic drugs either to inhibit antigen-induced activation of immune lymphocytes (site 1), or the release of lymphokines which such cells release (site 2), or the vascular effects of lymphokines (site 3) could account for their failure to arrest rheumatoid synovial swelling and articular damage (lymphocyte hypothesis[5]). A role for lysosomal enzymes (site 4) in addition to that for lymphokines in the development of inflammation caused by immune lymphocytes is not precluded by the lymphocyte hypothesis[49]

their inability to prevent either the antigen-induced activation of immune lymphocytes or the release of lymphokines.

Evidence in support of the lymphocyte hypothesis includes the fact that circulating RA lymphocytes show (a) increased RNA:DNA ratio[6] as do lymphocytes of patients with kidney homografts[7], (b) morphological features of mitogenically and antigenically stimulated lymphocytes[8], and (c) ability to kill autologous synovial lining cells[9]. However, the possibility that such lymphocytes may cause inflammation could not be seriously entertained until recently when several investigators[10,11] established that depletion of circulating RA lymphocytes by drainage of thoracic duct lymph improves joint pain, stiffness and swelling; whereas the intra-articular instillation of the harvested lymphocytes reprecipitates joint inflammation. More recent evidence[12–14] shows clearly that T-lymphocytes, capable of synthesizing lymphokines rather than antibodies predominate in the mononuclear cell infiltrate in the rheumatoid synovium, and that lymphokines are readily detectable in the joint fluid[15].

So although in 1968, when the present programme of research began, there was only scanty evidence in support of the lymphocyte hypothesis, today there would seem little doubt as to the importance of immune lymphocytes in the pathogenesis of rheumatoid inflammation.

To test whether drugs such as indomethacin and corticosteroids were unable to prevent inflammation caused by immune lymphocytes, it was necessary to resort to experimental studies. The homograft reaction, i.e. the inflammatory response stimulated by tissues transplanted from one individual to another of the same species[16], was chosen because it is known to be initiated by circulating immune lymphocytes[17]. Skin was preferred to synovium because of its accessibility for serial examination.

EXPERIMENTAL SYSTEM AND PROTOCOL

Skin graft model

The experimental system employed for the present investigations is referred to as the skin graft model because it involves the study of both homografts and autografts. As explained in Table 14.1, homografts consisted of skin transferred from a New Zealand White (NZW) donor rabbit to a Norfolk (NFK) recipient. Autografts consisted of similar pieces of NFK animal's skin sutured on to itself.

Immune lymphocytes infiltrate the homografts, but not the autografts and their entry is recognized by the onset of necrosis of the grafted cells and the rejection of the graft itself. In other respects homografts resemble autografts, in that they also develop initially a non-specific inflammatory reaction caused by the trauma of surgery.

Protocol

The experiments were designed, as described below, to overcome two major limitations.

(1) Since lymphocytic inflammation occurs together with non-specific inflammation in the homografts (Table 14.1) it was essential to distinguish

Table 14.1. Essential experimental features of the skin graft model and the basis for inflammation in auto- and homografts

	Rabbit	*Immune lymphocytes*	*Inflammation*
Homo-grafts	NZW → NFK	Present (necrosis)	Lymphocytic + non-specific
Auto-grafts	NFK → NFK	Not present (no necrosis)	Non-specific ONLY

between the effect of anti-inflammatory (AIF) drugs on lymphocytic inflammation and on non-specific inflammation. This was achieved by comparing the effect of each drug on the inflammatory response in homografts with that in autografts.

(2) Most AIF drugs interfere with immunization, i.e. they prevent or delay the emergence in the recipient animal of circulating or immune sensitized lymphocytes (CiSLs) which initiate inflammation, fibrin deposition and

necrosis in the homograft[18–20]. To measure activity against inflammation caused by immune lymphocytes it was therefore essential to avoid immunosuppression. This was achieved by adopting the protocol outlined in Figure 14.3.

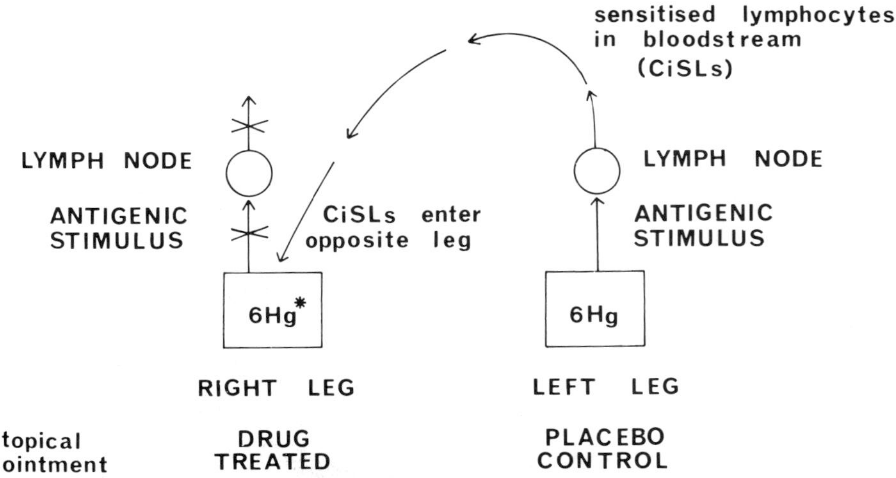

Figure 14.3 Protocol of experiments designed to measure activity against inflammation caused by immune lymphocytes without causing immunosuppression, i.e. avoiding interference by the drug with the emergence of circulating immune or sensitized lymphocytes (CiSLs). Six homografts (Hg) were transplanted on to each hind-limb of the recipient animal and the anti-inflammatory drug was applied topically to one set only, denoted by the asterisk. The placebo-treated set on the opposite leg provided the antigenic stimulus and so guaranteed the development of immune lymphocytes in the regional lymph node and their subsequent entry into the circulation via the femoral lymphatics and thoracic lymph duct. The immune lymphocytes (see Figure 14.4), then enter the homografts on the opposite leg, where the drug is tested. In this way, the activity of a drug against inflammation caused by immune lymphocytes can be tested even if it is capable of blocking immunization at various sites in the right leg

MATERIALS AND METHODS

Animals

Experiments were made using male New Zealand white (NZW) rabbits as donors and albino Norfolks (NFK) as recipients. The NFK rabbits were purchased from Morton Commercial Rabbits, Stanstead, Essex; whereas the NZW rabbits were obtained from several sources including Ranch Rabbits, Crawley Down, Sussex.

Anaesthesia was induced using pentobarbitone sodium (40 mg/kg) injected into the marginal ear vein and its level was maintained by further administration (10 mg/kg every 20 min) via a cannula inserted into the ear vein.

The donor rabbits were killed after removal of skin grafts and control skin;

the recipients were allowed to recover and were re-anaesthetized repeatedly for examination of the grafts. Mortality was around 10% and was solely due to overdose of the anaesthetic.

Operative procedures

With the animals fully anaesthetized the following operative procedures were carried out employing antiseptics and aseptic precautions described previously[21].

(1) *Homografts.* From the right leg of the donor animal 12 pieces of full-thickness skin (2.5 cm × 2.5 cm) were dissected free of the underlying connective tissue. The grafts were placed in a sterile petri dish on a gauze swab

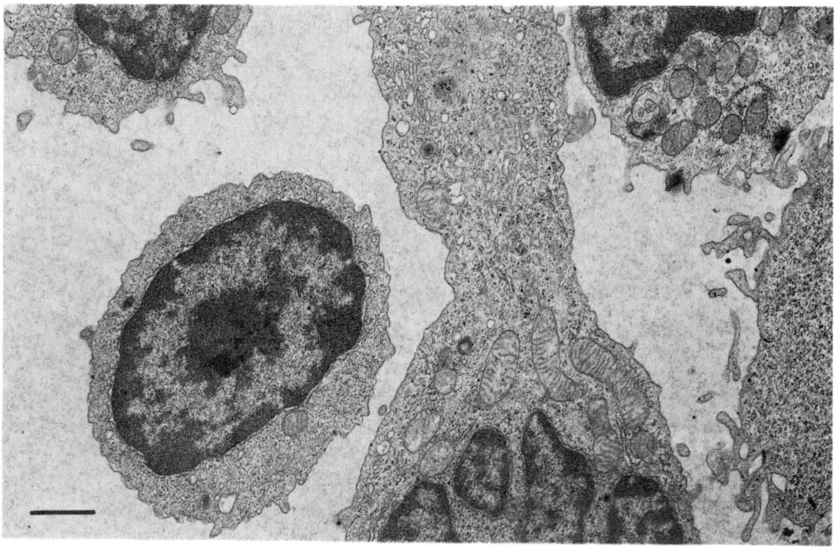

Figure 14.4 One type of immune or sensitized lymphocyte found in the femoral lymph draining right popliteal node of a NFK recipient bearing six homografts on the right leg and destined to enter the circulation via the thoracic lymph duct. Compared with the normal looking lymphocyte to the left, the immune lymphocyte exhibits several distinct morphological features including especially the long cytoplasmic protuberance called the uropod and shown by several investigators[62,63] to be characteristic of lymphocytes exhibiting *in vitro* cytotoxicity. The presence of such lymphocytes in the microvasculature of homografts was found to be intimately associated with the onset of necrosis of the epidermal and follicular cells[19] (× 8000) (by permission of *Cell Biology Reports*)

dampened with sterile physiological saline and kept at 4 °C for 15–30 min until weighed. Using sterile forceps, each graft was transferred singly to a tared sterile petri dish containing a damp swab, weighed and replaced in the storage petri dish. Once weighed, the grafts were bathed in ice-cold saline for 15–60 min. Each graft was held at one corner with dissecting forceps and any blood remaining on its surface removed by gently brushing the convex surface of a pair of tonsil forceps over the graft.

Six grafts were transplanted on to suitable beds prepared over various anatomical sites as shown in Figure 14.5 and Figure 14.6 in the right leg, and the remainder were transplanted over identical sites in the opposite leg of the same recipient. The grafts were secured into place with continuous 5/0 silk sutures, sprayed with Polybactrin powder (Calmic Ltd., Crewe, England) and

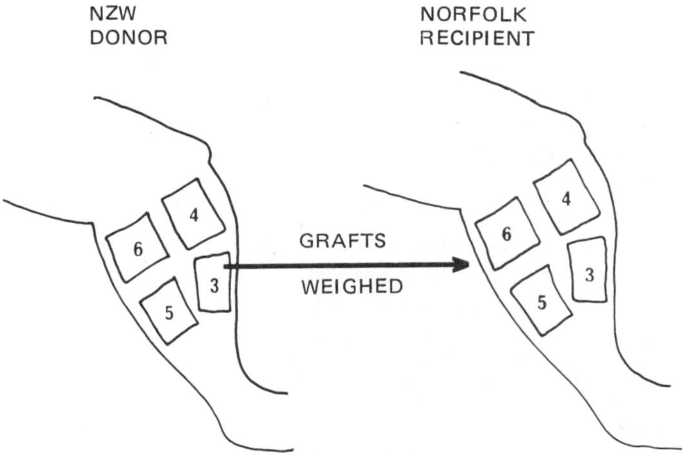

Figure 14.5 Sites 3 to 6 that were routinely employed for the transplantation of skin on to the lateral aspect of rabbit hind-limbs. Sites 1 and 2 were on the medial aspect (see Figure 14.6). Homografts were made by transfer of skin from a site on donor NZW rabbit on to a corresponding site on NFK recipients

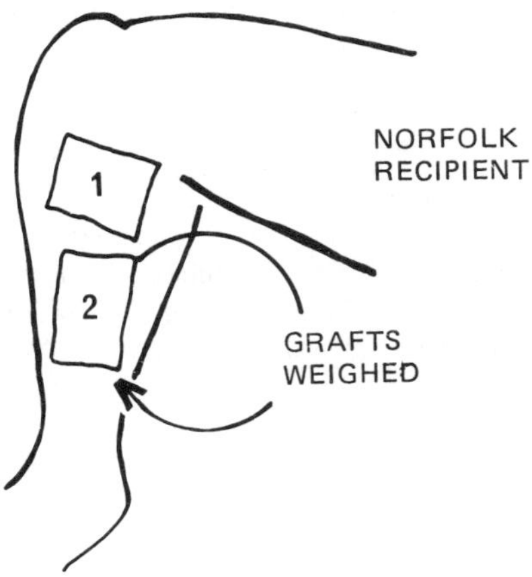

Figure 14.6 Autografts were made by re-suturing of skin on to the same site from which it had been dissected

covered with gauze swabs impregnated with liquid paraffin and Soframycin (Roussel), then dry dressings and finally elastoplast. The day of grafting is referred to as day 0.

(2) *Autografts*. From both hind limbs of a NFK rabbit full-thickness skin (2.5 cm × 2.5 cm) was dissected from each of six sites shown in Figures 5 and 6. They were weighed as described above, washed with sterile physiological saline and sutured on to the same site from which they were dissected.

Control skin

Control skin for homograft experiments was obtained by dissecting post-mortem the skin overlying the area between the left knee and ankle of each donor NZW rabbit. Control skin for autograft experiments was obtained by removal of an ellipsoid piece from the medial and lateral aspect of each leg of the NFK animal. The incision was then sutured, sprayed with Polybactrin powder and dressings in the same way as the skin grafts.

Control skin was used to measure indirectly the amount of DNA, protein and moisture content contained in each graft at the time of transplantation (initial value). It was also employed to estimate the dry weight of tissue transplanted in order to standardize the amount of drug applied to each graft.

Substances administered

A standard amount of the ointment (1 mg/mg dry weight of skin grafted) containing equimolar doses of one of six AIF compounds was applied to each graft immediately after operation (day 0) and once daily then onwards until the end of the experiment. The six AIF substances studied were: acetylsalicylic acid (ASA), indomethacin (INDO), phenylbutazone (PBZ), chlorflumethasone (CF), flumethasone pivalate (FP) and fluocinolone acetonide (FA).

Values shown in Table 14.2 indicate the average quantity of each drug applied daily for 6 days to each graft.

Table 14.2. The average total amount of drug received by each graft after six once daily applications of four anti-inflammatory compounds in the experiments of Figures 14.11, 12, 16 and 17. Values are mean ± SE*

	Dry weight of graft (mg)	*Mean Total amount of drug* (μg)
Fluocinolone acetonide (0.025%)	58.1 ± 1.1	8.7 ± 0.2
Indomethacin (0.02%)	63.0 ± 9.1	7.6 ± 1.1
Phenylbutazone (0.02%)	83.7 ± 5.4	10.0 ± 0.7
Acetylsalicylic acid (0.01%)	58.2 ± 8.4	3.5 ± 0.5

* The molar concentration of drug with respect to graft is the same in all experiments. This was possible through the choice of percentage concentration (w/v) of various ointments on the basis of the molecular weights of the four drugs and by application of a standard amount (1 mg/mg dry weight tissue grafted). Values for CF (0.025%) and FP (0.025%) were similar to those for fluocinolone acetonide

Grafts on the contralateral limb received an equivalent amount of the ointment base.

Routine examination of grafts

In order to inspect the grafts daily, the animals were re-anaesthetized with a full dose of pentobarbitone sodium and the dressings were removed under aseptic conditions. After inspection, Polybactrin and the standard amount of ointment, or ointment base, was reapplied to each graft and the leg bandaged once more in sterile dressings and elastoplast.

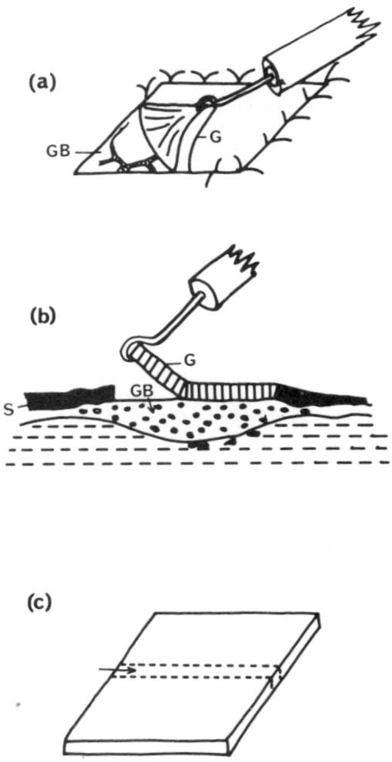

Figure 14.7 Removal and biopsy of skin grafts: (a) to show how, once the sutures were removed, it was easy to separate the graft (G) from the underlying vascular graft bed (GB); (b) to show the relationship of the graft (G) to the inflamed graft bed (GB) and the surrounding healthy skin (S); (c) to show the site of removal of tissue for histological examination (↓)

A homologous pair (grafts transplanted on to identical anatomical sites on the opposite legs) was removed daily for examination starting on day 3. Previously reported observations[22] show that the rate and extent of increase in various parameters is significantly influenced by the anatomical position of the graft; increases in the medial grafts (Figure 3) were earlier and lower than in the lateral grafts. Therefore, in all animals grafts belonging to the medial position 1 were removed on day 3, position 2 on day 4, lateral position 3 on day 5, etc.

Each graft was removed by separating it gently from its underlying connective tissue which then constituted the graft bed as illustrated in Figure 14.7a and b. Bleeding was stopped with a piece of sterile gauze pressed firmly over the graft bed. The dressings were then completed as described above.

After removal, the grafts were weighed wrapped in tared aluminium foil to minimize loss of moisture. Biopsies were taken as shown in Figure 14.7c. The graft including the inflammatory cellular and fibrinous exudate was dissected to yield a 3–4 mm wide strip of tissue which was fixed in 10% buffered formalin for histological examination. The remaining tissue was stored frozen (−20 °C) for the determination of DNA, protein and moisture content.

Qualitative assessments

Inflammatory vascular changes were assessed by visual inspection. Vasodilatation was assessed as degree of redness. Stasis in the homografts[23,24] was judged by a change in their colour from bright pink to reddish purple. Cyanosis which followed shortly after stasis was recognized by the appearance of blueness.

Presence or absence of lymphocytes, polymorphonuclear leukocytes, necrosis of grafted epidermal cells, venous congestion[25] and rupture of graft vessels in the homografts[26] were judged by light microscopic examination of sections ($<5\ \mu m$) made from paraffin-embedded tissue and stained with haematoxylin and eosin. Lymphocytes were recognized as mononuclear inflammatory cells and identified by examination of resin-embedded tissue by light and electron microscopy[19].

Measurements

Since little is still known about the *in vivo* effects of lymphokines[27], swelling of grafts and changes in their main constituents (moisture, protein, DNA and blood) were assessed gravimetrically using the chemical methods described below.

Swelling. It was measured as the increase in weight of the graft, i.e. as the difference in weight before suturing and after removal.

Hyperaemia. Regarded as the increase in blood content, it was assessed as described elsewhere[28] from the increase in haemoglobin content of the graft.

DNA. Grafts and control skin were chopped finely in the frozen state and portions (50–100 mg) were placed into tared glass centrifuge tubes (15 ml) and weighed. For dehydration and lipid extraction each portion was subjected to the Schneider procedure[29]. This involved treatment with 10% ice-cold trichloracetic acid, TCA (5 ml) for 30 min, frequent agitation of the suspension and centrifugation at 4 °C. This step was repeated and followed by extraction at 4 °C for 30 min in 70% alcohol (5 ml) containing 5% (w/v) sodium acetate to neutralize excess TCA. Then the tissues were stored overnight in the cold in absolute alcohol (5 ml). The following morning the tissues were centrifuged, extracted once more with absolute alcohol at room temperature and recentrifuged. The residues were then extracted once in alcohol: ether (3 : 1) and twice in ether before evaporation to dryness at room temperature.

This lipid-free, acid-insoluble residue was weighed, suspended in 0.5 M perchloric acid (5 ml) and stored at 4 °C for at least 24 h. It was then heated for 20 min at 70 °C in the water-bath, centrifuged and re-extracted. The two extracts were combined and DNA was estimated as described by Burton[30] using calf thymus DNA as a standard. Following two extractions only 2.1% DNA remained on average in the final sediment.

Total protein. This was measured as the weight of acid-insoluble, lipid-free dried proteinaceous residue obtained using the Schneider procedure described above. In this way it was possible to measure not only the changes in water-soluble proteins due to increased vascular permeability or synthesis of cytoplasmic proteins but also those due to increased synthesis of structural proteins such as collagen or deposition of water-insoluble proteins such as fibrin.

Water-soluble protein content. To solubilize the proteins, the chopped grafts (80–240 mg, wet weight) were homogenized individually with a Polytron Homogenizer (Northern Media Supply Ltd., Brough, North Humberside, UK) in ice-cold 0.15 M sucrose medium (5.0 ml) for 60 sec at maximum speed. This isotonic medium also contained the following electrolytes: $MgCl_2$ (9 mM), KCl (75 mM), Tris buffer pH 7.4 at 37 °C (35 mM). The homogenate was centrifuged (5000 *g* for 15 min) at 4 °C (MSE Major Centrifuge, 8 place rotor 6875) and the clear supernatant retained. The sediment was resuspended in 4.5 ml homogenizing medium and rehomogenized. Triton X-100 (0.5 ml, 2%) was added to the homogenate which was then agitated intermittently for 30 min before centrifugation at 1400 *g* for 10 min. The clear supernatant was combined with that obtained after the first homogenization and the pooled supernatants employed for the determination of water-soluble protein.

Control skin was homogenized similarly though in larger amounts (0.75–1.5 g in 9.0 ml).

To a portion (2.5 ml) of the pooled supernatants 20% TCA (2.5 ml) was added to denature the solubilized proteins. The ice-cold mixture was agitated and 30 min later centrifuged. The sediment was then subjected to the Schneider procedure. The lipid-free dried residue was weighed to measure the amount of water-soluble protein present in the graft. Schneider procedure was preferred to the method of Lowry[31] as it enabled a direct comparison to be made with the determinations of the total protein content.

Water-insoluble protein content. This was calculated as the difference between the total and the water-soluble protein in the graft.

Moisture content. This was measured as the difference between the wet and dry weight of each graft. This was possible because (a) the hind-limb skin of rabbit is virtually devoid of fat, (b) inflammation did not result in deposition of fat.

Simple dehydration. This was employed to determine the amount of dry weight transplanted in order to standardize the amount of ointment applied per graft. A portion of chopped control skin (400–600 mg) was placed in preweighed aluminium cups and dried in a hot air oven at 60 °C to constant weight.

Basis for quantification

Changes in all the parameters were estimated either as the difference between the initial and final values and expressed in the appropriate units (e.g. mg for weight, μg for DNA), or as % increase in initial value.

The initial value was estimated from the biochemical composition of control skin and the wet weight of each graft before suturing, e.g. initial DNA content = DNA (μg/mg control skin) × initial weight of graft. The final value was obtained from the analysis and weight of the graft on removal.

RESULTS

Inflammatory changes in control skin grafts

Outward appearance

Differences between changes in the outward appearance of the two types of graft were as described previously[21,26]. Essentially, up to day 5 the homografts resembled autografts. Then whilst the inflammation subsided in the autografts, it became more acute in the homografts. For instance between days 5 and 8, swelling in the autografts subsided and they became pale pink like the surrounding skin. By contrast, swelling in the homografts became more prominent and they felt firm (indurated) instead of soft on palpation. In addition, the healthy bright pink colour of the homografts changed to dull blue (cyanosis). In the majority of animals bearing 12 homografts this occurred on, or around, day 6. By day 8 the homografts appeared black, felt hard and were completely necrosed.

Light microscopy

The microscopical appearance of the homografts also differed from that of the autografts as reported previously by several investigators[25,26]. Apart from the intravascular localization of lymphocytes in only the homograft, the principal difference found between the two types of graft on day 6 was the fact (see Figure 14.8) that at a time when the epidermal and follicular cells of the autografts showed signs of active proliferation, the corresponding cells of the homografts were either necrotic or about to be necrosed (Figure 14.8).

As previously reported[19], necrosis of the epithelial cells in homografts was (a) preceded 2 to 3 days earlier by the intravascular localization of lymphocytes which showed morphological features found in lymphocytes activated by

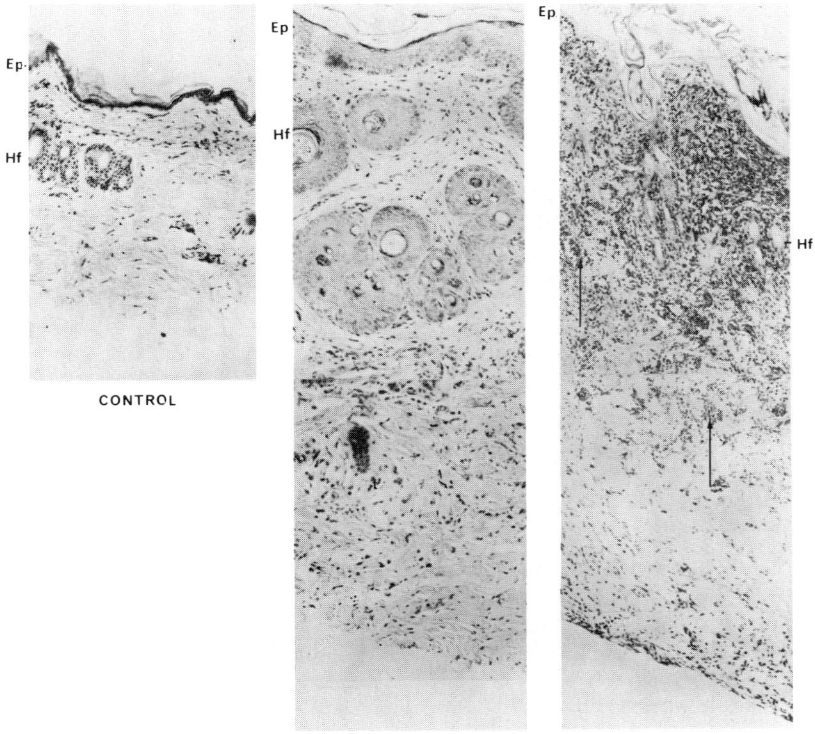

Figure 14.8 Presence of epidermal (Ep) and follicular (Hf) cell necrosis in the homograft (HG) but not autograft (AG) removed from NFK recipients on day 6, day 0 being the day of transplantation. Light microscope view (× 120) of sections (5 μm) of paraffin-embedded tissue stained with haematoxylin and eosin. Note the epidermal and follicular cells of autografts have proliferated several-fold compared with non-grafted control skin, and the connective tissue of the homograft but not that of the autograft is grossly cellular on account of the infiltration of inflammatory cells. Haemorrhages (↓) are also present only in the homograft.

phytohaemagglutinin, PHA[32], (b) associated with the presence of uropod-bearing lymphocytes (CiSLs) which developed in the popliteal lymph nodes (Figures 14.3 and 14.4), circulated in the femoral lymph[19] and entered the homografts via the systemic circulation.

Results of histological examination failed, however, to substantiate the impression gained from gross inspection that the degree of swelling in homografts was significantly greater than that of the autografts.

Swelling

Results summarized in Figure 14.9 show that when epithelial necrosis commenced in six out of nine animals and even 24 h before that, the degree of

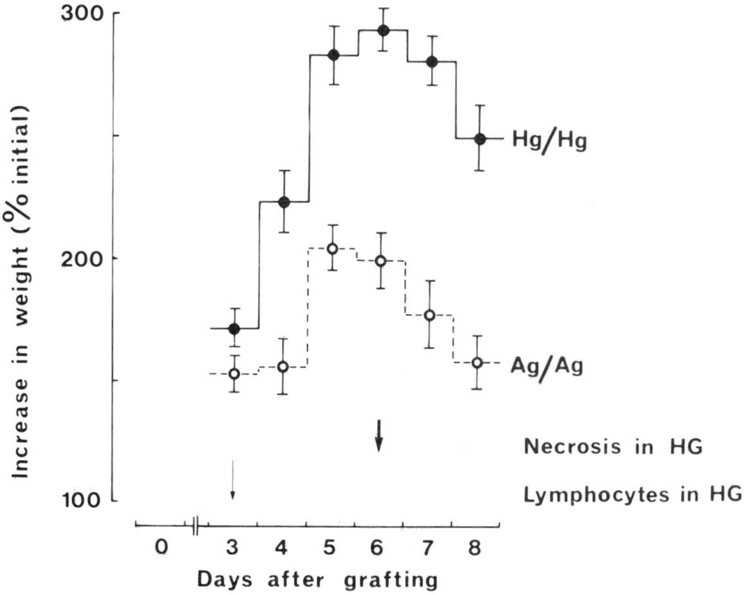

Figure 14.9 Comparison of swelling, measured as percentage increase in wet weight, of homografts (Hg/Hg) of nine NFK rabbits bearing six homografts on each hind-limb and autografts (Ag/Ag) of seven NFK rabbits bearing six autografts on each hind-limb. Arrows indicate the time when (a) the intravascular localization of lymphocytes and (b) necrosis of the donor epidermal cells first became evident in a majority of the homografts, day 0 being the day of transplantation

swelling measured as increase in the wet weight was at least 2-fold greater in homografts than in comparable autografts. The mean increase (final − initial) in the wet weight of day 6 homografts of nine rabbits was 377.1 ($\pm$21.9 mg, SE) compared with 184.4 $\pm$ 12.3 in comparable autografts of seven animals, the differences being highly significant ($p < 0.001$).

Hyperaemia

Increase in the blood content accounted for 234.8 $\pm$ 27.4 mg of the rise in the wet weight of day 6 homografts and 145.8 $\pm$ 19.5 mg in that of the corresponding autografts ($p < 0.02$).

DNA

Increase in the cellularity of day 6 homografts was nearly 7-fold the initial value, but in terms of the rise in their weight, DNA accounted for only 173.8 $\pm$ 13.1 μg ($p < 0.001$).

Protein

Accumulation of blood proteins and the synthesis of tissue proteins, including collagen, minus the degradation of blood and/or tissue proteins accounted for a net rise of 82.2 ± 6.1 mg; the corresponding value for autografts was statistically significantly lower: 28.5 ± 4.2 mg, $p < 0.001$. The increase in homografts comprised a rise of 49.4 ± 3.4 mg of water-soluble and 35.8 ± 3.8 mg of water-insoluble protein.

Moisture content

Accumulation of fluid due to (a) increase in the blood content, (b) increased cellularity, (c) exudation and retention of fluid[28], *minus* dehydration of the graft following onset of epidermal necrosis accounted for a mean rise of 301.6 ± 17.8 mg in the wet weights of day 6 homografts. By contrast, in day 6 autografts in all of which both the cuticle and the epidermis remained intact, the increase in moisture content accounted for a rise of 159.9 ± 12.1 mg in the wet weight; the value being significantly lower than that found in the homografts ($p < 0.001$).

In addition, whereas hyperaemia accounted for most of the rise in the moisture content of day 6 autografts, it accounted for only a part of the increase in the moisture content of the homografts of all the six animals which did not show evidence of epidermal necrosis on day 5. The mean difference between the rise in moisture and blood contents of the homografts was 132.7 ± 44.0 (SD) mg ($p < 0.001$); whereas that for similar autografts was only 14.5 ± 10.4 mg ($p < 0.01$).

However, in homografts of the three animals which developed epidermal necrosis on day 5 the corresponding individual values for the rise in moisture content not accounted for by hyperaemia were: -35.7, -35.7 and -124.2 mg; the negative signs indicating a deficit, presumably arising from loss of fluid through dehydration.

Conclusion

Taken together the results of gravimetric analysis show that the *extra* swelling of day 6 homografts as compared with that of the corresponding autografts (Figure 14.9) is due mainly to a rise in the moisture content. Hyperaemia and the rise in protein account for it to a lesser extent and DNA accounts for it to only a negligible extent.

Previously it has been shown that as long as cyclophosphamide (750 mg per animal, administered over 10 days) prevents the entry of CiSLs and the development of cyanosis, epidermal necrosis, intralymphatic fibrin deposition and haemorrhages, neither the degree of swelling, nor the increase in DNA, protein or moisture content of homografts differs significantly from the corresponding measurements in the comparable autografts[18,33]. The data indicate that changes in the various parameters in homografts due solely to non-specific inflammation caused by the trauma of surgery equals that of the autografts and therefore, the differences between the two types of graft measure the degree of change caused by activated immune lymphocytes.

Thus in physiological terms the results of gravimetric analysis suggest that the swelling of homografts associated with inflammation caused by immune lymphocytes is characterized by a rise in moisture content due, as explained elsewhere[28], to retention of fluid in the extravascular space. And, in pharmacological terms they provide two useful yardsticks: firstly, that drugs fully active against inflammation caused by immune lymphocytes ought to lower the increase in the weight of homografts to that of comparable drug-treated autografts and secondly that when they fail to do so it could be because they failed to prevent oedema, i.e. retention of fluid in the extravascular space.

Effect of topical drug treatment on inflammation caused by immune lymphocytes

Acetylsalicylic acid

Despite clear-cut evidence of intravascular localization of lymphocytes (Figure 14.10), mild venous congestion and cyanosis, aspirin applied once daily in amounts indicated in Table 14.2 depressed the increase in the wet weight of homografts (Hg*) to the level found in autografts (Ag*) (Figure 14.11) – the asterisk denotes the set which received the drug topically.

Results of gravimetric analysis summarized in Table 14.3 show that aspirin profoundly depressed the rise in the DNA content of the homografts. Histologically, as shown by Figure 14.10a, the lowering of DNA was associated not with the inhibition of epidermal hyperplasia but with inhibition of the migration of inflammatory cells from the blood vessels. Results of Table 14.3 show also that aspirin lowered the swelling associated with inflammation caused by immune lymphocytes largely through lowering of the moisture content but also to a lesser extent through depression of the protein content. Additional results of gravimetric analysis, including especially the measurement of hyperaemia, summarized in Table 14.4, indicate that in the four animals in which epidermal necrosis did not begin on day 5, i.e. group B, aspirin lowered the moisture content of the homografts partly through reduction of blood content and partly through reduction of the extravascular accumulation of fluid, i.e. oedema. In the remaining animal, A, dehydration and haemoconcentration following the onset of necrosis on day 5 resulted, as in the placebo-treated group A, in values for hyperaemia which exceeded the increase found in the wet weight of the homografts.

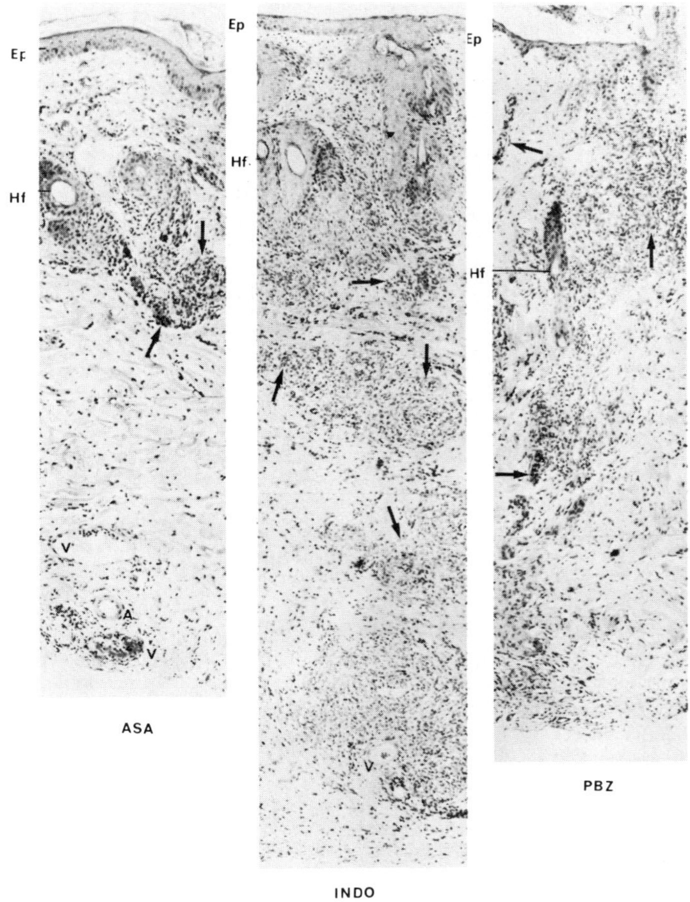

Figure 14.10 Presence of intravascular localization of inflammatory cells including lymphocytes (↓) in homografts which received six once daily applications of 0.01% acetylsalicylic acid (ASA), 0.02% indomethacin (INDO) and 0.02% phenylbutazone (PBZ) ointments. Degree of such localization of lymphocytes is mild in ASA-treated, severe in INDO-treated, and intermediate in PBZ-treated homografts. Note also that inhibition of the migration of inflammatory cells from vascular spaces is maximal in ASA, minimal in INDO and intermediate in PBZ homograft and that compared with control day 6 homograft (Figure 8c) epidermal necrosis (Ep) is patchy and mild in all the drug-treated homografts. The view (× 120) does not allow insight into whether the inflammatory cells occlude venules, or lymphatic spaces, or both, but clearly shows that arterioles (A) are not as prominently dilated as venules (V)

Indomethacin

When applied in a dose equimolar in amount to that of aspirin (Table 14.2), indomethacin depressed swelling of homografts to the level found in comparable

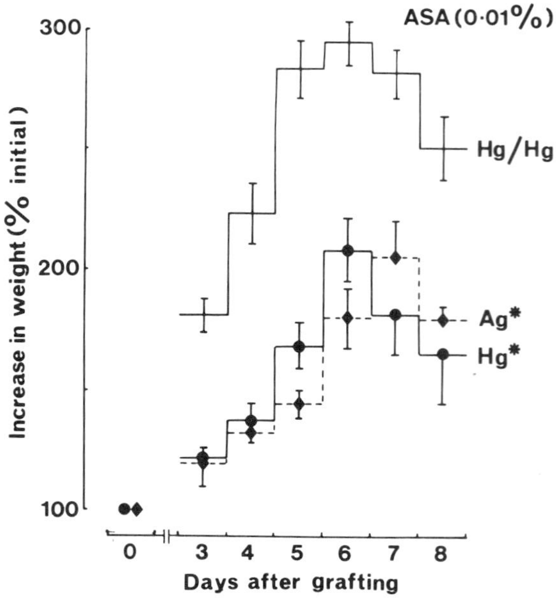

Figure 14.11 Effect of topical acetylsalicylic acid (0.01% w/v) on swelling, measured as percentage increase in wet weight, of homografts (Hg*) and autografts (Ag*) of rabbits bearing an equal number of placebo-treated homografts or autografts on the opposite leg. Results of drug-treated grafts are compared with those of control animals (Hg/Hg) bearing six placebo-treated homografts on each leg. ASA was applied immediately post-transplantation on day 0 and once daily thereafter

Table 14.3. Effect of three non-steroidal anti-inflammatory drugs on moisture, protein and DNA content of day 6 homografts; day 0 being the day of transplantation. Results shown are mean ± SE

Topical Treatment	*n*	*% Initial content*		
		DNA	*Moisture*	*Protein*
Placebo	9	648.0 ± 58.0	328.9 ± 14.7	250.4 ± 8.7
Aspirin	5	292.6 ± 47.5*	210.5 ± 19.3*	208.5 ± 16.5†
Indomethacin	6	455.8 ± 61.8†	245.6 ± 18.0‡	215.5 ± 13.4†
Phenylbutazone	5	421.9 ± 55.7§	257.5 ± 17.9‡	201.5 ± 8.9‡

* $p < 0.001$
† $p < 0.05$
‡ $p < 0.01$
§ $p < 0.02$

Table 14.4. Moisture content not accountable for by hyperaemia, i.e. rise in blood content, of day 6 homografts treated with non-steroidal anti-inflammatory drugs; day 0 being the day of transplantation*

Topical treatment		*n*	*Increase (Final–Initial; mg)* *Wet weight*	*Blood content*	*Moisture content*	*Extravascular moisture content* (mg)
Placebo	A	3	301.9 ± 21.3	300.2 ± 21.9	235.1 ± 15.4	−65.1
	B	6	414.6 ± 14.5	202.1 ± 19.2	334.8 ± 7.0	+132.7
Aspirin	A	1	109.5	319.1	59.6	−259.5
	B	4	238.8 ± 39.9	124.1 ± 26.7	188.2 ± 27.5	+64.1
Indomethacin	A	3	193.2 ± 19.2	NA	116.7 ± 9.6	NE
	B	3	325.3 ± 0.6	NA	257.4 ± 6.8	NE
Phenylbutazone	A	1	190.0	160.6	150.3	−10.3
	B	4	414.8 ± 15.3	157.1 ± 38.0	338.6 ± 13.2	+181.5

* Results shown are mean ± SE for animals with evidence of epidermal necrosis on day 5 (A) or day 6 (B). Negative values indicate dehydration, positive values indicate oedema

NA, not available; NE, not estimable

autografts, but only up to day 5 (Figure 14.12). On day 6 the mean increase in the wet weight of homografts treated with 0.02% (w/v) indomethacin (Hg*, Figure 14.12), though significantly lower than that of day 6 homografts of control Hg/Hg animals ($p < 0.05$), was definitely higher than that of the drug-treated autografts, Ag* (Figure 14.12, $p < 0.02$). This was associated with more severe, as well as more diffuse, intravascular localization of lymphocytes (Figure 14.10), venous congestion and cyanosis than in day 6 aspirin-treated homografts. Application of a 10-fold higher concentration of indomethacin (0.2% w/v) did not depress the weight of day 6 homografts to a greater extent than that found with the use of 0.02% ointment.

Several observations, detailed below, indicate that the failure of indomethacin to suppress the development of swelling caused by immune lymphocytes was not due to failure of absorption of the drug either into the inflamed skin or via the skin into the circulation. Firstly, in homografts such as that shown in Figure 14.10, an apparently greater number of intact, i.e. non-degranulated, polymorphonuclear leukocytes were present than in the control day 6 homografts such as that shown in Figure 14.8. In addition epidermal necrosis in the indomethacin-treated homografts was milder and patchy as compared with that in the comparable control homograft.

Secondly, as shown by results of gravimetric analysis (Table 14.3) indomethacin significantly depressed the rise in moisture and protein content, though as compared with aspirin, it depressed both DNA and the migration of inflammatory cells to a considerably lesser extent.

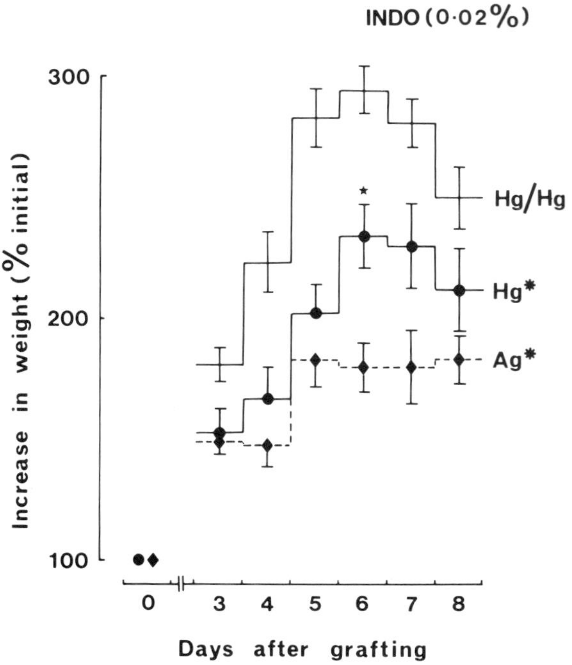

Figure 14.12 Effect of topical indomethacin (0.02% w/v) on swelling, measured as percentage increase in wet weight, of homografts (Hg*) and autografts (Ag*) of rabbits bearing an equal number of placebo-treated homografts or autografts on the opposite leg. Results of drug-treated grafts are compared with those of control animals (Hg/Hg) bearing six placebo-treated homografts on each leg. Indomethacin was applied immediately post-transplantation on day 0 and once daily thereafter; *, $p < 0.02$

Thirdly, although results for the degree of hyperaemia are not available, results summarized in Figure 14.13 show that indomethacin significantly lowered the rise which could have occurred in the water-soluble protein content due to accumulation of blood and extravasation of plasma proteins.

Finally, unlike acetylsalicylic acid, even 0.02% indomethacin depressed the swelling of homografts present on the opposite leg to almost the same extent as that of the homografts which received the drug topically. These results, summarized in Figure 14.14, suggested also that the percutaneously absorbed drug was more active against (a) swelling in homografts than in comparable autografts, (b) swelling which preceded rejection (day 6) as compared with that which occurred in association with it.

Another feature which distinguished the pharmacological action of indomethacin from that of aspirin was the fact that, as shown by the results summarised in Figure 14.15, the water-insoluble protein content of

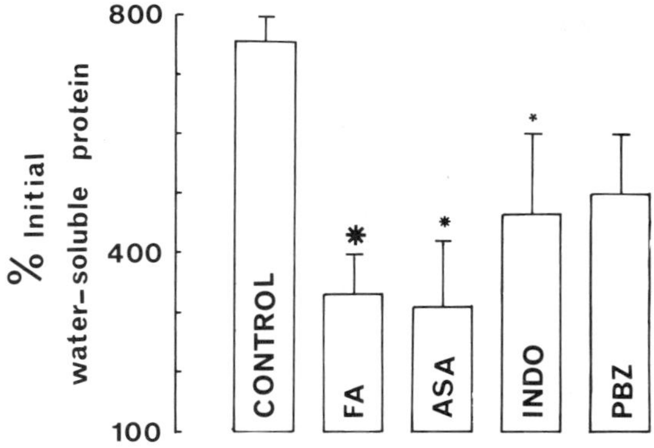

Figure 14.13 Effect of six once daily applications of various topical anti-inflammatory compounds: 0.025% (w/v) fluocinolone acetonide (FA), 0.01% acetylsalicylic acid (ASA), 0.02% indomethacin (INDO) and 0.02% phenylbutazone (PBZ), on the increase in water-soluble protein content of day 6 rabbit skin homografts, day 0 being the day of transplantation (*, $p<0.05$; *, $p<0.01$; *, $p<0.001$)

indomethacin-treated homografts tended to be higher than that of control homografts.

Phenylbutazone

Like indomethacin, doses of phenylbutazone equimolar in amount to 0.01% aspirin (Table 14.2) depressed the swelling of homografts to the level found in autografts up to day 5 only (Figure 14.16). The subsequent significantly greater increase in the wet weight of day 6 homografts despite continued treatment was associated with evidence of intravascular localization of lymphocytes (Figure 14.10) and venous congestion, both of which were more severe and more diffuse than in aspirin-treated but less severe than in the indomethacin-treated homografts. Phenylbutazone (0.02%) resembled acetylsalicylic acid (0.01%), but differed from indomethacin (0.02%) in being active only against the swelling of homografts which received the drug topically.

Gravimetric analysis of phenylbutazone-treated homografts revealed that the failure of this drug to arrest the development of swelling associated with inflammation caused by immune lymphocytes was due to its inability to prevent the extravascular accumulation of fluid, i.e. oedema (Table 14.4) and to lower the rise in the water-insoluble protein content (Figure 14.15).

Corticosteroids

As reported previously[20], fluocinolone acetonide applied in a dose equimolar to

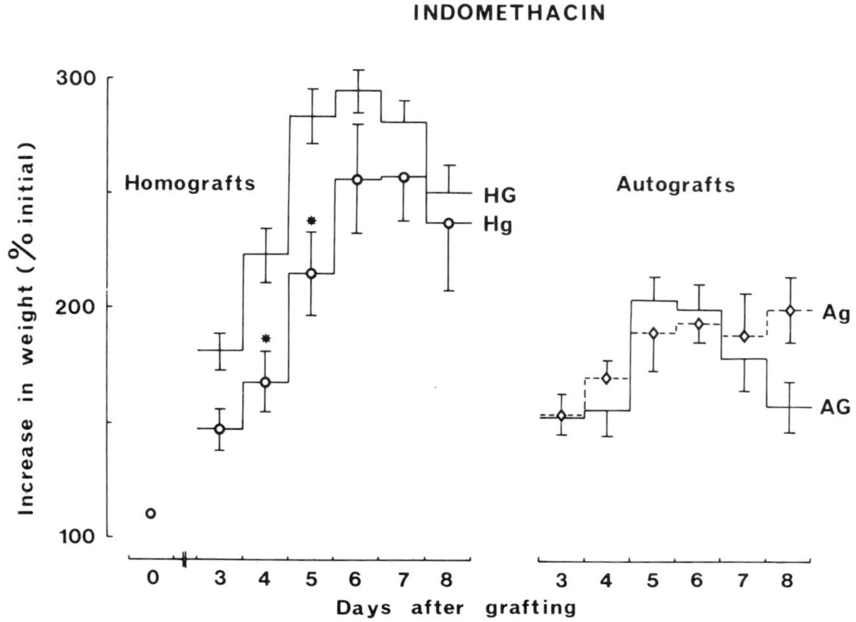

Figure 14.14 Percutaneous absorption of topical indomethacin. Experimental details and animals studied were the same as in the experiment of Figure 14.12. Results of placebo-treated set of homografts (Hg) and autografts (Ag) on the left leg of drug-treated animals are compared with those of homografts (HG) and autografts (AG) of control animals in which the grafts on both the legs received placebo (*, $p < 0.01$)

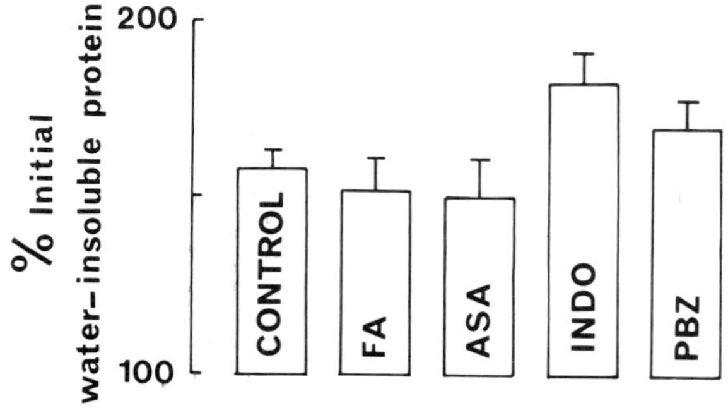

Figure 14.15 Effects of six once daily applications of various topical anti-inflammatory compounds: 0.025% (w/v) fluocinolone acetonide (FA), 0.01% acetylsalicylic acid (ASA), 0.02% indomethacin (INDO) and 0.02% phenylbutazone (PBZ), on the increase in water-insoluble protein content of day 6 rabbit skin homografts, day 0 being the day of transplantation. None of the differences was statistically significant, though results for indomethacin-treated day 7 homografts were significantly higher than in the control group ($p < 0.05$)

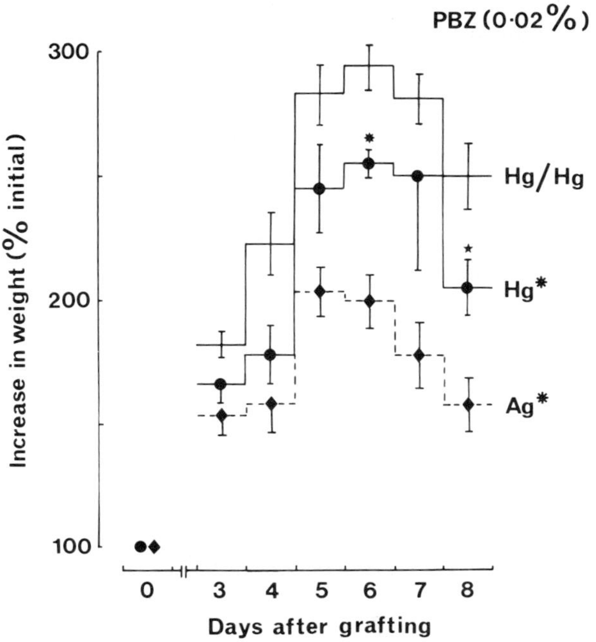

Figure 14.16 Effect of topical phenylbutazone (0.02% w/v) on swelling, measured as percentage increase in wet weight, of homografts (Hg*) and autografts (Ag*) of rabbits bearing an equal number of placebo-treated homografts or autografts on the opposite leg. Results of drug-treated grafts are compared with those of control animals (Hg/Hg) bearing six placebo-treated homografts on each leg. Phenylbutazone was applied immediately post-transplantation on day 0 and once daily thereafter; ⋆, $p < 0.02$; ✱, $p < 0.01$

aspirin, indomethacin or phenylbutazone, or even in doses one-tenth that amount (0.0025% w/v) depressed the degree of swelling in homografts to the level found in autografts but only up to day 5 when, as in the present experiments, a placebo-treated set of homografts was present on the opposite leg. Results for day 6 homografts treated with fluocinolone acetonide and two additional corticosteroids, namely chlorflumethasone and flumethasone pivalate, are summarized in Figure 14.17. They show that compared with the mean value for control homografts, the increase in the weight of steroid-treated homografts was significantly lower in all the instances except in the case of 0.0025% fluocinolone acetonide. But since the autograft values were also appreciably lowered by all the three corticosteroids the net reduction due to activity against lymphocytic inflammation was without exception less than 100%. In fact without exception it was not more than 60%. In other words, even the highest concentration of fluocinolone acetonide, chlorflumethasone or

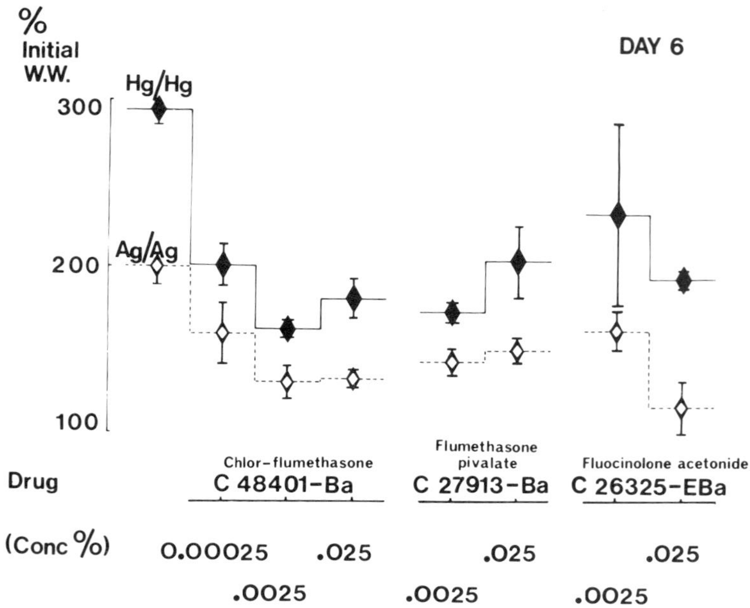

Figure 14.17 Effect of various concentrations of topical chlorflumethasone, flumethasone and fluocinolone acetonide on the swelling, measured as percentage increase in wet weight (W.W.) of homografts (Hg*) and autografts (Ag*) removed on day 6 from NFK recipients bearing six drug-treated skin grafts on R leg and six placebo-treated grafts on the L leg, day 0 being the day of transplantation. Results of drug-treated grafts are compared with those of control animals (Hg/Hg; Ag/Ag) bearing six placebo-treated grafts on each leg. Corticosteroid ointments were applied immediately post-transplantation on day 0 and once daily thereafter

flumethasone was less than fully active against inflammation caused by immune lymphocytes. Evidence of intravascular localization of lymphocytes (Figure 14.18), venous congestion and cyanosis was on the whole patchy and rather diffuse and the severity of the vascular changes was more variable in homografts receiving the lower as compared with the higher concentrations of the corticosteroids.

As in the case of indomethacin, the failure of corticosteroids to arrest the swelling associated with inflammation caused by immune lymphocytes was not due to failure of absorption of the drug either into the inflamed skin or, via the skin into the circulation. Besides depressing profoundly the epidermal and follicular hyperplasia as well as the increase in the connective tissue normally found in control autografts (cf Figure 14.18 with Figure 14.8), all three corticosteroids depressed thymic and/or adrenal weights as can be seen from results summarized in Table 14.5. Moreover, as indicated by results of

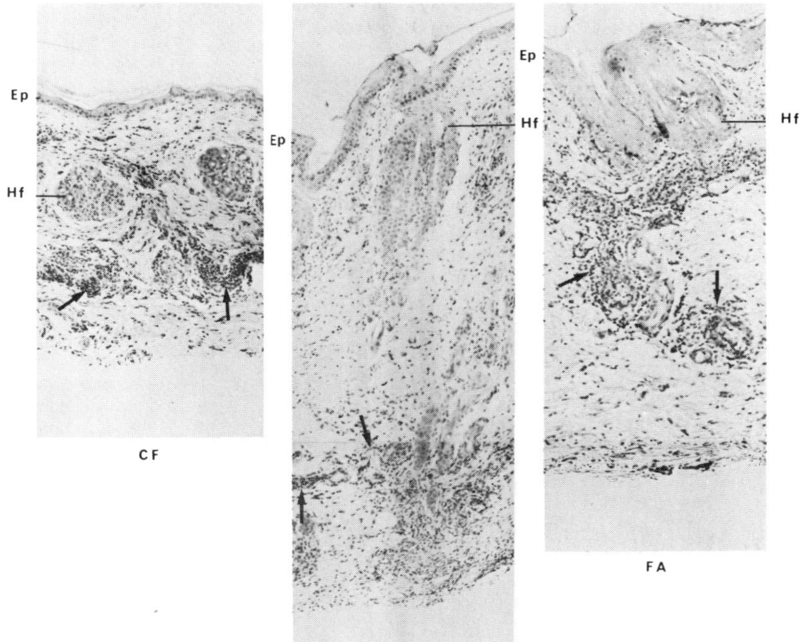

Figure 14.18 Presence of intravascular localization of inflammatory cells including lymphocytes (↓) in homografts which received five once daily applications of 0.025% chlorflumethasone (CF), flumethasone pivalate (FP) and fluocinolone acetonide (FA) ointments. Degree of such localization is similar in the three types of corticosteroid-treated homografts and as mild as in the aspirin-treated homografts shown in Figure 14.10a. Degree of epidermal hyperplasia is strikingly less pronounced than in INDO and PBZ homograft (Figure 14.10b, c) and control autograft (Figure 14.8b). The view (× 120) does not allow insight into whether the inflammatory cells occlude venules, or lymphatic spaces, or both

gravimetric analysis summarized in Table 14.6, at least two out of the three corticosteroids tested profoundly suppressed hyperaemia. However, as with aspirin and phenylbutazone, the failure of corticosteroids to arrest the swelling associated with inflammation caused by immune lymphocytes was also due to their failure to prevent the accumulation of extravascular fluid (see Table 14.6).

DISCUSSION

The homograft reaction being a typical example of a cellular hypersensitivity reaction was considered ideal for examining the effects of several commonly employed anti-rheumatic drugs against the overall end-result of biological

Table 14.5. Percutaneous absorption following application of topical anti-inflammatory corticosteroids*

Treatment	*n*	*Wet weight of organs* — *Thymus* (g)	*Adrenals* (mg)
Placebo	10	3.2 ± 0.3	307.4 ± 11.2
Chlorflumethasone			
0.00025%	(3)	4.0 ± 0.8	338.0 ± 37.9
0.0025%	(3)	2.0 ± 0.5	319.7 ± 16.9
0.025%	(6)	1.4 ± 0.1†	183.5 ± 17.7†
Flumethasone pivalate			
0.0025%	(3)	3.8 ± 0.6	363.0 ± 35.4
0.025%	(3)	1.3 ± 0.3†	299.2 ± 39.2
Fluocinolone acetonide			
0.0025%	(8)	3.3 ± 0.5	259.1 ± 14.4‡
0.025%	(6)	3.1 ± 0.5	249.1 ± 9.9§

* Results shown are for actual thymic and adrenal weights of animals bearing six homografts on each leg; one set having been treated from day 0. Total amount of drug received 4.9 μg in case of 0.00025%, 49.5 μg in 0.0025% and 495 μg in case of 0.025% ointment. Values shown are mean weights (± SE) expressed in appropriate units

† $p < 0.001$
‡ $p < 0.02$
§ $p < 0.01$

Table 14.6. Moisture content not accountable for by hyperaemia, i.e. the rise in blood content, of day 6 homografts treated with anti-inflammatory corticosteroids; day 0 being the day of transplantation*

Topical treatment		*n*	*Increase (final – initial; mg)* — *Wet weight*	*Blood content*	*Moisture content*	*Extravascular moisture content*
Placebo	A	3	301.9 ± 21.3	300.2 ± 21.9	235.1 ± 15.4	−65.1
	B	6	414.6 ± 14.5	202.1 ± 19.2	334.8 ± 7.0	+132.7
Chlorflumethasone						
0.00025%	B	3	269.3 ± 53.5†	35.9 ± 19.8‡	226.0 ± 39.3†	+190.1
0.0025%	B	4	188.8 ± 25.8‡	29.2 ± 21.5‡	147.2 ± 19.1‡	+115.4
0.025%	B	3	243.0 ± 51.0§	53.4 ± 21.1¶	183.6 ± 52.7†	+130.2
Flumethasone pivalate						
0.025%	B	3	262.2 ± 50.1†	69.8 ± 31.4¶	201.7 ± 57.1	+131.7
Fluocinolone acetonide						
0.025%	A	3	186.4 ± 13.3	224.4 ± 35.8	144.7 ± 32.6	−79.7

* Results shown are mean ± SE for animals with evidence of epidermal necrosis by day 5 (A) or day 6 (B). Negative values indicate dehydration, positive values indicate oedema

For comparisons between placebo and drug-treated B:

† $p < 0.05$
‡ $p < 0.001$
§ $p < 0.02$
¶ $p < 0.01$

effects of lymphokine-like factors released by invading CiSLs following their antigen-induced metabolic activation. Studies designed to simulate the clinical condition of rheumatoid arthritis experimentally ought ideally to have involved the use of orthoptic homografts of the synovium. However, skin grafts, particularly on comparable hind-limbs, were chosen because they were easily accessible for quantitative analysis.

Quantification of the inflammatory response

Inflammation leads to tissue swelling which, though customarily measured as increase in tissue volume, e.g. during the testing of anti-inflammatory compounds using the kaolin- or carrageenan-induced rat's hind-paw oedema[41,42], can also be measured as increase in tissue wet weight. Wet weight may increase not only due to extravascular accumulation of fluid, i.e. oedema, but also to a varying extent from increase in the cellularity and blood circulating through the inflamed tissue. As indicated by the data presented, these changes can be quantified by the measurement of appropriate parameters such as moisture and protein content, DNA and the haemoglobin content of the grafts. As already explained, the gravimetric approach was adopted for the quantification and distinction of lymphocytic from non-specific inflammatory response in skin homografts because little was known about the *in vivo* effects of lymphokines when the present study began in 1968.

Skin grafts were preferred because the study of intact skin, e.g. when using the tuberculin reaction, suffers from lack of availability of appropriate controls that can allow accurate assessment of the changes induced by inflammation. As explained under methods, this problem can be readily supervened in the case of skin grafts by recording the weight of the graft prior to transplantation and by analysis of the composition of representative non-grafted control skin. Changes in any parameter due to the postoperative inflammatory reaction can then be accurately evaluated at chosen time intervals by subtracting the final from the initial value, the final value being obtainable through analysis of the graft itself.

The quantitative approach presented is, however, time-consuming and is potentially subject to many inaccuracies because of its complexity. However, the inaccuracies can be, and have been, avoided by careful standardization of the operative as well as gravimetric analytical procedures in our laboratories. Some sources of error could not however be eliminated owing to the physiological changes characteristic of the inflammatory process in general and of the homograft reaction in particular. These remarks especially refer to both the dehydration and haemoconcentration which result from loss of the cuticle following epidermal necrosis in the homografts, a source of error which was avoided in the analysis of the results of Table 14.4 by separately assessing the grafts which became necrotic by day 5 instead of day 6, the day chosen for the routine assessment of the quantitative changes. It was not avoided, however, in the analysis of the results for hyperaemia reported on p. 206 and that could explain why a statistically significant difference was observed between the values for autografts and homografts in the present study of NFK recipients but not in that on the NZW recipients reported elsewhere[28]. As reported previously[21], several changes including the onset of epidermal necrosis occur earlier in NFK as compared with NZW recipients. The onset of epidermal necrosis is also accelerated by doubling the number of homografts per animal[21].

Distinction of lymphocytic inflammatory component

Interaction of CiSLs, or immune lymphocytes, with the donor histocompatible antigens in the homograft results in a complex series of metabolic changes which culminate in the release of pharmocologically active substances, presumably lymphokines, that elicit many biological effects besides necrosis of the grafted cells. Many of these effects have been defined during *in vitro* experiments[51,52]. Although their biological correlates can readily be visualized in the homografts[25], their quantification remains difficult. However, the availability of autografts as well as the choice of appropriate measurements already referred to has enabled us to quantitatively distinguish between lymphocyte-induced swelling, interstitial accumulation of fluid, increase in cellularity, water-soluble and water-insoluble protein content, hyperaemia, vascular permeability[28] and the accumulation of fibrin[18]. We can also distinguish the corresponding effects of non-specific inflammation simultaneously occuring in the homografts owing to the trauma of surgery. In turn this ability has enabled us to recognize the effectiveness of anti-rheumatic drugs against lymphocyte-induced inflammation.

Features characteristic of lymphocytic inflammation

The data obtained so far[18,19,28] and including that presented, indicate that of the seven features listed in Table 14.7, four have been found to characterize the lymphocytic component of the inflammatory response stimulated by rabbit skin homografts. These include venous congestion, interstitial and intra-lymphatic deposition of fibrin, extravascular retention of fluid and the presence of activated lymphocytes. This realization has several important pharmacological and therapeutic implications.

Pharmacological implications

The fact that hyperaemia occurs during lymphocytic inflammation as well as during non-specific inflammation (see Table 14.7) could explain why the potent vasoconstrictive agents such as the anti-inflammatory corticosteroids depressed the swelling of homografts as well as autografts (cf Figure 14.9 and 14.17) to a greater extent than the less vasoconstrictive and anti-erythemic agents such as

Table 14.7. Comparison of the vascular and cellular changes found to accompany inflammation in autografts and homografts*

Feature	*Inflammation*	
	Autografts	*Homografts*
Hyperaemia (erythema)	+	+
Exudation	+	+
Migration, etc.		
PMNs	±	+
Venous congestion	0	+
Interstitial and intralymphatic fibrin	0	+
Extravascular retention of fluid	0	+
Activated lymphocytes	0	+

* Whereas features common to both types of graft represent changes due to the non-specific inflammatory component, those present only in the homografts characterize the lymphocytic inflammatory component

phenylbutazone (cf Tables 14.4 and 14.6) or indomethacin. Likewise, the fact that retention of fluid and not exudation alone, accounts for the development of oedema during lymphocytic as opposed to non-specific inflammation could explain why indomethacin as well as the potent anti-exudative corticosteroids fail to prevent the extravascular accumulation of fluid in the homografts.

In other words, the data presented strongly suggest that the presence or absence of ability to suppress non-specific inflammation, is not a reliable guide for the recognition of compounds fully effective against the lymphocytic inflammatory component. Such suppression of non-specific inflammation can occur through vasoconstriction, or interference with the proliferation of grafted epidermal, follicular and fibrocytic cells, or the migration and degranulation of polymorphonuclear leukocytes, or inhibition of the synthesis of prostaglandins and other such pharmacological mediators known to be released during non-specific inflammation.

Since the non-specific vascular, cellular and metabolic processes such as those referred to above underlie many of the models of inflammation at present employed for the *in vivo* screening of anti-rheumatic drugs, it is not altogether surprising that agents which act on such non-specific processes, e.g. indomethacin[42], phenylbutazone[41] and corticosteroids[53,54], proved to be only partially active against swelling of rabbit skin homografts.

It was possible that some drugs, e.g. indomethacin and corticosteroids, were found to be only partially active against inflammation caused by immune lymphocytes because when topically applied they were not adequately absorbed into the inflamed skin, or via the skin into the circulation. However, the data summarized in Figure 14.14 leave little doubt that indomethacin was sufficiently well absorbed to depress the swelling of homografts present on the opposite leg to almost the same extent as those which received the drug topically. Likewise, the results of thymic and adrenal weight measurements summarized in Table 14.5 leave little doubt that the corticosteroids were also absorbed more than adequately into the circulation.

These as well as other observations[34,35] exclude the possibility that poor absorption of the drugs from the site of application accounted for the partial effectiveness of indomethacin or corticosteroids against lymphocytic inflammation. Instead they highlight the need to identify points in the inflammatory process at which the two classes of drugs were inactive against lymphocytic inflammation.

Indomethacin and phenylbutazone

Although results for blood content of indomethacin-treated homografts are not available, the fact that it lowered the rise in the water-soluble protein content to almost the same level as phenylbutazone (Table 14.3) suggests that indomethacin resembles phenylbutazone in being unable to reduce significantly the rise that occurs in the extravascular fluid content during lymphocytic inflammation due to the combined effect of fibrin-induced blockage of lymph flow and venous congestion[28]. This view is supported by the fact that both indomethacin and phenylbutazone augment the increase in the water-insoluble protein content of homografts (see Figure 14.15). Since such augmentation occurred in the homografts but not in comparable autografts and in spite of the lowering of DNA (Table 14.3), it seems probable that neither collagen nor cell debris is responsible for it. In the case of indomethacin data reported elsewhere[36] suggest that the augmentation in the water-insoluble protein is in part due to the inability of the drug to interfere with lymphocyte-initiated interstitial and intralymphatic deposition of fibrin.

Little is known as yet about the cellular basis for the interstitial and intralymphatic deposition of fibrin in rabbit skin homografts. If it should prove, however, to be mediated by a lymphokine as seems probable in the case of human kidney homotransplants[55] it could be interesting to investigate whether the presently reported augmentation of the increase in water-insoluble protein content and the previously reported augmentation of the increase in fibrin content[36] by indomethacin is related to its property to inhibit the biosynthesis of prostaglandins. The possibility arises from the observations[56,57] that E-type prostaglandins modulate the severity of lymphocytic inflammation through control of the release of lymphokines, either their deficiency or a lack of responsiveness to them[58] augmenting and perpetuating delayed-type hypersensitivity.

Corticosteroids

A basis for the failure of corticosteroids to prevent lymphocyte-induced extravascular accumulation of fluid (Table 14.6) requires to be investigated. Previously reported preliminary data[36] indicate that unlike indomethacin both chlorflumethasone and fluocinolone acetonide are capable of inhibiting, even if not preventing, the accumulation of fibrin in rabbit skin homografts. The data presented show, however, that in association with their failure to prevent the development of lymphocytic inflammation, the corticosteroids fail to prevent the intravascular localization of lymphocytes and the resultant venous and/or lymphatic congestion (Figure 14.18).

Since the intravascular locaiization of lymphocytes occurs as a result of the physical interaction between circulating immune lymphocytes and the histoincompatible antigens on the donor endothelial cells lining the post-capillary venules[25], the data imply that the corticosteroids are not capable of interfering either with the interaction between lymphocytes and the antigen, or with the resultant metabolic activation of lymphocytes and the attendant synthesis and release of lymphokines. The inference which is well supported by other observations[20,40] can explain (a) why necrosis of the grafted cells ensues in the experimental system, (b) why in rheumatoid arthritis the inflammatory process expresses itself again as soon as treatment is discontinued, (c) why at times the rheumatoid process shows signs of escape from control even in spite of continued treatment.

Aspirin

Contrary to results of foot-pad oedema tests[41,42] the u.v.-induced erythema tests[43] or the prostaglandin synthetase system[44], the relative efficacy of acetylsalicylic acid against lymphocytic inflammation equals, or is slightly greater than, that of indomethacin and phenylbutazone. Whether this is due to some important difference(s) between the activity spectrum of aspirin and indomethacin or phenylbutazone, or is simply due to the use of topical instead of oral route of administration requires to be investigated.

Although acetylsalicylic acid reduced the increase in the wet weight of homografts to levels found in comparable autografts, the data summarized in Table 14.4 show that it did not reduce the increase in the extravascular moisture content to levels characteristic of autografts[28]. This suggests that it does not differ from indomethacin and phenylbutazone in being unable to prevent the interstitial and intralymphatic deposition of fibrin. The basis for its failure requires to be formally investigated.

Since the oedema due to lymphatic blockage is more pronounced when venous congestion is also present[37] and since the immune lymphocytes appear to be capable of inducing both the vascular effects concomitantly[28], the question also arises as to whether aspirin moderated the swelling of homografts through its manifestly greater effectiveness against venous congestion (Figure

14.10a). Besides being more active when administered topically instead of orally[34], it is possible that aspirin may be intrinsically more active than indomethacin against fibrino-purulent exudation[38] and against inflammatory changes in the venules[39].

The data presented are also consistent with the possibility that acetylsalicylic acid is active against some metabolic processes underlying antigen-induced lymphocytic activation. The *in vitro* evidence in favour of such an explanation for the observed effect of aspirin on swelling of homografts though available[59,60] however remains disputed[61].

Practical implications

Apart from providing a rational basis for the selection of anti-rheumatic drugs, studies of the homograft reaction highlight a key role for fibrin in the development of lymphocytic inflammatory swelling. Since the clinical observations not only indicate that fibrin continues to be extravascularly deposited in RA synovium despite administration of maximally-tolerated doses of currently available drugs[45,46], but support also its key role in both the development and perpetuation of joint swelling[47,48], the data presented underline the need to develop compounds which can either prevent fibrin formation or promote its removal. For such a purpose it is possible that owing to its elaborateness the skin graft model may before long be superseded by a simpler testing procedure. The availability of the skin graft model is however likely to remain useful for (a) the elucidation of the cellular[20] and molecular aspects[49,50] of lymphocytic inflammation, (b) the pharmacological characterization of substances selectively active against them.

SUMMARY

1. The present investigation was designed to test the hypothesis that maximally-tolerated doses of currently available anti-rheumatic drugs, while relieving pain, fail to arrest rheumatoid inflammation because they are not capable of preventing the antigen-induced activation of circulating immune lymphocytes or the vascular effects which result from such activation.
2. Homograft reaction, i.e. the inflammatory response stimulated by tissues transplanted from one individual to another of the same species, was chosen because it is known to be initiated by circulating immune lymphocytes. Skin was preferred to synovium because of its accessibility for serial examination.
3. Twelve pieces of full-thickness skin removed from New Zealand white rabbits were transplanted on to Norfolk whites, six per hind-limb, and the anti-rheumatic drugs were applied topically to only one set. The placebo-treated contralateral set provided the antigenic stimulus leading to the development of circulating immune lymphocytes.

4. An equal number of autografts were made in another group of Norfolk rabbits in order to define the effect of topical anti-rheumatic medication on the non-specific inflammation caused by trauma of surgery.
5. The effect of anti-rheumatic drugs on swelling, hyperaemia, moisture, protein and DNA content as well as on the intravascular accumulation of lymphocytes, venous congestion, migration of inflammatory cells and degranulation of polymorphonuclear leukocytes was examined. Whereas results of drug-treated homografts measured the effect against both lymphocytic and non-specific inflammation, those of the autografts measured the effect solely against non-specific inflammation. The difference between the two measured the extent to which a drug was effective against lymphocytic inflammation.
6. Of six compounds tested so far only acetylsalicyclic acid depressed the swelling of homografts to the level found in comparable autografts. It failed however to prevent intravascular localization of immune lymphocytes and also to reduce the extravascular increase in moisture content to levels characteristic of autografts.
7. Although highly active against both non-specific inflammation and the migration of inflammatory cells, all three corticosteroids tested (chorflumethasone, flumethasone and fluocinolone acetonide) failed to prevent intravascular localization of lymphocytes and venous congestion.
8. Although active against non-specific inflammation and the degranulation of polymorphonuclear leukocytes, indomethacin was virtually inactive against the intravascular localization of lymphocytes, venous congestion and extravascular fibrin formation and only partially active against the extravascular retention of fluid. The activity profile of phenylbutazone was similar to, but possibly not identical to, that of indomethacin.
9. The observations indicate that the presence or absence of ability to suppress non-specific inflammation, e.g. through vasoconstriction, or interference with proliferation of epithelial and connective tissue cells, or the migration and degranulation of polymorphonuclear leukocytes, or the inhibition of the synthesis and release of prostaglandins, is not a reliable guide for the selection of compounds fully effective against the lymphocytic inflammatory component of homograft reaction and by implication also that of rheumatoid arthritis.

ACKNOWLEDGEMENTS

The authors wish to thank Mr R. Parsons for the illustrations.

References

1. Zvaifler, N. J. (1974). Rheumatoid synovitis an extravascular immune complex disease. *Arthr. Rheum.*, **17**, 297

2. Weissmann, G. (1972). Lysosomal mechanism of tissue injury in arthritis. *N. Engl. J. Med.*, **286,** 141
3. Ignarro, L. J. (1974). Regulation of lysosomal enzyme secretion: role in inflammation. *Agents Actions*, **4,** 241
4. Arigonni-Martelli, E. and Restelli, A. (1972). Release of lysosomal enzymes in experimental inflammations: effect of anti-inflammatory drugs. *Eur. J. Pharmacol.*, **19,** 191
5. Jasani, M. K. (1975). The importance of ACTH and glucocorticoids in rheumatoid arthritis. In: *Clinics in Rheumatic Diseases*, Vol. 1(2), p. 335 (London and Philadelphia: W. B. Saunders Co. Ltd.)
6. Glen, A. C. and Jasani, M. K. (1968). Lymphocyte DNA and RNA content in rheumatoid arthritis. *Ann. Rheum. Dis.*, **27,** 170
7. Glen, A. C., Cooper, W. C., Boak, J. L., Murray, R. C. and Munro, H. N. (1970). DNA and RNA measurements on thoracic duct lymphocytes of patients undergoing renal transplantation *Transplantation*, **9,** 83
8. Delbarre, F., LeGo, A. and Kahan, A. (1975). Hyperbasophilic immunoblasts in circulating blood in chronic inflammatory rheumatic and collagen diseases. *Ann. Rheum. Dis.*, **34,** 422
9. Person, D. A., Sharp, J. T. and Lidsky, M. D. (1976). The cytotoxicity of leukocytes and lymphocytes from patients with rheumatoid arthritis for synovial cells. *Arthritis Rheum.*, **58,** 690
10. Wegelius, O., Laine, V., Lindström, B. and Klockars, M. (1970). Fistula of the thoracic duct as immunosuppressive treatment in rheumatoid arthritis. *Acta Med. Scand.*, **187,** 539
11. Pearson, C. M., Paulus, H. E. and Machleder, H. I. (1975). The role of the lymphocyte and its product in the propagation of joint disease. *Ann, N.Y. Acad. Sci.*, **256,** 150
12. Boxal, J. A. van and Paget, S. A. (1975). Predominantly T-cell infiltrate in rheumatoid synovial membranes. *N. Engl. J. Med.*, **293,** 517
13. Bankhurst, A. D., Husby, G. and Williams, R. C. Jr. (1976). Predominance of T-cells in the lymphocytic infiltrates of synovial tissues in rheumatoid arthritis. *Arthritis Rheum.*, **19,** 555
14. Meijer, C. J. L. M., Putte, L. B. A. van de, Eulderink, F., Kelinjan, R., Lafeber, G. and Bots, Th. A. M. (1977). Characteristics of mononuclear cell populations in chronically inflamed synovial membranes. *J. Pathol.*, **121,** 1
15. Stastny, P., Rosenthal, M., Andreis, M., Cooke, D. and Ziff, M. (1975). Lymphokines in rheumatoid synovitis. *Ann. N.Y. Acad. Sci.*, **256,** 117
16. Medawar, P. B. (1958). The homograft reaction. *Proc. R. Soc., Ser. B.*, **149,** 145
17. Brent, L. and Medawar, P. B. (1967). Cellular immunity and the homograft reaction. *Br. Med. Bull.*, **23,** 55
18. Bach, C. S. and Jasani, M. K. (1976). Role of lymphocytes in accumulation of fibrin in rabbit skin homografts. *Br. J. Pharmacol.*, **58,** 292
19. Bullock, G. R., Jasani, M. K. and Lewis, G. P. (1977). Morphology of immune lymphocytes in homograft lymph. *Cell. Biol. Intl. Reports*, **1,** 123
20. Jasani, M. K. (1977). Anti-inflammatory steroids: mode of action in rheumatoid arthritis and homograft reaction. In *Inflammation and Anti-inflammatory Drugs* (ed. S. H. Ferreira and J. R. Vane), Handbook of Experimental Pharmacology Series, Vol. 50 (in press) (Heidelberg: Springer Verlag)
21. Jasani, M. K. and Lewis, G. P. (1971). Lymph flow and changes in intracellular enzymes during rejection of rabbit skin homografts. *J. Physiol. (Lond.)*, **219,** 525
22. Bitterli, E. and Jasani, M. K. (1972). A quantitative assessment of tissue changes accompanying homograft reaction: changes in tissue dry weight, DNA and moisture content in rabbit skin homografts. *Br. J. Pharmacol.*, **45,** 138
23. Taylor, A. C. and Lehrfeld, J. W. (1953). Determination of survival time of skin homografts in rat by observation of vascular changes in graft. *Plast. Reconstr. Surg.*, **12,** 423
24. Edgerton, M. T., Peterson, H. A. and Edgerton, P. J. (1957). The homograft rejection mechanism. *Arch. Surg. (Chicago)*, **74,** 238

25. Wiener, J., Lattes, R. G. and Pearl, J. S. (1969). Vascular permeability and leukocyte emigration in allograft rejection. *Am. J. Pathol.*, **55,** 295
26. Medawar, P. B. (1944). The behaviour and fate of skin autografts and skin homografts in rabbits. *J. Anat.*, **78,** 176
27. David, J. R. (1972). Lymphocyte mediators and cellular hypersensitivity. *N. Engl. J. Med.*, **288,** 143
28. Bach, C. S., Jasani, M. K., Lockwood, K. and Roberts, J. M. (1977). Role of hyperaemia and vascular permeability in lymphocyte-mediated inflammation (see Chapter 8 of the present book).
29. Schneider, W. C. (1945). Phosphorus compounds in animal tissues. I. Extraction and estimation of deoxypentose nucleic acid and of pentose nucleic acid. *J. Biol. Chem.*, **161,** 293
30. Burton, K. (1956). A study of the conditions and mechanism of the diphenylamine reaction for the colorimetric estimation of deoxyribonucleic acid. *Biochem. J.*, **62,** 315
31. Lowry, O., Rosebrough, N. J., Farr, A. L. and Randall, R. J. (1951). Protein measurement with the Folin phenol reagent. *J. Biol. Chem.*, **193,** 265
32. Elves, M. W., Gough, J., Chapman, J. A. and Israels, M. C. G. (1964). Electron microscope studies of lymphocytes. Transformation under the influence of P.H.A. *Lancet*, **i,** 306
33. Jasani, M. K. (1973). The usefulness of enzyme measurements for evaluation of pharmacological agents which modify the homograft reaction. *Biochem. Soc. Trans.*, **1,** 1043
34. Law, E. and Lewis, A. J. (1977). The effect of systemically and topically applied drugs on ultraviolet induced erythema in the rat. *Br. J. Pharmacol.*, **59,** 591
35. Walz, D. T., Dolan, M. M., DiMartino, M. J. and Yankell, S. L. (1971). Effects of topical hydrocortisone and acetylsalicylic acid on the primary lesion of adjuvant-induced arthritis. *Proc. Soc. Exp. Biol. Med.*, **137,** 1466
36. Bach, C. S. and Jasani, M. K. (1977). On the ineffectiveness of indomethacin against rheumatoid swelling. *Br. J. Pharmacol.*, **59,** 473P
37. Rusznyak, I., Foldi, M. and Szabo, G. (1960). *Lymphatics and lymph circulation* p. 235 (Oxford: Pergamon Press)
38. Walters, W. N.-I. and Willoughby, D. A. (1965). Indomethacin, a new anti-inflammatory drug; its potential use as a laboratory tool. *J. Pathol. Bact.*, **90,** 64
39. Spector, W. G. and Willoughby, D. A. (1959). Experimental suppression of the acute inflammatory changes of thermal injury. *J. Pathol. Bact.*, **78,** 121
40. Butterworth, A. E. (1975). Non-specific cytotoxic effects of antigen-transformed lymphocytes. *Cell. Immunol.*, **16,** 60
41. Domenjoz, R. (1960). The pharmacology of phenylbutazone analogues. *Ann. N.Y. Acad. Sci.*, **86,** 263
42. Winter, C. A., Risley, E. A. and Nuss, G. W. (1963). Anti-inflammatory and anti-pyretic activities of indomethacin, 1-(*p*-chlorobenzoyl)-5-methoxy-2-methyl-indole-3-acetic acid. *J. Pharm. Exp. Ther.*, **141,** 369
43. Lewis, A. J. (1977). Evaluation of the ability of anti-rheumatic drugs to suppress hyperaemia and increased vascular permeability. (Chapter 7 in this volume).
44. Flower, R. J. (1974). Drugs which inhibit prostaglandin biosynthesis. *Pharm. Rev.*, **26,** 33
45. Bullock, G. R., Jasani, M. K. and Roberts, J. M. (1976). Tissue localization of fibrin in homograft reaction and its relevance to the pathophysiology of rheumatoid synovial swelling. *Proc. R. Microsc. Soc.*, **11,** (suppl) 65
46. Rennie, J. A. N., Protheroe, K. and Jasani, M. K. (1977). Intrasynovial accumulation of ^{125}I-human fibrinogen (^{125}I-HFg) as fibrin in rheumatoid arthritis (RA) (In preparation)
47. Lipson, R. L., Baldes, E. J., Anderson, J. A. and Polley, H. F. (1965). Osmotic pressure gradients and joint effusions. *Arthritis Rheum.*, **8,** 29
48. Dumonde, D. C. and Glynn, L. E. (1962). The production of arthritis in rabbits by an immunological reaction to fibrin. *Br. J. Exp. Pathol.*, **43,** 473
49. Jasani, M. K. (1976). Lysosomal enzymes in diagnosis and assessment of joint disease. In

Clinics in Rheumatic Diseases, Vol 2(1) p. 273 (Philadelphia and London: W. B. Saunders and Co.)

50. Jasani, B., Jasani, M. K. and Talbot, M. D. (1978). Characterization of two acid proteinases in rabbit skin homografts. *Biochem. J.*, **169,** 287
51. Dumonde, D. C., Wolstencroft, R. A., Panayi, G. S., Mathew, M., Morley, J. and Howson, W. T. (1969). Lymphokines: non-antibody mediators of cellular immunity generated by lymphocyte activation. *Nature (London)*, **224,** 38
52. Bloom, B. R., Stoner, G., Fischetti, V., Nowakowski, M., Mushel, R. and Rubenstein, A. (1974). Products of activated lymphocytes (PALs) and the virus plaque assay. In *Progress in Immunology*, II. 3 (Ed. L. Brent and J. Holborow) (Amsterdam: North-Holland Publishing)
53. Meier, R., Schuler, W. and Desaulles, P. (1950). Zur frage des mechanismus der hemmung des bindegewebswachstums durch cortisone. *Experientia* **6,** 469
54. Sutton, P. M., Feldmann, R. J. and Maibach, H. I. (1971). Vasoconstrictor potency of corticoids: Intradermal injection. *J. Invest. Dermatol.*, **57,** 371
55. Hattler, B. G., Rocklin, R. E., Jr., Ward, P. A., Rickles, F. R. (1973). Functional features of lymphocytes recovered from a human renal allograft. *Cell. Immunol.*, **9,** 289
56. Smith, J. N., Steiner, A. L., Newbury, N. M. and Parker, C. W. (1971). Cyclic adenosine 3′,5′-monophosphate in human lymphocytes. Alterations after phytohaemagglutinin stimulation. *J. Clin. Invest.*, **50,** 432
57. Morley, J. (1974). Prostaglandins and lymphokines and arthritis. *Prostaglandins*, **8,** 315
58. Kirby, P. J., Morley, J., Ponsford, J. R. and McDonald, W. I. (1976). Defective PGE reactivity in leukocytes of multiple sclerosis patients. *Prostaglandins*, **11,** 621
59. Crout, J. E., Hepburn, B. and Ritts, R. E. (1975). Suppression of lymphocyte transformation after aspirin ingestion. *N. Engl. J. Med.*, **292,** 221
60. Opelz, G., Terasaki, P. I., Hirata, A. A. (1973). Suppression of lymphocyte transformation by aspirin. *Lancet*, **ii,** 478
61. Duncan, M. W., Person, D. A., Rich, R. R. and Sharp, J. T. (1977). Aspirin and delayed type hypersensitivity. *Arthritis Rheum.*, **20,** 1174
62. Biberfeld, P. and Johansson, A. (1975). Contact areas of cytotoxic lymphocytes and target cells. An electron-microscopic study. *Exp. Cell Res.*, **94,** 79
63. Sanderson, C. J. and Glauert, Audrey M. (1977). The mechanism of T cell mediated cytotoxicity V. Morphological studies by electron microscopy. *Proc. R. Soc. Lond. B.*, **198,** 315

15
The Contribution of Adjuvant Arthritis to the Recognition of Anti-Rheumatic Drugs

C. M. PEARSON and T.-Y. CHANG

INTRODUCTION

Many years ago[1] it was observed that laboratory rats, especially of certain strains, could develop a polyarthritis after a single injection of Freund's complete adjuvant (FCA) containing mycobacteria into either the tail (s.c.) or the paw (subplantar). The model which cannot be induced in mammals other than the rat, and which is referred to as adjuvant-induced arthritis, presents a clinical picture that closely resembles rheumatoid arthritis[2].

Unlike the arthritis associated with rheumatoid disease, adjuvant arthritis has a clear-cut starting point (the time of injection of FCA), followed by a well-defined latent period of 10 to 16 days. The almost explosive appearance of polyarthritis thereafter is associated with lesions in many other tissues. These include especially the vasculature of areas such as the ears, the tip of the nose and all over the tail. Histologically the erythematous nodules which develop over the ears show evidence of perivascular infiltrates of inflammatory cells and endothelial proliferation. Occasionally, granulomas appear in the liver, spleen and lungs and in male animals also in the prostate and surrounding connective tissue. A further study of adjuvant-induced arthritis has unfolded a number of additional interesting though complex aspects of this model[3].

PATHOGENESIS OF POLYARTHRITIS

The pathogenesis of polyarthritis following the injection of FCA remains perplexing, provocative and, as yet, not fully explained. The disease is thought to result from activation of delayed hypersensitivity to the tubercle bacilli or their components[3]. Much of the recent work in our laboratory has centered on investigations into the nature of the initiating 'immunogen' and Dr Kohashi and others have succeeded in sub-fractionating cell wall peptidoglycans, capable of inducing adjuvant arthritis, from the tubercle bacilli as well as other bacteria including *Staph. aureus*, various streptococcus strains and *L. plantarum*. Corynebacteria, which are closely related to the tubercle bacilli, have also been shown by others[5] to contain within their cell walls an arthritogenic factor.

It had been shown by us and others that many components of these bacterial cell walls, especially the peptidoglycans, are remarkably resistant to degradation by mammalian lysosomal enzymes. In this regard it is not unreasonable to speculate that such non-digestible material may persist in macrophages, including phagocytic synovial lining cells and therefore serve as a constant source of the immunogen[7].

Alternatively, it is possible that adjuvant disease may result from the development of auto-antibodies and, or, specifically sensitized lymphocytes which act against the animals' tissues, thereby inducing an auto-immune phenomenon[3,8].

A third possibility is that the development of adjuvant-induced arthritis may depend upon the activation of a latent infectious agent such as a virus which has the capacity to initiate a series of hypersensitivity reactions in the host. Such speculations, made as far back as 1963 [9] are quite tenable in view of the experimental data I have reviewed later on (p. 363).

EFFECTS OF ANTI-RHEUMATIC AND OTHER DRUGS

The effects of different doses of six classes of compounds upon the severity of adjuvant-induced polyarthritis is itemized in Tables 15.1–15.6. The data are largely based on the literature and show on an all-or-none basis (using appropriately chosen abbreviations) whether the drugs reduced or aggravated the severity of disseminated polyarthritis or whether they were ineffective against it. Data on their effect on the incidence of adjuvant-induced arthritis, regarding whether they prevented the development of disseminated polyarthritis, are not included mainly in the interest of clarity but also because such activity is clinically less relevant than their ability to modify the severity of established joint inflammation.

Essentially the data summarized in Tables 15.1–15.6 show the following. First, aspirin-like non-steroidal anti-inflammatory agents (Table 15.1) reduce the severity of joint inflammation irrespective of whether they are administered throughout the period after injection of FCA or given, in sufficient doses, within a few days before and during the expected time of onset of polyarthritis. If judged on that basis, the activity of corticosteroids summarized in Table 15.2 resembles that of the non-steroidal anti-inflammatory drugs. Some in-

Table 15.1 Effect of non-steroidal anti-inflammatory drugs on disseminated adjuvant-induced polyarthritis in the rat. Freund's complete adjuvant (FCA) containing dead mycobacteria was injected either in the tail (i.d.) or into the paw (sub-plantar) on day 0. Drugs were administered via the route indicated either from day 0, *or* several days before day 0 (minus sign precedes the number of day), *or* after day 0 (plus sign before the number of day is omitted for the sake of clarity). Activity of the drug, shown in column 6 is graded on all or none basis as follows: +, to indicate a statistically significant depression of the polyarthritis; 0, to indicate lack of significant depression compared with values found in matched non-treated controls.

Drug	*Daily dose mg/kg*	*Route*	*Time of administration day*	*Days when arthritis assessed*	*Activity*	*Reference*
Aspirin	200.0	p.o.	0→18	18	+	10
	200.0	p.o.	1→ 4	18	+	10
	200.0	p.o.	10→14	18	0	10
	200.0	p.o.	14→18	18	+	10
	200.0*	p.o.	22→28	28	+	11
Sulfinpyrazone	200.0	p.o.	−1→12	12	+	12
Phenylbutazone	50.0	p.o.	0→18	18	+	10
	50.0	p.o.	0→ 4	18	0	10
	50.0	p.o.	10→14	18	+	10
	50.0	p.o.	14→18	18	+	10
	30.0	p.o.	0→21	21, 28	+	13
	10.0*	p.o.	22→28	28	+	11
	100.0	p.o.	−1→15	16	+	14
	100.0	p.o.	0→ 4	16	0	14
	100.0	p.o.	13→15	16	+	14
Indomethacin	1.0	p.o.	0→18	18	+	10
	1.0	p.o.	10→14	18	+	10
	1.0	p.o.	14→18	18	+	10
	1.0	p.o.	17→24	24	+	15
	1.0	p.o.	0→21	21, 28	+	13
Indoxole	10.0*	p.o.	1→14	14	+	16
Flufenamic acid	3.1	p.o.	0→16	17	+	15
	3.6	p.o.	0→22	22	+	17
	3.0	p.o.	18→28	28	+	17
Mefenamic acid	25.0	p.o.	0→16	17	+	15
	21.6	p.o.	0→22	22	+	17
	15.0	p.o.	18→28	28	+	17

* twice daily

vestigators tend, however, to emphasize that since the corticosteroids additionally modify the response of the regional lymph nodes draining the site of injection, the mechanism(s) underlying the corticosteroid-induced reduction of joint inflammation may differ from those underlying depression of joint inflam-

Table 15.2 Effect of corticosteroids on disseminated adjuvant-induced polyarthritis in the rat. (Experimental protocol, numbering of days and the grading of activity were as in Table 15.1)

Drug	*Daily dose mg/kg*	*Route*	*Time of administration day*	*Days when arthritis assessed*	*Activity*	*Reference*
Hydrocortisone acetate	10.00	s.c.	0→21	21, 30	+	11
	2.50	s.c.	21→35	35	+	11
	12.50*	p.o.	22→28	28	+	11
	5.00*	p.o.	15→22	23	+	16
	4.00	p.o.	1→14	15	+	16
Prednisolone	20.00	p.o.	0→18	18	+	10
	20.00	p.o.	0→ 4	18	+	10
	20.00	p.o.	10→14	18	+	10
	20.00	p.o.	14→18	18	+	10
	4.00	p.o.	0→21	21	+	1
6α-methyl prednisolone	1.00*	p.o.	15→22	23	+	16
Fluoroprednisolone	1.00*	p.o.	15→22	23	+	16
Dexamethasone	0.02	p.o.	0→16	17	+	15
Paramethasone	0.50	p.o.	−1→12	20, 35	+	18
Oestradiol	0.50	s.c.	−1→12	20, 35	+	18
Testosterone	10.00	s.c.	0→20	21	+	11

* twice daily

mation by non-steroidal anti-inflammatory drugs. Both classes of drugs also inhibit the weight loss found to occur after the onset of disseminated polyarthritis.

Compounds commonly referred to as 'immunosuppressives' (Table 15.3) usually exert their effects early, i.e. when administered either before and/or at the time of injection of FCA and in some instances for a few days immediately post-injection. Although they also delay the development of polyarthritis, presumably via alteration of the immune responsiveness of the injected host, none of them prevents it altogether. Nor do they cure established polyarthritis. In the case of at least some of the cytotoxic immunosuppressive drugs listed in Table 15.3 the depressive effect of the drugs on disseminated polyarthritis might be attributable to an anti-inflammatory action which they exhibit in non-immunological models of inflammation such as (a) cutaneous inflammation caused by fresh egg white[22] or turpentine[23] (b) pleural exudate caused by turpentine[24], or (c) chronic granuloma induced by the subcutaneous implantation of sterile cotton pellets[24].

The reports on the effects of the slow-acting 'anti-rheumatic' drugs including especially gold preparations and chloroquine (Table 15.4) on adjuvant-induced arthritis have not been consistent. Gold preparations have been found to be either ineffective or effective, whereas most investigators have found chloroquine to be ineffective. In the few instances when chloroquine was found to be effective, the amount of the drug employed was so high as to aggravate the loss in body weight known to occur after the onset of disseminated polyarthritis. Although DL-penicillamine has been reported to significantly depress the established joint inflammation[30], the clinically employed D-penicillamine has been uniformly found to be without effect on the experimental model. If anything, like levamisole, D-penicillamine is known instead to aggravate the severity of disseminated adjuvant-induced arthritis[28,29].

The clinical relevance as well as the pharmacological significance of the inhibitory effect of miscellaneous agents on disseminated adjuvant-induced polyarthritis referred to in Table 15.5 requires much further investigation. Many of these agents are used for the treatment of various clinical conditions in humans but seem to have no anti-rheumatic activity, at least none has been

Table 15.3 Effect of cytotoxic and immunosuppressive agents on disseminated adjuvant-induced polyarthritis in the rat. (Experimental protocol, numbering of days and the grading of activity were as in Table 15.1.)

Drug	*Daily dose mg/kg*	*Route*	*Time of administration day*	*Days when arthritis assessed*	*Activity*	*Reference*
6-Mercaptopurine	10.0	p.o.	−1→10	16	+	14
	10.0	p.o.	−1→ 5	16	+	14
	10.0	p.o.	5→15	16	+	14
	10.0	p.o.	13→15	16	0	14
	25.0	i.m.	0→13	14	+	19
	35.0	p.o.	−1→12	20, 35	+	18
Methotrexate	0.1	i.m.	0→13	14	+	19
5-fluorouracil	0.5	s.c.	0→14	16	+	11
Cyclophosphamide	5.0	p.o.	0→18	18	+	10
	5.0	p.o.	0→ 4	18	+	10
	5.0	p.o.	10→14	18	0	10
	5.0	p.o.	14→18	18	0	10
	10.0	p.o.	−1→15	16	+	20
	10.0	p.o.	5→15	16	+	20
	10.0	p.o.	15→21	22	+	20
	20.0	p.o.	0→ 2	16	+	21
	20.0	p.o.	14→16	16	0	21
Anti-lymphocyte serum	8.0 ml	i.p.	0→ 2	16	+	21
	8.0 ml	i.p.	14→16	16	0	21

Table 15.4 Effect of miscellaneous slow-acting 'anti-rheumatic' drugs on disseminated adjuvant-induced polyarthritis in the rat. (Experimental protocol, numbering of days and the grading of activity were as in Table 15.1; AA, arthritis aggravated.)

Drug	*Daily dose mg/kg*	*Route*	*Time of administration day*	*Days when arthritis assessed*	*Activity*	*Reference*
Gold sodium thiomalate	2.5*	i.m.	−14→21	14→21	0	25
	5.0*	i.m.	−14→21	14→21	0	25
	10.0*	i.m.	−14→21	14→21	0	25
	10.0	i.m.	− 5→15	18, 30	+	26
	10.0	i.m.	15→30	30	+	26
Chloroquine diphosphate	25.0	p.o.	0→16	17	+	15
	10.0	i.p.	0→21	21	0	13
Hydroychloroquine sulphate	10.0	i.p.	0→21	21	0	13
DL-penicillamine	50.0	p.o.	−5→15	25	+	30
D-penicillamine	50.0	p.o.	15→30	30	0	21
	50.0	p.o.	− 5→15	18	0	26
	200.0	p.o.	− 4→20	15	0	27
Levamisole	25.0	p.o.	6 schedules	21	0	28, 29

* alternate days

observed so far. We must say, however, that compounds such as these have not been systematically tested in diseases such as human rheumatoid arthritis. Besides, it is possible that one or more of them might be acting against adjuvant-induced arthritis via pathways we know little or nothing of at the present time. For instance, most of these compounds are not inhibitors of prostaglandin synthetase but they could affect the arthritis through some other pathways of the immunological–inflammatory circuit so as to be beneficial in adjuvant-induced arthritis.

Administration of prostaglandin E has been reported to suppress adjuvant arthritis[31]. It is noteworthy, however, that the amounts of PGE_1 required for this effect were far in excess of those which could either be expected, or attained, *in vivo*.

Finally, attention has to be drawn to the ability of interferon and agents capable of inducing its synthesis (Table 15.6), to reduce the severity of disseminated adjuvant-induced polyarthritis. In our laboratories we have been deeply engaged in studies of the effects of tilorone HCl and interferon generated *in vitro* using the method of Tan *et al.*[34] on the incidence and severity of adjuvant-induced polyarthritis. Detailed results of these studies are now available as is the evidence to support the role of tilorone HCl as an interferon inducer[35,36].

Table 15.5 Effects of miscellaneous pharmacological agents on disseminated adjuvant-induced polyarthritis in the rat. (Experimental protocol, numbering of days and the grading of activity were as in Table 15.1.)

Drug	*Daily dose mg/kg*	*Route*	*Time of administration day*	*Days when arthritis assessed*	*Activity*	*Reference*
Dimethyl sulfoxide (DMSO)	2 ml/rat	p.o.	0→16	17	+	15
Epsilon amino caproic acid (EACA)	500.00	p.o.	0→16	17	+	15
Amethopterin	0.50	p.o.	−1→12	20, 35	+	18
Actinomycin D	0.04	i.p.	0→14	16	+	11
Puromycin	0.20	i.p.	0→14	16	+	11
d-amphetamine	20.00	p.o.	0→16	16	+	10
L-ephedrine	9.00	p.o.	0→16	16	+	10
Tranylcypromine	2.80	p.o.	0→16	16	+	10
Imipramine	50.00	p.o.	0→16	16	0	10
Chlorpromazine	10.00	p.o.	0→16	16	+	10
Chlordiazepoxide	10.00	p.o.	0→16	16	+	10
Chlorothiazide	15.00	p.o.	0→16	16	+	10

CONTRIBUTION TO THE SEARCH FOR BETTER ANTI-RHEUMATIC DRUGS

The model of adjuvant-induced polyarthritis which is so reproducible, especially in certain strains of inbred rats such as the Lewis rat, has been extensively used as a screening procedure to discover new and more potent drugs useful for the treatment of rheumatoid arthritis. The choice is based on the fact that as shown by observations summarized in Table 15.7, there is a greater similarity than dissimilarity between features characteristic of adjuvant-induced polyarthritis and RA.

The prevention of development of adjuvant-induced polyarthritis by the use of adequate doses of immunosuppressive drugs indicates that immunological factors are important to the development of joint inflammation following intra-cutaneous injection of FCA. This is directly supported by the fact that

Table 15.6 Effect of interferon and agents which may stimulate interferon synthesis on disseminated adjuvant-induced polyarthritis in the rat. (Experimental protocol, numbering of days and the grading of activity were as in Table 15.1.)

Drug	*Daily dose mg/kg*	*Route*	*Time of administration day*	*Days when arthritis assessed*	*Activity*	*Reference*
Interferon	0.2 ml*	i.p.	−1→15	16	+	14
Pyran copolymer	NS**	i.p.	−1, 7, 14	21	+	32
	NS	i.p.	−1	21	+	32
	NS	i.p.	7	21	+	32
	NS	i.p.	14	21	0	32
	NS	i.p.	18	21	0	32
Tilorone HCl	10.0	p.o.	−1→ 3	16	+	14, 33
	10.0	p.o.	−1→15	16	+	14, 33
	10.0	p.o.	−3	16	+	14
	10.0	p.o.	0	16	+	14
	10.0	p.o.	3	16	+	14
	10.0	p.o.	10	16	0	14
	10.0	p.o.	10→15	16	0	14, 33

* 1560 U/ml prepared *in vitro*; ** NS, not stated

surgical resection of all the lymph nodes draining the area of injection of FCA, e.g. the left popliteal, inguinal and para-aortic nodes in the case of FCA injected into the left-hind-paw, will prevent altogether the appearance of polyarthritis and other secondary lesions. The resection of lymph nodes prevents polyarthritis only if carried out before the fifth post-injection day; thereafter it is either without any effect, or it lessens the severity of polyarthritis.

The fact that drugs such as D-penicillamine and levamisole which, though clearly benefiting some patients with RA, are either uniformly without effect on adjuvant-induced polyarthritis or aggravate it, is often used to question the adequacy of the experimental system as a model of the human disease. It should, however, be noted that compounds of this class act slowly in RA and it is reasonable to consider that, until disproven experimentally, a similar type of slow reactivity may also occur in the rat. No studies, to our knowledge, have been undertaken in adjuvant arthritis to test the effect of 'pre-dosing' the animals with D-penicillamine or levamisole for 30, 60 or even 90 days prior to the injection of FCA, and then continuing the administration of the drug for a further period of four weeks.

With regard to the question whether studies of the effect of chemicals on adjuvant-induced polyarthritis can provide a positive lead for novel types of anti-rheumatic drugs, we can only speculate that if interferon, when it becomes available in quantities sufficient to test it clinically in humans, may prove to have as beneficial an effect in RA as it has in the experimental model. Pending approval by agencies for drug licensure, it would be equally interesting to investigate the therapeutic effects of interferon-inducers such as tilorone HCL and pyran copolymer.

CONCLUDING REMARKS

Similarity between the histopathological and clinical features of adjuvant-induced polyarthritis and RA, makes the former a fairly suitable experimental model for detection of compounds useful for the treatment of RA as well as for investigations into the sequence of cascading events responsible for the development of immunologically-mediated joint inflammation.

Table 15.7 Comparison of human rheumatoid arthritis with adjuvant-induced polyarthritis in the rat

	Human RA	*Rat AA*
Initiating insult	? stress	FCA, stress
Persistence of antigen	?+	+ (indigestable cell wall fragments)
Latent period	?	10–16 days
Genetic effects	Ir genes, HLA DW4	++
Activation of microbial (? viral) agent	?	?+
Inhibition by anti-viral agents	ND*	++
Partial or complete suppression by immunosuppressive drugs	+	++
Inhibition by lymphocyte depletion (thoracic duct drainage) (refs 37 and 38)	++	++
Transfer by lymphocytes	ND	++ (ref 37)
Transfer by serum	–	–
Partial or complete suppression by anti-inflammatory drugs	+→++	++
Effect of D-penicillamine or levamisole	+	**

* ND — not done
** Needs further testing

References

1. Pearson, C. M.: (1965). Development of arthritis, periarthritis and periostitis in rats given adjuvants. *Proc. Soc. Exp. Biol. Med.*, **91,** 95
2. Pearson, C. M.: (1964). Experimental models in rheumatoid disease. *Arthr. Rheum.*, **7,** 80
3. Pearson, C. M., Waksman, B. H. and Sharp, J. T. (1961). Studies of arthritis and other lesions induced in rats by injection of mycobacterial adjuvants. V. *J. Exp. Med.*, **113,** 485
4. Kohashi, O., Watanabe, Y., Beck, F. W. J. and Pearson, C. M. (1976). Studies on adjuvant arthritis in rats. III. Antigenic requirements for arthritogenicity of peptidoglycans from S. aureus and L. plantarum. (In press)
5. Paronetto, F. (1972). Studies on experimental arthritis induced by *Corynebacterium rubrum.* I. Localization of the arthritogenic factor in the cell walls. *Arthr. Rheum.*, **15,** 36
6. Adler, E., Heller, H., Weiner, E., *et al.* (1973). Degradation of ^{14}C-labelled group A streptococci and micrococci in muscular lesions, in the mouse. *Isr. J. Med. Sci.*, **9,** 483
7. Hadler, N. M. (1976). A pathogenetic model for erosive synovitis. *Arthr. Rheum.*, **19,** 256
8. Ryzewska, A. G. (1967). Influence of lymphatic tissue on the development of adjuvant-induced polyarthritis in rats. *Ann. Rheum. Dis.*, **26,** 506
9. Jones, R. S. and Ward, J. R. (1963). Studies on adjuvant-induced polyarthritis in rats. II. Histogenesis of joint and visceral lesions. *Arthr. Rheum.*, **6,** 23
10. Walz, D. T., DiMartino, M. J., and Misher, A. (1971). Adjuvant-induced arthritis in rats. II. Drug effects on physiologic, biochemical, and immunologic parameters. *J. Pharmacol. Exp. Ther.*, **178,** 223
11. Glenn, E. M. (1966). Adjuvant-induced arthritis: Effects of certain drugs on incidence, clinical severity and biochemical changes. *Am. J. Vet. Res.*, **27,** 339
12. Piliero, S. J. and Colombo, C. (1969). *J. Clin. Pharmacol.*
13. Ward, J. R. and Cloud, R. S. (1966). Comparative effect of anti-rheumatic drugs on adjuvant-induced polyarthritis in rats. *J. Pharm. Exp. Ther.*, **152,** 116
14. Pearson, C. M. and Chang, Y.-H. (1977). Adjuvant arthritis: Immune responses and effects of Tilorone or interferon in partially suppressing the disease. In D. A. Willoughby J. P. Jiroud and G. P. Velo (eds.), p. 131. *Perspectives in Inflammation* (Lancaster: MTP).
15. Winter, C. A. and Nuss, G. W. (1966). Treatment of adjuvant arthritis in rats with anti-inflammatory drugs. *Arthr. Rheum.*, **9,** 394
16. Glenn, M. E. and Kooyers, W. M. (1966). Plasma Inflammation units: An objective method for investigating effects of drug on experimental inflammation. *Life Sci.*, **5,** 619
17. Winder, C. V., Lembke, L. A. and Stephens, M. D. (1969). Comparative bioassay of drugs in adjuvant-induced arthritis in rats: Flufenamic acid, mefenamic acid, and phenylbutazone. *Arthr. Rheum.*, **12,** 472
18. Graeme, M. L., Fabry, E. and Sigg, E. D. (1969). Mycobacterial adjuvant periarthritis in rodents and its modification by antiinflammatory agents. *J. Pharm. Exp. Ther.*, **153,** 373
19. Ward, J. R., Cloud, R. S., Krawitt, E. L. and Jones, R. S. (1964). Studies on adjuvant-induced polyarthritis in rats. III. The effect of "immunosuppressive agents" on arthritis and tubercular hypersensitivity. *Arthr. Rheum.*, **7,** 654
20. Chang, Y.-H. (1977). Adjuvant polyarthritis. I. Incorporation of quantitative measures of humoral and cellular immune response. *J. Pharmacol. Exp. Ther.* **201,** 1
21. Currey, H. L. F. (1964). A comparison of immunosuppressive and anti-inflammatory agents in the rat. *Clin. Exp. Immunol.*, **9,** 879
22. Page, A. R., Condie, R. M. and Good, R. A. (1962). Effect of 6-mercaptopurine on inflammation. *Am. J. Pathol.*, **40,** 519
23. Hurd, E. R. and Ziff, M. (1968). Studies of the anti-inflammatory action of 6-mercaptopurine. *J. Exp. Med.*, **128,** 785
24. Stevens, J. E. and Willoughby, D. A. (1969). The anti-inflammatory effect of some immunosuppressive agents. *J. Pathol.*, **97,** 367

25. Jessop, J. D. and Currey, H. L. F. (1968). Influence of gold salts on adjuvant arthritis in the rat. *Ann. Rheum. Dis.*, **27**, 577

26. Arrigoni-Martelli, E. and Bramm, E. (1975). Investigation on the influence of cyclophosphamide, gold sodium thiomalate, and D-penicillamine on nystatin oedema and adjuvant arthritis. *Agents Actions*, **5**, 264

27. Liyanage, S. P. and Currey, H. L. F. (1972). *Ann. Rheum. Dis.*, **31**, 521

28. Kapusta, M. A. and Mendelson, J. (1967). Inhibition of adjuvant arthritis by statolon. *Proc. Soc. Exp. Biol. Med.*, **126**, 496

28. Willoughby, D. A. and Dieppe, P. A. (1976). The effects of D-penicillamine in animal models. In *Penicillamine Research in Rheumatoid Disease*, pp. 45–49 (E. Munthe ed.)

29. Huskinsson, E. C., Dieppe, P. A., Scott, J., Terappnell, J., Balme, H. W. and Willoughby, D. A. (1976). Rheumatoid arthritis. *Lancet*, i, 393

30. Klamer, B., Kimura, E. T. and Makstenieks, M. (1968). Effects of oral cysteine, penicillamine and N-acetyl-penicillamine on adjuvant arthritis in rats. *Pharmacology*, **1**, 283

31. Zurrier, R. B. and Quagliata, F. (1971). Effect of prostaglandin E, on adjuvant arthritis, *Nature* (*London*), **234**, 304

32. Kapusta, M. A. and Mendelson, J. (1969). The inhibition of adjuvant disease in rats by the interferon-inducing agent pyran copolymer. *Arthr. Rheum.*, **12**, 463

33. Chang, Y.-H. (1977). Adjuvant polyarthritis. II. Suppression by tilorone. *J. Pharmacol. Exp. Ther.*, (in press)

34. Tan, Y. H., Armstrong, J. A., Ke, Y. H. and Ho, M. (1970). Regulation of cellular interferon production: enhancement by antimetabolites. *Proc. Nat. Acad. Sci. U.S.A.*, **67**, 464

35. Krueger, R. F. and Jayer, G. D. (1970). Tilorone hydrochloride: An orally active interferon inducer. *Science*, **169**, 1213

36. Mayer, G. D. and Krueger, R. F. (1970). Tilorone hydrochloride: Mode of action. *Science*, **169**, 1214

37. Whitehouse, D. J., M. W. Whitehouse and C. M. Pearson. (1969). Passive transfer of adjuvant-induced arthritis and allergic encephalomyelitis in rats using thoracic duct lymphocytes. *Nature* (*London*), **224**,1322

38. Pearson, C. M., Paulus, H. E. and Machleder, H. L. (1975). The role of the lymphocyte and its products in the propagation of joint disease. *Ann. N.Y. Acad. Sci.*, **256**, 150

Discussion V

Control Mechanisms in Cell-Mediated Immunity (Chapter 12)

R. R. A. COOMBS: Professor Turk showed a slide of immune complex disease and he showed arthritis. Were they clinical observations?

J. L. TURK: Yes.

W. CARSON DICK: The metabolism of cyclophosphamide is an extremely complex series of events. Has anybody looked to see whether there is any particular metabolite, or a group of metabolites, that is most effective in either suppressing or enhancing cellular activity?

J. L. TURK: We have not looked at breakdown products of cyclophosphamide, though there is much evidence that it has no action *in vitro*. It needs to be used *in vivo*.

The only compounds we have found to resemble cyclophosphamide are melphalan and ICRF-159, a very interesting compound, I believe now marketed by ICI (although I do not know what it is called). It is interesting that we find melphalan active, and cyclophosphamide active, both being mustards. However, the other mustards that we have looked at, such as busulfan and chlorambucil, do not seem to be at all effective in our model, and we should be very interested if anybody has any ideas on this because we have asked people in the field and they do not understand why we get this differentiation between the two groups of compounds.

Azathioprine has a very marginal effect. We have also looked at methotrexate and procarbazine; both were ineffective.

The Rheumatological Significance of Lymphokines (Chapter 13)

C. M. PEARSON: That was a very nice discussion.

I have noticed that Dr. Dumonde has not stressed, or mentioned, a role for the macrophage or monocyte. In various discussions at recent symposia, etc. the monocyte or macrophage has assumed a significant role in the activation of lymphocytes.

How does Dr. Dumonde place it into his system?

Secondly, are monocytes necessary for the *in vitro* lymphocyte–endothelial interactions and would anti-monocyte antibody moderate the process in any way?

Third, why not culture some human vascular endothelium and take normal and rheumatoid lymphocytes and/or macrophages or monocytes to investigate whether they have a more aggressive approach against the endothelium that is being cultured in the monolayer.

D. C. DUMONDE: At Federation meetings it is customary to answer the last question first. We have not yet done it, but we are aware that the vascular surgeons can provide us with the raw materials, in more ways than one, and the rheumatologists can provide us with some of the other raw materials. We await characterization of the mixed cell system before extending it to the patients.

Secondly, what about the macrophage. We may well come back to it later, but over the years we, as a group, have thought a lot about the macrophage. Dr. John Morley has developed ideas on the possibility that lymphokine production by lymphocytes may activate macrophages to produce E-type PGs which could switch off lymphokine production by lymphocytes, and so provide a homeostatic mechanism that might be relevant to rheumatoid disease (*Prostaglandins*, **8**, 315; 1974).

Perhaps I might sow a seed which we might also come back to later. With the help of Dr. T. J. Williams of the Royal College of Surgeons we have been assaying PG production by culture of vascular endothelial cells and have shown that they produce substantial quantities of E-type PGs in monolayer culture in quantities that could be expected to switch off any potential activation of the circulatory lymphocytes that might take place during the orgasmic process of endothelial and vascular penetration.

J. R. VANE: Were only E-type PGs found in the vascular-endothelial cultures, or was 6-keto-PG-F_1-alpha found too?

D. C. DUMONDE: We are not quite such molecular wizards, but Dr. Williams might have further information.

T. J. WILLIAMS: We only found E-type PGs because we only looked for E-type PGs.

Recognition of Anti-Rheumatic Drugs using the Homograft Reaction (Chapter 14)

J. L. TURK: When one goes to rheumatological meetings one hears a lot about the joints. That hand that was shown had a massive rheumatoid nodule. Many people tend to forget the importance of the rheumatoid nodule. One wonders whether there should not be more models of chronic immunological granuloma investigated, and that one should be looking for a different group of compounds, perhaps, those which might be active in reducing the intensity of a nodule of that type. How often do we give Freund's complete adjuvant, which produces a chronic granuloma, and then look at the effect of drugs on the size of an adjuvant granuloma?

M. K. JASANI: In the light of our observations of the skin graft model we became most interested in what might happen during inflammation stimulated by the sub-plantar injection of mycobacterial antigen as in the adjuvant-induced arthritis model. On reviewing the literature we were impressed by evidence indicating that the currently available anti-rheumatic drugs are much less effective, or even ineffective, against swelling in the paw which received the adjuvant (see *J. Pharmacol. Exp. Ther.*, **178**, 223; 1971).

I. F. SKIDMORE: Could the apparent anamolous action of aspirin in the skin graft model be attributed to its action as an acetylating agent for cells? Local administration of an acetylating agent would maximise the chance of its acting on a cell in the local inflammatory response.

M. K. JASANI: It is a very attractive hypothesis which we should like to keep in mind and to test appropriately.

J. WEBB: It is obvious to all the clinicians that Dr. Jasani showed dorsal tenosynovitis.

M. K. JASANI: Dr. Webb is the first person to have spotted it, but that in no way detracts from the argument for the patient also shows definite sign of rheumatoid arthritis including swan-neck deformity of the fifth digit. I put it in to emphasize to those who are not familiar with rheumatoid arthritis how large the swelling can be. Additionally, the pathogenesis of tenosynovitis may not differ from that of synovitis.

The Contribution of Adjuvant Arthritis to the Recognition of Anti-Rheumatic Drugs (Chapter 15)

K. TRNAVSKY: I should like to add levamisole to the list. We recently tested levamisole

(5 mg/kg daily) starting on day zero till day 18. It had no effect, or even an aggravating effect on the clinical . . .

C. M. PEARSON (*interrupting*): We have confirmed the aggravating effect.

K. TRNAVSKY: So have we confirmed it.
On the other hand, we had interesting results with the thymic extract prepared in Bucharest by Dr. Mircowicz; it was very efficient when administered from day zero until day 18.

C. M. PEARSON: That is very interesting. I hope to be able to add that to my series.

A. A. J. GOLDBERG: Would Dr. Pearson, speaking as a clinician, care to comment on the natural history of adjuvant arthritis in the absence of any drug treatment.

I believe I have seen somewhere that it is self-limiting and that it disappears after a number of weeks, and no permanent lesions can be detected in the animal afterwards.

Is that correct?, and if it is, would that not complicate its use when examining for drugs of the penicillamine type which have to be administered for a long period of time before any effect on the disease manifestations become apparent.

C. M. PEARSON: As you know, customarily once disseminated adjuvant-induced polyarthritis becomes established, the result is noted and, within days, the animals are disposed of in some fashion or another. Consequently the long-term events are not really well-known.

However, in collaboration with Dr. F. Wood (unpublished observations) I have had an opportunity to follow up the course of the disseminated polyarthritis for up to 150 days. We found that after the first wave of arthritic lesions, which appeared at around day 18 and plateaued between days 25 and 30, there was a second wave of generalized arthritis at about day 60; and even a third wave — albeit not very severe, but very definite — at about day 120. Therefore, I believe that adjuvant-induced arthritic disease is not a one-shot type of disorder, though I agree that in general people have not taken the time to look at its full natural history in any detail. Dr. Goldberg is to be thanked for raising this rather interesting point.

J. L. TURK: One of the points that comes out from the discussion is that there is a spectrum of clinical manifestations in rheumatoid arthritis. One sees patients with self-limiting disease, and then the whole range to the very severe chronic patient who becomes very debilitated and disabled. The co-chairman mentioned that there are now strains of rats with self-limiting disease, and strains of rats with chronic disease. This points to the type of investigation that has been done in mouse leprosy where there is a similar spectrum and there are now two strains of mice, one which develops tuberculoid leprosy, and the other which develops lepromatous leprosy. In such situations one can begin to do genetic experiments and one can begin to get some insights into the genetics of these conditions.

A. T. A. DOBLE: If we are using this model for selecting drugs for anti-rheumatic use, as many of us are, it is worth looking at the histology, particularly of the disseminated arthritic lesions. The earliest changes to be seen are not in the joint space, nor even in the joint synovium, but they are in the subcutaneous tissue. They show what looks typically like mast-cell degranulation followed by oedematous reaction which then draws in mononuclear cells which the literature suggests are lymphocytes, but which come in such vast numbers that that has to be questioned. It should also be noted that the mononuclear cells change through several different morphological types, ending up almost like fibroblasts.

Secondly, some secondary lesions occur in the soft tissues, away from the bones, and these tend to reach their maximum severity at about 2 or 3 weeks, and then subside. They are self-limiting. When inflammation occurs against the bone, it appears that the lesions cannot undergo resolution, but progress all the way through the bone until fibrous tissue replaces what used to be the bone. Two things can bring that inflammation to an end: either the inflammatory front sweeps right through the bone, or it seems to run out of steam — perhaps because of interference with supplies of nutrients.

But, if we are testing anti-rheumatic drugs, then we may be doing the wrong thing in assuming that the chronicity is due to the lymphocytes acting against some antigen. It may be that there is antibody mediation only, and that there are geographical considerations.

C. M. PEARSON: I would only support the comment about the very active early lesion being present in the subcutaneous tissues with profound activation of what appear to be fibroblasts, osteoclasts, and osteoblasts, and perhaps degranulation of mast cells. Whether that is unique to the rat or not is certainly not clear. There are not enough biopsies done in human rheumatoid arthritis to clarify that.

Some of the secondary lesions are not too dissimilar to those described by Dr. Dumonde since they appear in the vascular endothelium and in the perivascular regions. One sees, for instance, nodules in the ears in these rats at about the second or third week, and they all appear to be around blood vessels with swollen endothelium.

J. L. TURK: One of the points that Dr. Doble raised was the large numbers of mononuclear cells that he thought were perhaps different from lymphocytes. Of course a lot of these cells will be macrophages, and in various forms of activation, perhaps going on to taking on an epitheloid cell appearance which may be why he says some of the cells have a fibroblast-like appearance. It is often very difficult to distinguish early macrophages from lymphocytes without using histocytochemical methods for the presence of lysosomal acid phosphatase. Large numbers of lysosomes are found in the cytoplasm of activated macrophages.

C. M. PEARSON: If I might respond. I remain very impressed with Dr. A. C. Allison's speculation concerning the possibility that a granuloma could be an ongoing response of macrophages secreting some of their substances, recruiting additional macrophages, and inflammatory cells, into an area to give rise to a granuloma. That is not too dissimilar, obviously, to what one sees in sarcoid, or in leprosy, or conceivably, with a little imagination, in adjuvant arthritis.

A. T. A. DOBLE: That is precisely my point. It is so often said that adjuvant arthritis relies on cell-mediated immunity for its chronicity, but since Dr. Allison and others have shown that macrophages are quite capable of perpetuating a lesion without the involvement of lymphocytes, the evidence supporting a role for cell-mediated immunity requires to be carefully re-examined.

K. WHALEY: Pyran copolymer, apart from being an interferon inducer, also activates the alternative complement pathway. Is cobra venom effective against adjuvant arthritis?

C. M. PEARSON: To my knowledge cobra venom has not been utilized in this model.

A. R. MACKENZIE: With regard to Dr. Whaley's question, there are reports (Copusto and Nelson) — some years ago now — which suggest that depletion of complement with cobra venom factor delayed the onset of disseminated adjuvant-induced polyarthritis by 2 or 3 days. It had no impressive effect on the arthritic lesions themselves.

Dr. Pearson made the comment that immune complexes might have a role in the pathogenesis of adjuvant arthritis. I would suggest that they play a crucial role in the initiation of adjuvant arthritis. We have been able to show by treating rats with a single large dose of cyclophosphamide in the way described by Professor Turk, and then injecting them with adjuvant that there is a total inhibition of adjuvant arthritis. More important, we have been able to show that we can induce polyarthritis in the cyclophosphamide-treated, adjuvant-injected animals by transferring passively small amounts of immune serum collected from arthritic rats.

We should like to propose that the initial lesions are caused by soluble immune complexes deposited in the joints, and that the cellular mechanisms only become important at a later stage. The serum reconstitution experiments show a very strict dose requirement. Large amounts of serum consistently fail to reconstitute the effect. We have used very small amounts, and this suggests that we are looking at a situation of soluble immune complexes formed in antigen excess.

I am not quite sure where the comments made earlier by Dr Perper fit in, but this is another mechanism whereby perhaps complexes, antibody, or some other serum factor may be important.

C. M. PEARSON: There certainly seems to be some evidence, generated by my colleague Dr. Chang, that there are circulating humoral factors combined with cell-mediated factors, and perhaps others that are involved in this latency period in order to induce the disease. Certainly giving large quantities of serum from animals at varying stages does not seem to initiate the disease by itself.

J. L. TURK: To go back to the point on the cobra venom factor. Elizabeth Lewis and I (*J. Pathol.*, **115**, 87–125; 1975) have compared the anti-inflammatory effect of cobra venom factor with that of depletion of circulating complement induced by use of immunological reagents including the immune complexes. We found cobra venom to be as effective as the immunological reagents against non-specific inflammation caused by turpentine but not against allergic inflammation caused by the Arthus or Swartzmann reactions in the guinea pig.

GENERAL DISCUSSION

W. CARSON DICK: My question is addressed to Dr. Pearson. We have the macrophage. We have other cell types, and most recently we have the vascular endothelial cell. But it seems to me that Dr. Pearson's observations of the beneficial effects of the depletion of circulating lymphocytes by drainage of thoracic duct lymph in patients with rheumatoid arthritis (*Ann. N.Y. Acad. Sci.*, **256**, 150; 1975), the re-precipitation of joint inflammation by re-injection of the drained autologous lymphocytes into a quiescent joint and other evidence must focus attention on the pathogenetic importance of lymphocytes. Would Dr. Pearson defend the lymphocyte?

C. M. PEARSON: Yes. I most assuredly would. I feel that the lymphocyte plays a crucial role in human rheumatoid arthritis, in adjuvant arthritis, and very likely in a number of the other models that we deal with; and probably it functions in conjunction with the humoral responses, perhaps immune complexes, perhaps the vascular endothelium, and unquestionably the monocyte-derived macrophage. They are all working in concert, and they have lost their regulatory capabilities in a number of disorders due to something that we have done, for instance to the rat in adjuvant arthritis, and something we do not know that is the inciting agent in human rheumatoid arthritis.

W. WATSON BUCHANAN: If the lymphocyte is so important, then the observation of Dr. Jasani are even more relevant, more germane to our therapy. Can he tell us whether once lymphocytes are recruited to the homograft, if salicylates are then given can these lymphocytes be dispersed?

Secondly, could he tell us the effects of topical administration of these various compounds in the recruitment of lymphocytes in, for instance, the tuberculin reaction.

M. K. JASANI: The homograft reaction, so far as we know, is a one-way process, probably because it has a lot of antigen it it. My straight answer, both on the basis of the homograft model and on the basis of other models that I know, is no. In fact the activated immune lymphocyte will deliver its damaging potential though topically applied aspirin might be able to moderate the vascular effects induced by its products. The process is self-limited, so in that sense there may be recovery.

R. J. PERPER: I would agree that the lymphocyte is probably important in the pathogenesis of rheumatoid arthritis, but to try to approach treatment of the disease through the lymphocyte appears to me like using a sledge-hammer. Drugs such as penicillamine and levamisole have no overt effect on lymphocyte activity *per se*, and yet they seem to work in rheumatoid arthritis. To account for their effectiveness I would like to suggest that in rheumatoid arthritis there is an imbalance in the immuno-regulatory mechanism, perhaps involving hyperactivity of suppressor cells, and resulting in immunodepression.

J. L. TURK: I wanted to ask Dr. Pearson whether he had any ideas on how levamisole might be working, if he believes it works, and I also wondered whether anyone else might have any ideas.

C. M. PEARSON: One of the characteristic responses is that it stimulates T-suppressor cells, thereby slowing down the response of B-cells, or some interaction such as that. I would generally tend to agree with that general concept as observed *in vitro*. I believe that in a number of instances it clearly does work in patients with rheumatoid arthritis, although the toxicity of both levamisole and penicillamine are such that it makes the use of either of them in the human somewhat suspect to my mind.

J. L. TURK: Has Dr. Jasani any ideas on levamisole?

M. K. JASANI: Whatever I say regarding levamisole will be too speculative and I would prefer to avoid it.

I have however, a general comment particularly addressed to the problem raised by Dr. Perper.

If I understood him correctly, he is asking how we can explain the clinical benefit that we observe in RA, not only with penicillamine, but with other drugs which do not show activity against the lymphocyte.

If we visualize that the activated immune lymphocytes operate not only via the direct vascular effects of lymphokines but also via the effects of lymphokines upon the macrophages, polymorphonuclear leukocytes, endothelial cells, etc. (see *J. Exp. Med.*, **133,** 1242; 1971; and *Clinics Rheum. Dis.*, **1,** (2), p354; 1975), then the clinical usefulness of drugs which inhibit non-lymphocytic factors but which do not show activity against lymphocytes *per se* becomes readily understandable. Treatment with a drug effective against non-lymphocytic factors will provide clinical improvement only in direct proportion to the pathogenetic importance of the cell-type or vascular phenomenon it inhibits. It will not arrest the inflammatory disease process, some manifestations of which will persist.

As you all by now know, in my own investigations of the effect of anti-rheumatic drugs against the homograft reaction, the emphasis has not been on the lymphocyte itself as much as on the elucidation of tissue changes which persist despite inhibition of the role of polymorphs and macrophages; for I believe that existing therapy of the lymphocytic component of rheumatoid inflammation could be improved by additional use of agents which may, to take but one example, be fully active against fibrin-induced blockage of lymphatics.

W. CARSON DICK: I have some data on levamisole which is important to support the points made by Dr. Jasani and by Dr. Pearson.

We have had 2½ years' experience in two different kinds of study and I shall not go into the details now other than to say that — as Dr. Pearson has indicated — it is a highly toxic drug, without any doubts whatsoever. It is very much more effective in a few individuals within a group of patients, though when judged by group response (mean ± SE.) it is only marginally effective as compared with non-steroidal analgesic/anti-inflammatory drugs.

The other important point is that when levamisole is stopped in a patient in whom it is successful, the disease immediately re-appears. In that respect it is only palliative.

R. J. PERPER: I might be able to shed a little light on the mechanism of action of levamisole — from some of our own data and from some that has been reported.

In rheumatoid patients with depressed PHA reactivity, levamisole restores the PHA reactivity to normal, but has no measureable effect in those patients who have normal PHA reactivity to begin with. In other words, it seems to work in immuno-depressed patients only. Penicillamine seems to have a similar clinical effect and it is possible that like levamisole it is working through eliminating this excessive suppressor T-cell activity, but that has yet to be tested directly.

J. L. TURK: But there is no evidence that the suppressor cell is a T cell. It could be either T- or B-lymphocyte.

R. J. PERPER: There is no evidence that levamisole has any activity at all on lymphocytes. It certainly does not alter normal immune response. It does not have an effect on any of the lymphocyte-mediated events. We have tested it on lymphokine release and cytotoxic activity. So as far as I am concerned, there is no evidence that levamisole works at all on the lymphoid system other than to stimulate the subnormal lymphoid system back to normal. Where it acts is certainly an open question.

J. L. TURK: But it could be doing it through the depression of a suppressor cell population.

R. J. PERPER: That seems the most logical place.

Z. BENTWICH: There are more than a few reports in support of Dr. Perper's views. Dr. Martin Jerry and Dr. Steitz have done studies in cancer patients and have shown some enhancement of recall-antigen response. We too have done studies, the results of which tend to support the idea that in case of patients who improve with levamisole we are dealing with a subset of immunosuppressed or severely suppressed patients.

If one can accept the histamine receptor as a marker for suppressor T lymphocytes, then there is some preliminary evidence to suggest that the levamisole does affect that population.

W. WATSON BUCHANAN: Referring back to Dr. Jasani's work regarding the deposition of fibrin in relation to mononuclear cells, is Dr. Jasani suggesting that without these cells there will be no fibrin deposition, and that in some way perhaps the lymphocytes are secreting a lymphokine that is causing fibrin accumulation?

M. K. JASANI: Yes. When we have all the evidence, that could well turn out to be the case.

Section: VI
The Severity of Inflammatory Rheumatic Disease: Clinical and Laboratory Assessment

Chairman: W. W. Buchanan

Co-Chairman: E. V. Barnett

16
Standardization in Clinical Measurement

G. P. BALINT, M. E. MAVRIKAKIS, P. LEE, P. J. ROONEY and W. W. BUCHANAN

INTRODUCTION

The methods of assessment of efficacy of non-steroidal, aspirin-like, anti-rheumatic drugs is reviewed. The desirability of objective measurement is emphasized but the insensitivity of such measurements is compared with that of the more subjective but clinically more useful methods. The dependence on measurements based on the cardinal signs of inflammation emphasizes the lack of real progress in the management of inflammatory joint disease.

Inflammation was defined by Celsus as: rubor, calor, dolor, tumor and functio laesa. These five cardinal features of inflammation are present to varying degree in different forms of inflammatory joint disease. Thus, for example, rubor is seen commonly in inflamed joints in acute gouty arthritis or septic arthritis, but is rare in rheumatoid arthritis. Calor is common in rheumatoid arthritis, but its measurement, by either skin temperature recording or by thermography, requires the environmental temperature to be constant. Dolor, tumor and functio laesa are the three features which are most frequently assessed in clinical therapeutic trials in rheumatoid arthritis, and are the basis of this short review.

MEASUREMENT OF TUMOR

Measurement of joint swelling in rheumatoid arthritis has proved extremely difficult. Hart and Clark[1] introduced jewellers' rings to measure the circumference of the interphalangeal joints of the thumbs and the proximal interphalangeal joints of the hands. The Geigy plastic spring gauge has been found more convenient than jewellers' rings, although both give comparable results ($r = 0.948$)[2]. An arthrocircameter, consisting of a spring gauge incorporating a fully flexible polyethylene loop, has been introduced and claimed[3] to be more accurate than the more simple Geigy spring gauge, but without evidence to support this claim.

Boardman and Hart[2] showed a significant reduction in digital joint circumference with prednisone and high doses of aspirin, 3 g daily or more, in patients with rheumatoid arthritis. They were unable to demonstrate any

Table 16.1 Digital joint circumference measurement (mm). Intra- and inter-observer error, diurnal variation and effect of hospitalization for one week

Observer and observations	*No. of patients*	*First measurement Mean ± SE*	*Second measurement Mean ± SE*	*Difference Mean ± SE*	*Significance t*	*p*
A versus A within 30 min	18	*569.6* ± 14.9	*568.9* ± 14.7	*2.7* ± 1.0	*2.7*	<0.01
A versus B within 30 min	34	559.8 ± 8.1	570.4 ± 7.8	10.6 ± 1.4	7.8	<0.001
A versus A 7 a.m. to 9 p.m.	11	592.2 ± 15.2	594.4 ± 16.3	2.2 ± 1.7	1.3	NS
A versus A 1 week interval	11	578.0 ± 16.3	574.9 ± 15.8	3.1 ± 2.6	1.4	NS

Reproduced by kind permission of the Editor of the *Scandinavian Journal of Rheumatology*.

reduction with low doses of aspirin, less than 3 g per day, or paracetamol. The authors concluded that less than 3 g of aspirin per day was without anti-inflammatory effect, but this dose of aspirin might be anti-inflammatory if a more sensitive method of demonstrating anti-inflammatory effect were available.

We[4] have investigated the measurement of 'ring size' using the Geigy apparatus, and found the intra-observer error to be quite acceptable (2.7 mm). This confirms the observations of Hart and his colleagues[1,2]. However, the important finding, as can be seen from Table 16.1, is that the inter-observer error is considerable (10.6 mm), and emphasizes the need for serial measurements to be made by the one observer. It should be noted that although intra-observer errors may be small they can be statistically significant using the commonly employed Student's t test for paired variables[4,5], and could easily be mistaken for drug effect. It is vital that the actual decrease in joint circumference be interpreted in clinical therapeutic trials rather than the p value. Figure 16.1 illustrates what was statistically a significant reduction in digital joint circumference, but if the authors[6] had examined the scale of the ordinate they would have concluded that the reduction (1.64 mm) was not of any clinical significance. Diurnal variation of digital joint circumference has been recorded[2, 7],

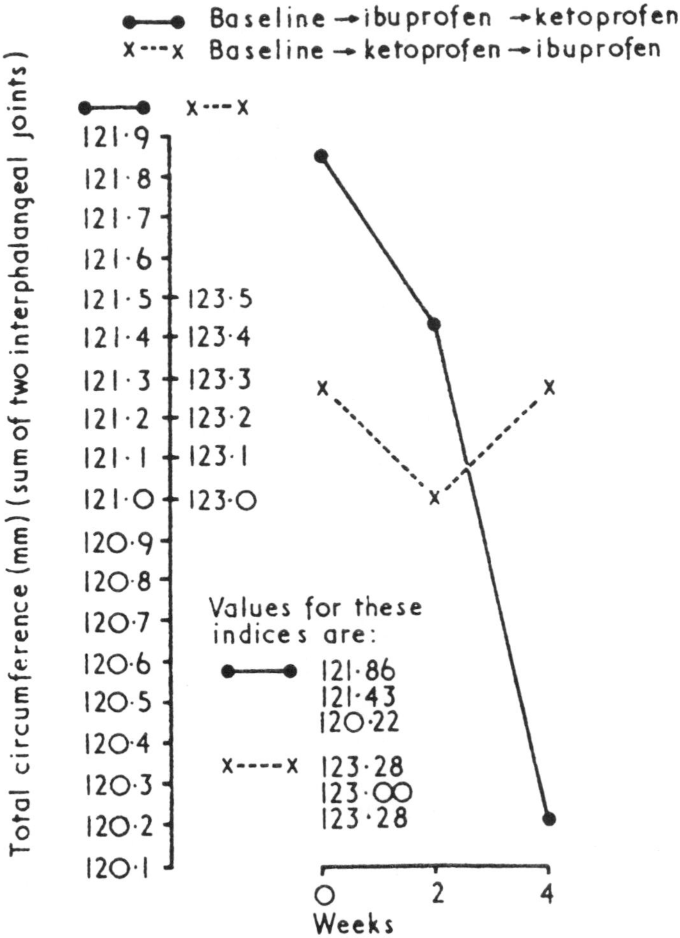

Figure 16.1 Statistically significant reduction in digital joint circumference of doubtful clinical significance (Reproduced by permission of the authors and by the Editor of the *British Medical Journal*)

but we[4] were unable to demonstrate this in a group of patients with rheumatoid arthritis.

From Table 16.2, it can be seen that reduction in digital joint circumference occurs especially where there is soft tissue swelling. Clearly joint size cannot be reduced if swelling is due to bony changes! In many publications of trials of

Table 16.2 Digital joint circumference measurements (mm) during aspirin and prednisone therapy

Drugs		*No. of patients*	*Placebo score Mean ± SE*	*Drug score Mean ± SE*	*Difference Mean ± SE*	*Significance t*	*p*
Aspirin versus	All joints	12	*599.5* ± 7.5	*593.1* ± 8.4	*6.4* ± 2.3	2.8	<0.01
Pacebo	'Soft' Joints	11	419.9 ± 29.8	410.6 ± 29.0	9.3 ± 1.6	5.7	<0.0005
	'Hard' joints	12	214.6 ± 43.6	216.7 ± 44.2	2.1 ± 1.0	2.2	<0.05
Prednisone versus	All joints	12	599.5 ± 7.5	586.2 ± 8.2	13.3 ± 2.5	5.3	<0.0005
Placebo	'Soft' joints	11	419.9 ± 29.8	402.9 ± 29.1	17.0 ± 1.4	11.9	<0.0005
	'Hard' joints	12	214.6 ± 43.6	216.8 ± 44.2	2.2 ± 0.7	3.0	<0.01

Reproduced by kind permission of the Editor of the *Scandinavian Journal of Rheumatology*.

anti-rheumatic drugs, no significant reduction in digital joint circumference is found. This, of course, does not mean that the active drugs have no anti-inflammatory effect, but implies merely that such an effect could not be measured. Government licensing agencies place a great deal of importance on whether a new anti-rheumatic agent has anti-inflammatory effect. However, this seems to us not of particular importance, since if the drug relieves the patient's pain this is all the physician and patient desire.

To our knowledge, anti-inflammatory effect of anti-rheumatic drugs has not been ascertained in joints other than the finger joints, although Deodhar *et al.*[8] did assess swelling in a clinical knee 'score' which included joint pain and tenderness.

MEASUREMENT OF FUNCTIO LAESA

Loss of function is common in rheumatoid arthritis but has proved remarkably difficult to measure. In 1949, the Committee for Therapeutic Criteria of the American Rheumatism Association (Steinbrocker *et al.*)[9] produced a simple classification consisting of four classes based on the matching descriptive method of Taylor[10]. The Joint Committee of the Medical Research Council and Nuffield Foundation used a five point scale. Other similar classifications have been employed by Savage[11]; the Empire Rheumatism Council[12]; and by Copeman[13]. Functional capacity has also been recorded as the patient's own estimate of his percentage fitness[12].

These functional indices employing four or five grades of incapacity have been found useful in monitoring the long-term course of a patient's illness, but have proved too insensitive to detect changes in functional status in short-term clinical trials[11,14–16]. In rehabilitation centres, more elaborate scoring systems have been employed using as many as a 100 or more separate activities of daily living[17–19]. However, these methods are time-consuming and have not proved popular to the busy rheumatologist.

Lee and his colleagues[16] have recently described a simple and reproducible method of recording functional status. This consists of 17 questions and can be filled in by the patient himself (Table 16.3). However, the method has not proved sensitive enough to record changes in short-term clinical therapeutic trials, although it is useful in monitoring change after major joint reconstructive surgery[16].

Table 16.3. Questionnaire used by Lee *et al.*[16]

Questions	*Yes with no difficulty*	*Yes but with difficulty, e.g. pain, stiffness or weakness*	*No score*	*Total*
1. Can you turn your head from side to side?	0			0
2. Can you comb your hair at the back of your head?			2	2
3. Can you close drawers (with arms only)?		1		1
4. Can you open doors?		1		1
5. Can you lift a full teapot?		1		1
6. Can you lift a cup with one hand to drink of it?		1		1
7. Can you turn a key in a lock?		1		1
8. Can you cut meat with a knife?			2	2
9. Can you butter bread?			2	2
10. Can you wind a watch?		1		1
11. Can you walk?		1		1
12. Can you walk without:				
a) someone's help?	0			0
b) crutches?	0			0
c) a walking stick?	0			0
13. Can you walk up a flight of stairs?		1		1
14. Can you walk down a flight of stairs?		1		1
15. Can you stand up with your knees straight?		1		1
16. Can you stand on your toes?			2	2
17. Can you bend down to pick something up off the floor?		1		1
			Total score:	19

The timing of a variety of manoeuvres related to various 'activities of daily living' such as tying knots, picking up pins, hopping on one foot, and walking a set distance have been employed to measure functional ability[11,15,20–23]. However, with the exception of the time to walk 50 feet, all of these methods have been discarded as they are considerably influenced by learning and their frequent repetition is boring to both patient and physician (Copeman, W.S.C., cited by Hollander and McCarty)[15]. We have found the time to walk 50 feet to be of little value in short-term clinical trials[16].

Goniometry has been used by orthopaedic surgeons to record changes after joint surgery, but although it is useful when performed carefully[24] the method has little place in short-term clinical drug trials.

Grip strength has been measured by a variety of dynanometers over the past 150 years[25], and has been frequently employed in clinical therapeutic trials.

The method of grip strength determination is based on the ability of the patient to squeeze an inflated rubber bag connected to a mercury manometer. The problem of lack of consistency in the shape and size of the bag has been eliminated by the introduction of the Davis bag, a rubber bag measuring 6 by 3 inches (see Savage[11]). A sphygmomanometer cuff folded and sewn to maintain a cylinder of constant dimensions has also been widely employed in clinical practice[21,22,26]. A 'mercurial ergometer' has been introduced which consists of a thin walled rubber bag which can be moulded to suit the individual patient's hand (Mandel[23]). This has not, however, been widely adopted in clinical practice. Spring dynanometers (Dresner *et al.*[27]) and calibrated tensiometers (Cousins[28]) have not proved to be any more accurate than the standard cuff-mercury column method in recording grip strength in patients with rheumatoid arthritis.

Several workers have made efforts to assess the intra- and inter-observer error in grip strength determination. Cousins[28], for instance, found a high degree of intra- and inter-observer agreement in grip strength measurement. Copeman (see Lansbury[29]) likewise found the method reliable and repeatable, but produced no data to substantiate this view. Mikkelsen, on the other hand, found a highly significant physician–patient interaction, and in our own studies we have observed mean variations of up to 20 mmHg between different physicians (Table 16.4). Clearly it is important for one observer to perform all serial measurements in the same patients. From Table 16.5, it can be seen that intra-observer variation of up to 10 mmHg can be expected[30].

A diurnal variation in grip strength ranging from 70 to 230 mmHg has been reported by Wright[31] in both normal subjects and in patients with rheumatoid arthritis. We[32] could not confirm the presence of a statistically significant diurnal variation in patients with rheumatoid arthritis, but nevertheless, we consider it important to carry out serial measurements at the same time of day.

Grip strength determination, although showing changes with variations in clinical disease activity, nevertheless is a relatively insensitive parameter in assessing anti-rheumatic drugs in patients with rheumatoid arthritis[8,32]. It is salutary to be reminded that in one controlled trial improvement in grip strength after one week's therapy with sodium salicylate was no greater than might have occurred due to intra-observer error![8]

We have had no experience with the Winthrop torquometer (De Choisy[33]) which is claimed not only to test grip strength but also ability to carry out rotational movements at the elbow and wrist, such as would occur in opening a tap or bottle top. The test is simple to perform and is claimed to detect changes with anti-rheumatic drug therapy, but to date no reproducibility or observer error studies have been reported, and the usefulness of the instrument remains, in our opinion, to be proven.

Table 16.4 Inter-observer error in grip strength determination in 20 patients by four observers

	Observers (mmHg Mean ± SE)			
	A	B	C	D
Right hand	100.1 ± 8.0	112.0 ± 10.4	117.2 ± 12.0	109.7 ± 11.6
Left hand	100.8 ± 9.5	115.7 ± 14.3	120.5 ± 14.8	105.1 ± 11.2

	Difference in means		*p*	
	Right	*Left*	*Right*	*Left*
A versus B	11.9	14.9	0.5	<0.025
A versus C	17.1	19.7	0.01	<0.01
A versus D	9.6	4.3	N.S.	N.S.
B versus C	5.2	4.8	N.S.	N.S.
B versus D	2.3	10.6	N.S.	<0.025
C versus D	7.5	15.4	0.005	<0.01

Reproduced by kind permission of the Editor of the *Scandinavian Journal of Rheumatology*[32].

Table 16.5 Intra-observer error in grip strength determination in 21 patients

	Grip strength mmHg (Mean ± SD)		*Difference of means*	*p*
	1st reading	*2nd reading*		
Right hand	88.1 ± 11.3	97.2 ± 11.9	9.1	<0.0005
Left hand	75.5 ± 8.9	80.8 ± 10.1	5.3	<0.05

Reproduced by kind permission of the Editor of the *Scandinavian Journal of Rheumatology*[16].

MEASUREMENT OF DOLOR

Beecher[34] has aptly stated that 'pain is measured in terms of its relief' and it can be argued that the only relevant feature of an aspirin-like or first-line anti-rheumatic drug is to relieve the patient's pain. Numerous clinical therapeutic trials have been reported testifying the validity of using the patient's pain response in assessing the efficacy of anti-rheumatic drugs. Indeed, the studies of Deodhar and his colleagues[8] clearly showed that the patients' own assessment of their pain relief was the most sensitive parameter of anti-rheumatic drug efficacy. During the recent decade there has been a craving for objective measurements in assessing the clinical status of patients with rheumatoid arthritis[35]. In a withering review of clinical trials of indomethacin O'Brien[36] showed that in those studies in which objective measurements were performed, only 25 per cent of patients had good or excellent responses, compared with an average of 60 per cent in studies where subjective indices were employed. However, it is to be noted that the clinical trials which employed subjective methods were poorly designed and lacked control observations, and cannot therefore be regarded as indicating the invalidity of subjective assessments. Indeed, as Joyce[37] has stated '... the point is not that objective measures are better than subjective but that sensitive measures are better than insensitive'.

Innumerable methods have been proposed for recording pain but none is ideal. Analogue scales of pain intensity, varying from four to nine set divisions, have been widely employed[38–43]. It is generally assumed in calculating the response in such scales that the divisions are of equal magnitude, but this assumption may be erroneous[40] since, as Lasagna has pointed out[44], a fall from 'severe' to 'moderate' pain may be greater than a fall from 'mild' to 'none'. Copeman[21] employed a percentage scale where patients began at 100% and moved up and down. However, unlike the visual analogue scales, this method has no descriptive limits and patients with the same apparent intensity of pain may choose widely varying levels on the scale[35].

It has been suggested that if the various pain categories do not bear a linear relationship then each category could be weighted in order to increase sensitivity, but this does not seem in practice to make a significant difference to the outcome[35,45]. Those who consider that pain rating where only three or four grades are recorded are too insensitive, have employed a nine-point scale[26]. However, on scrutinizing their data it is clear that their four point scale also discriminated between placebo and aspirin and ibuprofen, and we[43] have found a five point scale quite adequate in demonstrating differences between placebo, aspirin and prednisolone. It is important in assessing such a complex problem as pain not to become too philosophical and to keep the method as simple as possible. It seems of little importance whether an adjectival or numerical scale is used to delineate the patient's response as far as the final outcome is concerned[34,46]. Indirect methods of measuring pain such as assessment of pain threshold or pain tolerance[34,41,47] are too tedious in clinical practice, and measurement of irrelevant laboratory data such as catecholamine excretion[48] cannot be too strongly condemned.

We have recently used a new method for assessing anti-rheumatic drug therapy[43]. The method is single-blind and non-crossover in design. The

Table 16.6 Example of pain chart with instructions given to the patient

	DEGREE OF PAIN				
	Nil	Mild	Moderate	Severe	Very Severe
0				X	
1				X	
2					X
3				X	
4				X	
5				X	
6			X		
7			X		
8			X		
9			X		
10		X			
11			X		
12		X			
13		X			
14	X				

Assess the amount of your joint pain every day before going to bed. Indicate in the appropriate space above with a cross (x).

patients receive the drug for a period of 14 days and each evening record their pain on a chart (Table 16.6). The patients are also requested at the end of the 14-day treatment period to record their overall satisfaction rate on a five point scale: totally ineffective, ineffective, moderately effective, effective and highly effective. If the patient had to stop the drug, they were requested to indicate whether this was due to side effects or lack of effect. The number of days withdrawn were also recorded. For statistical purposes both the five grades of pain and global grades of satisfaction were allocated the numerical scores one to five.

Table 16.6 Results of studies of ten drugs in 605 patients with rheumatoid arthritis

Trial reference no.	*Drug and daily dosage*	*Number of patients*	*Withdrawals number (%)*	*Mean days withdrawn Mean SE*	*IPR* Mean SE*	*ATPR† Mean SE*	*Adjusted ATPR Mean SE*	*Ranking‡*	*Mean satisfaction score Mean SE*
	Calcium Lactate 2 g	41	28 (68)	6.4 ± 0.7	3.0 ± 0.2	3.5 ± 0.1	3.5 ± 0.1	14	1.7 ± 0.2
37	Aspirin (enteric coated 3.9 g	42	14 (33)	3.0 ± 0.7	2.9 ± 0.2	3.0 ± 0.1	3.1 ± 0.1	1	3.7 ± 0.2
	Prednisone 15 mg	45	6 (13)	1.3 ± 0.7	3.0 ± 0.2	2.6 ± 0.1	2.6 ± 0.1	8–9–10	2.4 ± 0.2
	Aspirin (enteric coated) 3.9 g	44	26 (59)	4.9 ± 0.7	2.8 ± 0.2	3.1 ± 0.1	3.3 ± 0.1	8	2.4 ± 0.2
38									
	Paracetamol 4 g	38	20 (53)	4.5 ± 0.7	2.7 ± 0.2	3.4 ± 0.1	3.5 ± 0.1	13	2.0 ± 0.2
	Indomethacin 100 mg	41	13 (32)	2.0 ± 0.7	2.6 ± 0.2	2.8 ± 0.1	2.9 ± 0.1	3–4	2.8 ± 0.2
	Ketoprofen 100 mg	44	15 (34)	2.8 ± 0.7	3.0 ± 0.1	3.2 ± 0.1	3.2 ± 0.1	11–12	2.3 ± 0.2
1	Ketoprofen 200 mg	46	17 (37)	2.7 ± 0.7	2.8 ± 0.1	3.1 ± 0.1	3.2 ± 0.1	6–7	2.5 ± 0.2
	Ibuprofen 1.2 g	45	16 (36)	3.0 ± 0.7	2.9 ± 0.1	3.1 ± 0.1	3.2 ± 0.1	8–9–10	2.4 ± 0.2
	Indomethacin 100 mg	41	14 (34)	2.2 ± 0.6	2.6 ±0.1	2.7 ± 0.1	2.9 ± 0.1	2	2.9 ± 0.2
	Flurbiprofen 150 mg	45	13 (28)	2.1 ± 0.6	2.8 ± 0.1	2.7 ± 0.1	2.8 ± 0.1	3–4	2.8 ± 0.2
39	Mefenamic acid 1.5 g	46	12 (26)	2.3 ± 0.6	2.8 ± 0.1	2.6 ± 0.1	2.7 ± 0.1	5	2.7 ± 0.2
	Alclofenac 3 g	45	17 (38)	3.1 ± 0.6	2.7 ± 0.1	3.1 ± 0.1	3.0 ± 0.1	11–12	2.3 ± 0.2
	Benorylate 8 g	42	15 (36)	3.6 ± 0.6	3.0 ± 0.1	3.0 ± 0.1	3.0 ± 0.1	6–7	2.5 ± 0.2

* IPR = Initial Pain Rating

† ATPR = Average Treated Pain Rating

‡ Ranking of each drug on the basis of the mean satisfaction scores

The three variables which are used in assessing response to therapy in this method are: the patient's assessment of his satisfaction with the drug, the number of days withdrawn from the trial, and the average treated pain rating (ATPR). This last rating is calculated as the average of daily pain rating ignoring missing values. Statistical comparisons of different treatment groups are made using analysis of variance and co-variance using the initial observations on the patients as concomitant variables[49]. One problem in such a study method is that patients when they enter the trial vary considerably in disease activity, and we have found it necessary to make adjustments to correct for initial differences between the different treatment groups. We have found[43] that the inclusion of the initial pain rating (IPR) as a covariate significantly increases the precision of the analysis of between-treatment differences in ATPR After allowing for the IPR the effects of other pretreatment observations, such as age, sex, duration of arthritis etc. (concomitant variables) on the analyses were surprisingly not significant[43].

The method allows for adjustment of the ATPR to give a mean ATPR at a specific IPR level. We have accordingly adjusted the initial ATPRs to an IPR value of 3.0, which corresponds to the mid-point of the pain scale rating, i.e. moderate pain. The effects of the IPR on the patient's satisfaction rating and withdrawal from the trial are not significant[43].

The results of several trials are shown in Table 16.7 of the 605 patients who participated in these trials, 381 (63%) returned their completed forms. Active drugs could be differentiated statistically from placebo, but somewhat surprisingly some of the drugs e.g. indomethacin, flurbiprofen and mefenamic acid could not be shown to be significantly different from prednisone. Paracetamol was found to be no better than placebo.

When compared with the double-blind crossover method, this technique clearly has advantages: it is simple and rapid in performance and is economical in both time and costs. It also allows comparison between different treatment groups studied at different times. What is still not known is how the technique would work in different countries: would, for instance, the method work with Italian, Greek or Spanish patients? We have recently shown that our colleagues in Edinburgh, Dundee and Aberdeen obtain similar results to ourselves with aspirin, ibuprofen and flurbiprofen.

JOINT TENDERNESS

Both Savage[11] and Copeman[13] considered joint tenderness to be the most reliable clinical parameter of joint inflammation. However, to date no entirely satisfactory method of assessing joint tenderness has been evolved. This is due to the fact that the degree of joint tenderness is not only dependent on the severity of the underlying inflammatory process in the joint, but also on the amount of pressure applied by the examining physician and the patient's pain threshold. Clearly different observers will apply different pressures to the joints and the patient's reaction to the same stimulus will also vary. In addition, the side of joint to which this is applied may vary not only between different physicians but also with the same observer, and the inflammatory process within a joint may also vary considerably at different sites. Presumably this is why we found[50] the inter- and intra-observer error differences in eliciting joint tenderness to be variable.

Various instruments have been proposed to overcome these difficulties and provide more objective estimates of joint tenderness [23,26,51–54], but the problem with them is that they cannot be generally applied to all the joints.

Most methods for estimating joint tenderness have simply used digital pressure[20–22,50,55]. Lansbury and his colleagues[56,57] included an estimate of joint size in assessing an articular index, but despite the high degree of precision and close correlation with the systemic index the method has proved tedious to perform. The Co-operating Clinics' Committee of the American Rheumatism Association[58] recorded the number of active joints, i.e. whether tender on pressure, painful on passive movement or swollen (other than due to bony deformity), and this index correlates well with our own articular index[50]. The latter has the advantage that it is simple to perform and takes only 2–2½ mins. We have attempted to increase the sensitivity of the Ritchie index[50] by increasing the number of joints scored, but in practice we have found this no better than the simple index. Both the American Co-operating Clinics[58] and our own articular index[50] show significant differences during placebo and aspirin and prednisolone therapy. The only advantage in the Ritchie index and the reason why it has proved popular is its simplicity.

CONCLUSIONS

The most sensitive index for recording change in disease activity in patients with rheumatoid arthritis when treated with an anti-inflammatory analgesic drugs is the patient's response. The patient is the only person who can evaluate his or her pain. In all the therapeutic trials we have done we have consistently found the patient's own assessment to be the most sensitive index, followed by the articular index of joint tenderness. Grip strength is relatively insensitive and measurement of joint circumference is extremely crude in determining anti-inflammatory effect. Changes in functional status are only of value in long-term clinical trials.

ACKNOWLEDGEMENTS

As usual, we are grateful for financial support from the Arthritis and Rheumatism Council for Research in Great Britain. One of us (G.P.B.) was in receipt of a Robins European Research Fellowship, and another (P.L.) of a Merck, Sharp and Dohme Fellowship in Clinical Pharmacology.

References

1. Hart, F. D. and Clark, C. J. M. (1951). Measurement of digital joint swelling in rheumatoid arthritis. *Lancet*, **i**, 775
2. Boardman, P. L. and Hart, F. D. (1967). Clinical measurement of the anti-inflammatory effects of salicylates in rheumatoid arthritis. *Br. Med. J.*, **4**, 264
3. Wilkens, R. F., Gleichert, J. E. and Gade, E. T. (1973). Proximal interphalangeal measurement by arthrocircameter. *Ann. Rheum. Dis.*, **32**, 585

4. Webb, J., Downie, W. W., Dick, W. C. and Lee, P. (1973). Evaluation of digital joint circumference measurement in rheumatoid arthritis. *Scand. J. Rheumatol.*, **2,** 127
5. Mills, S. B., Bloch, M. and Bruckner, F. E. (1973). Double-blind crossover study of ketoprofen and ibuprofen in management of rheumatoid arthritis. *Br. Med. J.*, **4,** 82
6. Gyori, A. N., Bloch, M., Burry, H. C. and Grahame, R. (1972). Orudis in management of rheumatoid arthritis and osteoarthritis of the hip: comparison with indomethacin. *Br. Med. J.*, **4,** 398
7. Fremont-Smith, F., Harter, J. G. and Halberg, F. (1969). Circadian rhymthacity of proximal interphalangeal/pip/joint circumference in patients of rheumatoid arthritis. *Arthr. Rheum.*, **12,** 294
8. Deodhar, S. D., Dick, W. C., Hodgkinson, R. and Buchanan, W. W. (1973). Measurement of clinical response to anti-inflammatory drug therapy in rheumatoid arthritis. *Q. J. Med. N.S.*, **387**
9. Steinbrocker, O., Traeger, C. H. and Battermann, R. C. (1949). Therapeutic criteria in rheumatoid arthritis. *J. Am. Med. Assoc.*, **140,** 659
10. Taylor, S. (1937). Table for degree of involvement in chronic arthritis. *Can. Med. Assoc. J.*, **36**
11. Savage, O. (1958). *Criteria for Measurement in Chronic Diseases.* In Report of a Symposium on Clinical Trials (Kent: Pfizer)
12. Empire Rheumatism Council (1961). Gold therapy in rheumatoid arthritis. Final report of a multicentre controlled trial. *Ann. Rheum. Dis.*, **20,** 315
13. Copeman, W. S. C. (1964). *Textbook of the Rheumatic Diseases,* 3rd Edition. (Edinburgh and London: A. and S. Livingstone)
14. Lansbury, J. (1968). Clinical appraisal of the Activity Index as a measure of rheumatoid activity. *Arthr. Rheum.*, **11,** 599
15. Hollander, J. L. and McCarty, D. J., Jr. (1972). *Arthritis and Allied Conditions,* 8th Edition. (Philadelphia: Lea and Febiger)
16. Lee, P., Jasani, M. K., Dick, W. C. and Buchanan, W. W. (1973). The evaluation of a functional index in rheumatoid arthritis. *Scand. J. Rheumatol.*, **2,** 71
17. Lowman, E. W. (1958). Rehabilitation of the rheumatoid cripple: a five year study. *Arthr. Rheum.*, **1,** 38
18. Verhaeche, A. and Lebeurre, R. (1961). Presentation d'un bareme decimal a quatre criteriums (le T.A.P.I.) permettant l'evaluation d'un faux synthetique de capacites functionelles en rhumatologie. *Rev. Rhum.*, **28,** 145
19. McEwen, C. (1968). Evaluation of the patient as a whole and evaluation of the individual functional units of musculo-skeletal system. In L. Preston and C. McEwen (eds.) *Surgical Management of Rheumatoid Arthritis* (London: W. B. Saunders Co.)
20. Bywaters, E. G. L., Dixon, A. St. J. and Wild, J. B. (1950). Deoxycortone and ascorbinic acid in the treatment of rheumatoid arthritis. *Lancet*, **i,** 951
21. Copeman, W. S. C., Savage, O., Bishop, P. M. F., Dodds, P. M. F., Dodds, E. C., Gohlieb, B., Glynn, J. H. H., Henly, A. A. and Kellie, A. E. (1950). A study of cortisone and other steroids in rheumatoid arthritis. *Br. Med. J.*, **2,** 849
22. Quin, C. E., Mason, R. M. and Knoweldon, J. (1950). Clinical assessment of rapidly acting agents in rheumatoid arthritis. *Ann. Rheum. Dis.*, **22,** 91
23. Mandel, L. (1956). Assessment of therapeutic agents in rheumatoid arthritis. *Can. Med. Assoc. J.*, **74,** 515
24. Mitchell, W., Miller, J. and Sturrock, R. D. (1974). An evaluation of goniometry as an objective method for measuring joint motion. (To be published)
25. Hunsicker, P. A. and Donelly, R. V. (1955). Instruments to measure strength. *Res. Q.*, **26,** 408
26. Duthie, J. J. R. (1950). Clinical trials of ACTH: preliminary report. *Edinburgh Med. J.*, **57,** 341
27. Dresner, E., Pugh, L. G. C. and Wild, J. B. (1950). ACTH in rheumatoid arthritis compared

with intramuscular adrenaline, with deoxycortone and ascorbinic acid. *Lancet*, **i,** 1149

28. Cousins, G. F. (1955). Trained and untrained testers upon the administration of grip strength tests. *Res. Q.*, **26,** 273
29. Lansbury, J. (1966). Methods for evaluating rheumatoid arthritis. In J. L. Hollander (ed.) 7th Edition. *Arthritis and Allied Conditions.* (Philadelphia: Lea and Febiger)
30. Lee, P., Watson, M., Webb, J. and Buchanan, W. W. (1975). The therapeutic effectiveness of paracetamol in rheumatoid arthritis. *Int. J. Clin. Pharmacol.*, **11,** 68
31. Wright, V. (1959). Some observations on diurnal variation of grip. *Clin. Sci.*, **18,** 17
32. Lee, P., Baxter, A., Dick, W. C. and Webb, J. (1974). As assessment of grip strength measurement in rheumatoid arthritis. *Scand. J. Rheumatol.*, **3,** 17
33. De Choisy, J. (1973). A new method of assessing grip strength and wrist and arm movement in the arthritic patient. *Rheumatol. Rehabil. Suppl.*, vol. 81
34. Beecher, H. K. (1959). *Measurement of Subjective Responses.* (New York: Oxford University Press)
35. Hart, F. D. and Huskisson, E. C. (1972). Measurement in rheumatoid arthritis. *Lancet*, **i,** 28
36. O'Brien, W. H. (1968). Indomethacin: a survey of clinical trials. *Clin. Pharmacol. Ther.*, **9,** 94
37. Joyce, C. R. B. (1968). Psychological factors in the controlled evaluation of therapy. In M. Balint (ed.) *Mind and Medicine Monographs.* (Philadelphia: J. B. Lippincott Co.)
38. Keele, K. D. (1948). The pain chart. *Lancet*, **ii,** 6
39. Hewer, A. J. H., Keele, C. A., Keele, K. D. and Nathan, P. W. (1949). A clinical method of assessing analgesics. *Lancet*, **i,** 431
40. Houde, R. W. and Wallenstein, S. L. (1953). A method for evaluating analgesics in patients with chronic pain. *Drug Addiction Neurotics Bull., Appendix B:*, 1383
41. Houde, R. W. Wallenstein, S. L. and Beaver, W. T. (1965). Clinical measurements of pain. In G. De Stevens (ed.) *Analgesics.* (New York: Academic Press)
42. Huskisson, E. C., Shenfield, G. M., Taylor, R. T. and Hart, F. D. (1970). A new look at ibuprofen. *Rheumatol. Phys. Med.*, **10** (Suppl.), 88
43. Lee, P., Webb, J., Anderson, J. A. and Buchanan, W. W. (1973). A method of assessing the therapeutic potential of anti-inflammatory, anti-rheumatic drugs in rheumatoid arthritis. *Br. Med. J.*, **2,** 685
44. Lasagna, L. (1960). The clinical measurement of pain. *Ann. N. Y. Acad. Sci.*, **86,** 28
45. Wilks, S. J. (1938). Weighting systems for linear functions of variables when there is no dependent variable. *Psychometrics*, **3,** 23
46. Stevens, S. S. and Galanter, E. H. (1957). Ratio scales and category scales for a dozen perpetual continue. *J. Exp. Psychol.*, **54,** 377
47. Kast, E. C. (1968). Clinical measurement of pain. *Med. Clin. N. Am.*, **52,** 23
48. Huskisson, E. C. (1974). Catecholamine excretion and pain. *Br. J. Clin. Pharmacol.*, **1,** 80
49. Cochrane, W. C. and Cox, G. M. (1957). *Experimental Designs.* (London: Wiley)
50. Ritchie, D. M., Boyle, J. A., McInnes, J. M., Jasani, M. K., Dalakos, T. G., Grieveson, P. and Buchanan, W. W. (1968). Clinical studies with an articular index for assessment of joint tenderness in patients with rheumatoid arthritis. *Q. J. Med., N.S.*, **37,** 393
51. Steinbrocker, O. (1949). A simple pressure gauge for measured palpation in physical diagnosis and therapy. *Arch. Phys. Med.*, **30,** 284
52. Jonus, O. (1950). Objective assessment of rheumatoid arthritis. *Br. Med. J.*, **2,** 1244
53. Hollander, J. L. and Young, D. C. (1963). The palpameter, an instrument for quantification of joint tenderness. *Arthr. Rheum.*, **6,** 277
54. McCarty, D. J., Getter, R. A. and Phelps, P. (1965). A dolorimeter for quantification of articular tenderness. *Arthr. Rheum.*, **8,** 551
55. Hench, P. S., Kendall, E. C., Slociemb, C. H. and Polley, H. F. (1950). Effects of cortisone acetate and pituitary ACTH on rheumatoid arthritis, rheumatic fever and certain other conditions: study in clinical physiology. *Arch. Intern. Med.*, **85,** 545
56. Lansbury, J. and Hant, D. D. (1956). Quantitation of the manifestation of rheumatoid

arthritis. IV. Area of joint surfaces as on index of total joint inflammation and deformity. *Am. J. Med. Sci.*, **232**, 150, 150

57. Lansbury, J. (1958). Report of a three year study on the systemic and articular indexes in rheumatoid arthritis. *Arthr. Rheum.*, **1,** 505

58. Co-operating Clinics' Committee of the American Rheumatism Association (1967). A three month trial of indomethacin in rheumatoid arthritis with special reference to analysis and interference. *Clin. Pharmacol. Ther.*, **8,** 11

17
Criteria for Clinical Usage of New Diagnostic Laboratory Tests (Abstract)

EUGENE V. BARNETT

Currently clinical laboratory tests provide an extension of physical diagnosis rather than ultimate diagnostic tools. Few diseases are the result of a single pathophysiological process and most diseases, particularly inflammatory diseases, share common pathogenetic pathways. Most laboratory tests in current use reflect abnormalities in multiple physiological processes. We therefore, must define a clinical laboratory test as an extension of physical diagnosis rather than an ultimate diagnostic tool.

Only a minority of published reports describing new test methods define the accuracy and precision of the procedures. Rarer still are the descriptions of non-disease factors which can effect test results and indeed produce false-positive or negative results. As enumerated by Robert S. Galen they include: (1) genetic factors; (2) physiological intra-individual status; (3) influence of drugs; (4) speciman collection variables; and (5) specimen handling variables. Sensitivity of a particular test for detecting an index disease is usually given in such reports, e.g. 90% true positive in disease A. The authors frequently report the percent of false positives in healthy subjects the reciprocal of which equals the specificity of the new test. The particular value of a positive laboratory result can be calculated by the reader by dividing the true positive percentage by the sum of true positives plus false positives and multiplying by 100. The appropriate application of a new test depends not only on its sensitivity and specificity for single disease but also on its prognostic value, that is its positivity in the pre-clinical state and in its response to therapy. A new test of high sensitivity is of value in excluding a particular disease but should not be applied as part of a multiphasic screen of healthy people when the incidence of the index disease in the general population is lower than the false positive rate in the general population. Such inappropriate application results in detecting more false positives than true positive, and if the information is applied to all the prospective patients, those individuals with false positive results may be needlessly alarmed. The seminar on this subject will review several published reports of new diagnostic laboratory tests and evaluate (on the basis of the above criteria) their sensitivity, specificity, accuracy, predictive value and appropriate application.

18
The Usefulness of Radioisotopes in the Assessment of Inflammation of the Diarthrodial Joint

W. S. MITCHELL, I. J. ZEITLIN, D. M. GRENNAN, P. J. ROONEY and W. C. DICK

INTRODUCTION

The cardinal signs of the inflammatory response, so clearly defined by Celsus, are heat, redness, pain, swelling and loss of function. The importance of applying a quantitative approach has been stressed by Lord Kelvin. The goals are clear. However, despite the dramatic advances in technology of the last century, our progress towards the achievement of these goals has been frustratingly slow. Measurements of pain and loss of function remain imprecise and contentious[1–3]. Some progress in the measurement of local heat has been achieved using direct temperature recording or indirectly by thermography or through the use of liquid crystals[4–6]. However, no satisfactory solution to the problem of quantifying the inflammatory response has emerged.

The physiological changes underlying the production of pain, swelling, warmth, redness and loss of function include (a) increased flow through existing vascular channels; (b) increased permeability of these vessels (particularly the postcapillary venules) to fluid, (c) emigration of inflammatory cells, (d) cellular proliferation including the formation of new blood vessels. The present report reviews the manner in which in the last decade the unique properties of radionuclides have been exploited for the study of some of the vascular and cellular components of the inflammatory response.

INTRAVENOUSLY INJECTED RADIOISOTOPES

In the earliest studies various radiochemicals were injected intravenously and the inflamed joints were then examined. Such studies revealed that the accumulation of intravenously administered radionuclide, whether monitored by scanning of the joint or by the more simple method involving the use of a collimator placed over pre-selected areas of the joint was considerably greater over the inflamed joint or joints as compared with non-inflamed controls. For joints to be scanned it is necessary to administer millicurie doses of the radionuclide, whereas external directional counting demands much smaller doses of the radionuclide in the microcurie range. Important technical points to be observed include (a) strict standardization of counting geometry (b) standardization of repositioning and environmental conditions (c) the correction both for physical and biological decay, (d) expression of the results as a percentage uptake with reference to both external and internal standards.

Elevated uptakes or 'scan positivity' have been recorded with many different radioisotopes including pertechnetate (^{99m}Tc), radioiodinated serum proteins including albumin or fibrinogen, radioactive calcium, strontium, yttrium, and gold[7–12].

Although studies with each have shown elevated values when compared to normals the mechanism and pathophysiological process reflected by each radionuclide vary. Thus radioactive calcium provides an expression of the enhanced calcium movement both into and out of bone adjacent to the inflamed joint, radioactive iodinated serum albumin provides an expression of vascularity and of vascular permeability, ^{99m}Tc, reflects enhanced uptake due to a multiplicity of factors including tissue volume, protein binding in tissue and synovial fluid, vascularity and enhanced flow through the scanned segment and perhaps even a component of the synoviocyte anion concentration.

From the point of view of the clinician the radionuclide most commonly used in clinical practice is ^{99m}Tc. This has the advantage of a short physical half life and is primarily a gamma emitter. Following intravenous injection equilibration produces a rise to a peak count rate (5–20 min after injection) followed by a plateau succeeded by a fall. Routinely we relate the count rate over a joint, or a group of joints, 14–16 min after injection to the count rate of the injected dose in order to estimate the percentage of radionuclide localized in the inflamed tissue[2,3,7,13].

The percentage uptake is elevated over inflamed joints in proportion to the activity of the inflammatory process regardless of whether the underlying cause is a specific infection (gonococcal, staphyloccocal or tuberculous), one of the sero-negative spondyloarthritides, a crystal-induced arthropathy (urate or calcium pyrophosphate), a metabolic arthropathy (e.g. hyperlipidaemic polyarthropathy) or rheumatoid arthritis[2,3,7,21].

The percentage uptake is related to the clinical assessment of severity of joint inflammation but discrepancies occur[2,3,7,13]. The correlation coeficient (r) lies in the range of 0.4–0.7 with an index of determinancy of only between 16 and 49%. In practical terms this implies that although a severely painful, tender or swollen joint is usually associated with a high uptake, the high uptake is the composite end-result of physiological processes only partly responsible for each of the clinically observed indices. This may explain why a point-to-point correlation cannot be observed between results of radioisotopic measurements and those of thermographic measurements in the same group of individuals, a realization which renders futile the debate on whether clinical assessment is to be preferred to radioisotopic or thermographic measurement. Each approach is measuring different though inter-related, or overlapping, aspects of the inflammatory process and therefore each method must be regarded as adjunctive to and not a substitute for the other. A combination of properly controlled, quantifiable, subjective as well as objective indices is required to obtain a more meaningful overall assessment of disease than is possible using any method singly.

Discrepancies between clinical and radioisotopic measurements may also arise when apparently non-involved joints of patients with polyarticular disease are examined radioisotopically. Uptake values are higher than those found in the non-inflamed joints of non-arthritic controls, even in the absence of any clinical signs or symptoms of inflammation[7,13]. Although conclusive evidence based upon histology has not to our knowledge been produced in humans, results from animal studies and follow-up studies of our own and other workers suggest that these enhanced uptake results denote subclinical involvement. Accepting Popperian constraints it would nevertheless be reassuring if definitive evidence could be produced to support this contention which may yet prove to have some predictive importance.

Finally, lower uptake results are often encountered in late chronic arthritis in the presence of obvious signs of disease. These signs, however, on close inspection are usually those associated with subluxation destruction and fibrosis but little active inflammatory activity.

Elevated uptake values may be reduced by synovectomy, by local corticosteroid injection, by treatment with second-line drugs such as gold, penicillamine or levamisole and by corticosteroids[7–13]. The position with first-line drugs is more complicated. Where the initial disease activity is marked and is considerably reduced by for example, indomethacin, aspirin or a propionic acid derivative, both clinical and radioisotopic results will reflect that change. Where the degree of change is less marked, clinical indices may demonstrate a significant difference and radioisotopic uptake may not. The most sensitive arbiters of changes found with first-line symptom-relieving drugs are indices which reflect symptoms such as pain relief or patient opinion–hardly a surprising observation![13]

INTRA-ARTICULARLY INJECTED RADIOISOTOPES

In studies with intra-articularly injected radioisotopes the radionuclide is injected directly into the synovial cavity. It has to penetrate the synovial membrane, and is cleared by subsynovial blood vessels. Attempts have been made to exploit this system to measure synovial blood flow and vessel permeability[7,20].

Synovial blood flow

The inert gamma emitting gas ^{133}Xe is removed from the circulation during its passage through the lungs. There being no recirculation, disappearance of ^{133}Xe from the articular cavity provides an indirect measure of functional status of the capillary microcirculation and, following correction for diffusion and partition coefficients, an estimate of synovial blood flow[7].

The exponential clearance of ^{133}Xe from the joint cavity between 5 and 40 min after a careful intra-articular injection is significantly more rapid in the case of inflamed than in non-inflamed human or canine diarthrodial joints. The clearance rate of ^{133}Xe can be consistently altered by intra-articular injection of a variety of pharmacological substances known to mediate the inflammatory process. Judged by such alterations induced in normal synovial membrane, prostaglandins of the E series were found to be the most potent vasodilators. In decreasing order of potency serotonin, bradykinin and histamine were less active than postaglandin E_1[15]. In addition, results of the effects of suitable agonist and antagonist combinations on ^{133}Xe clearance rate demonstrate the presence of adrenergic, cholinergic and histamine (H_2) receptors in both normal and inflamed synovial membrane[15].

Clinical studies have revealed that the ^{133}Xe clearance rate, as an index of synovial tissue perfusion, remained elevated in synovectomized patients to levels similar to those encountered in unoperated patients with rheumatoid arthritis[16], correlated with clinical indices (though less will than did the ^{99m}Tc uptake), and was responsive to some, but not all anti-rheumatic drugs[7]. A correlation between ^{133}Xe clearance rate and severity of joint inflammation judged both clinically and biochemically has been reported by Goetzl *et al.*[17]

Synovial vascular permeability

Customarily the changes in vascular permeability accompanying experimentally induced inflammation have been assessed by measurement of the accumulation in the inflamed tissue of intravenously administered indicator dyes such as Evan's blue which bind to plasma proteins or radioiodinated serum proteins such as albumin or globulins[18,19]. Recently, we have shown that it is also possible to assess synovial vascular permeability in the dog by measurement of the intra-articular accumulation of intravenously administered radiolabelled dextran of known molecular size[20]. The method has shown that in the order of decreasing potency bradykinin, prostaglandin E and histamine are all capable of increasing the permeability of synovial vessels. The permeability response to intra-articular infusion of prostaglandin E together with bradykinin, or histamine, was found to be greater than that which could be expected on the basis of the summation of their effects when administered individually; a synergism which although previously reported[21] was not demonstrable by measurements of ^{133}Xe clearance rate. We interpret the discrepancy between the two methods to indicate that whereas ^{133}Xe clearance rate provides a measure of synovial blood flow, the accumulation of radiolabelled dextran reflects increased vascular permeability.

ASSESSMENT OF JOINT INFLAMMATION USING ^{133}Xe AND ^{99m}TC

During a survey of patients with Type II hyperlipoproteinaemia we had an opportunity to study prospectively the development of joint inflammation characteristic of the metabolic disorder in four individuals. The patients, all of whom were fully documented genetically and phenotypically, gave a past history of similar episodes following excessive physical exertion, and gave also a similar history during the prospective episode. In all four patients the arthropathy was acute and characterized by swollen, red and hot knee or ankle joints. It was asymmetrical, migratory and non-destructive and its onset was not preceded, nor associated with, clinical evidence of rheumatic fever, bowel disorder, skin eruption, mouth ulcers or urethritis.

Radioisotopic assessment of the inflamed joints revealed a grossly elevated uptake of ^{99m}Tc but a ^{133}Xe clearance rate characteristic of a non-inflamed normal joint. Synovial fluid analysis was also normal and negative for the presence of crystals and microorganisms. We interpret the radioisotopic data to indicate the occurrence of an acute periarthritis and not a synovitis in Type II hyperproteinaemia and recommend more extensive use of a combination of techniques for the further characterization as well as assessment of the severity of inflammation underlying different types of joint disease.

References

1. Huskisson, E. C. (1974). Measurement of pain. *Lancet*, **ii**, 1127
2. Levy, J. and Dick, W. C. (1975). Detection of change in disease activity. *Clin. Rheumat. Dis.*, **1**, (2), 1975
3. Lee, P. and Dick, W. C. (1976). Assessment of disease activity and drug evaluation. *Recent Adv. Rheumatol.*, **1**, Part III
4. Horvath, S. M. and Hollander, J. L. (1949). Intra-articular temperature as a measure of joint reaction. *J. Clin. Invest.*, **28**, 469
5. Ring, E. F. H. and Cosh, J. A. (1968). Skin temperature measured by radiometry. *Br. Med. J.*, **4**, 448
6. Collins, A. J., Ring, E. F. J., Cosh, J. A. and Bacon, P. A. (1974). Quantitation of thermography in arthritis using multi-isothermal analysis. *Ann. Rheumat. Dis.*, **33**, 113
7. Dick, W. C. (1972). The use of radioisotopes in normal and diseased joints. *Sem. Arthr. Rheum.*, **1**, 301
8. Green, F. A. and Hays, M. T. (1972). The pertechnetate joint scan. II. Clinical correlations. *Ann. Rheumat. Dis.*, **31**, 278

9. Weiss, R. E., Mayfield, W. S., Murison, P. J. and Hidalgo, J. V. (1965). Iodinated human serum albumin (^{131}I) localisation studies of rheumatoid arthritis joints by scintillation scanning. A preliminary report. *Arthr. Rheumatol.*, **8,** 976
10. Hashimoto, H., Okada, T., Sato, H. and Shiokana, Y. (1969). Studies with ^{131}I-labelled human plasma fibrinogen in rheumatoid arthritis. In: *12th International Congress of Rheumatology* (Prague: Geigy) (Abstract)
11. Bauer, G. C. H. (1968). The use of radionuclides in orthopaedics. *J. Bone Jnt. Surg.*, **50A,** 1681
12. Bauer, G. C. H. and Smith, E. M. (1969). ^{85}Sr scintimetry in osteoarthritis of the knee. *J. Nucl. Med.*, **10,** 106
13. Dick, W. C. and Grennan, D. M. (1976). Radioisotopes in the study of normal and inflamed joints. *Clin. Rheum. Dis.*, **2,** (1), 1976
14. Grennan, D. M., Rooney, P. J., St. Onge, R. A., Brooks, P. M., Zeitlin, I. J. and Dick, W. C. (1975). Histamine receptors in the synovial microcirculation. *Eur. J. Clin. Invest.*, **5,** 75
15. Grennan, D. M., Zeitlin, I. J. and Dick, W. C. (1975). Effects of inflammatory mediators on synovial blood flow. *Prostaglandins*, **9,** 799
16. Dick, W. C., Doedhar, S. D., Provan, G. J., Nuki, G. and Buchanan, W. W. (1971). Isotope studies in normal and diseased knee joints. *Clin. Sci.*, **40,** 327
17. Goetzl, E. J., Falchuk, K. H., Zeiger, L. S., Sullivan, A. L., Herbert, C. L., Adams, J. D. and Decker, J. L. (1971) A physiological approach to the assessment of disease activity in rheumatoid arthritis. *J. Clin. Invest.*, **50,** 1167
18. Williams, T. J. and Morley, J. (1974). Measurement of rate of extravasation of plasma protein in inflammatory responses in guinea pig skin using a continuous recording method. *Br. J. Exp. Pathol.*, **55,** 1
19. Soria-Herrera, C. (1973). Accumulation of ^{125}I-labelled albumin as a measure of the inflammatory response in experimental arthritis. *Rheumatol. Rehabil.*, **12,** 148
20. Grennan, D. M., Mitchell, W., Miller, W. and Zeitlin, I. J. (1977). The effects of prostaglandin E_1, bradykinin and histamine on canine synovial permeability. *Br. J. Pharmacol.*, **60,** 251
21. Rooney, P. J., Madkour, M., Kennedy, A. C., Third, J. and Dick, W. C. (1978). The arthropathy of type II hyperlipoproteinaemia. *J. Med.* (in press)

19 Thermography in the Assessment of Rheumatic Inflammation

P. A. BACON

INTRODUCTION

Thermography, which detects the infra-red radiation from the skin surface, can be used to assess the vascular component of the inflammatory process. In rheumatoid arthritis (RA) it detects cutaneous changes which result from increase in the vascularity of the inflamed synovium. Thermographic measurements in RA also correlate well with other indices of the inflammatory process, e.g. intra-articular temperature, synovial fluid white cell and protein content, and the gross synovial pathology detected at operative synovectomy[1].

Thermography has the advantage to the patient in that it is harmless and painless, and to the operator in that it can be quantified to produce an objective thermographic index[2]. We have produced a range of normal values for standardized joint areas which includes most of the joints involved in rheumatoid arthritis. With this knowledge it is possible to examine quantitatively the effects of anti-rheumatic drugs. We have looked in particular at intra-articular steroid injections, at oral non-steroidal anti-inflammatory drugs over a short period, and at slowly-acting anti-rheumatic drugs such as penicillamine and cyclophosphamide over a longer time-scale.

INTRA-ARTICULAR CORTICOSTEROIDS

Intra-articular steroid injections have remained popular since their first introduction[3] because of their obvious beneficial effect. Many steroids have been proposed as alternatives to the original hydrocortisone but there has been little evidence to show that one preparation has advantages over another, or that some preparations are really longer-acting than others, as claimed. We have recently investigated the comparative effects of the three analogues of a single compound, prednisolone. Their action on injected and non-injected joints was assessed using quantitative thermography. Their solubility and ability to leak into the plasma was assessed both by the measurement of plasma prednisolone and as depression of circulating level of endogenous cortisol[4].

Effect on the injected knee

A single intra-articular injection of 50 mg each of the three analogues into a group of patients induced a rapid suppression of inflammation by 48 hours (Figure 19.1). The soluble prednisolone acetate group showed an early return towards pre-injection values, which in many cases was reached by 7 days. The less soluble prednisolone pivalate showed a longer duration of action, of approximately 3 weeks. The least soluble prednisolone tertiary butyl acetate showed the maximum and the most sustained fall in thermographic index. The differences between the acetate and the tertiary butyl acetate groups were increasingly significant at 1, 2 and 3 weeks.

A single intra-articular injection of 100 mg of the three analogues, results for which are also shown in Figure 19.1, did not depress the thermographic index to a greater extent, except in the case of the soluble prednisolone acetate.

Plasma prednisolone level

As shown in Figure 19.2, the plasma prednisolone levels reached a peak at 24 hours and the rise was most pronounced after the instillation of the most soluble prednisolone acetate. The plasma curves for the less soluble prednisolone tertiary butyl acetate was flatter and more sustained.

Depression of circulating cortisol

All the three intra-articular preparations of prednisolone depressed profoundly the circulating level of endogenous cortisol. The effect was observed with both the 50 mg and 100 mg dose level.

Effect on the contralateral non-injected knee

The rise in the plasma level of prednisolone was also associated with a fall in the thermographic index of the contralateral non-injected knee. As shown in Figure 19.2, the maximal fall in the non-injected joint was seen after the injection of the most soluble prednisolone acetate. In fact at 24 hours the thermographic indices of the opposite knees in the case of prednisolone acetate were virtually comparable.

Conclusion

This investigation has shown not only that thermography can be used to detect the clinically observable beneficial effect of intra-articular steroid injection in

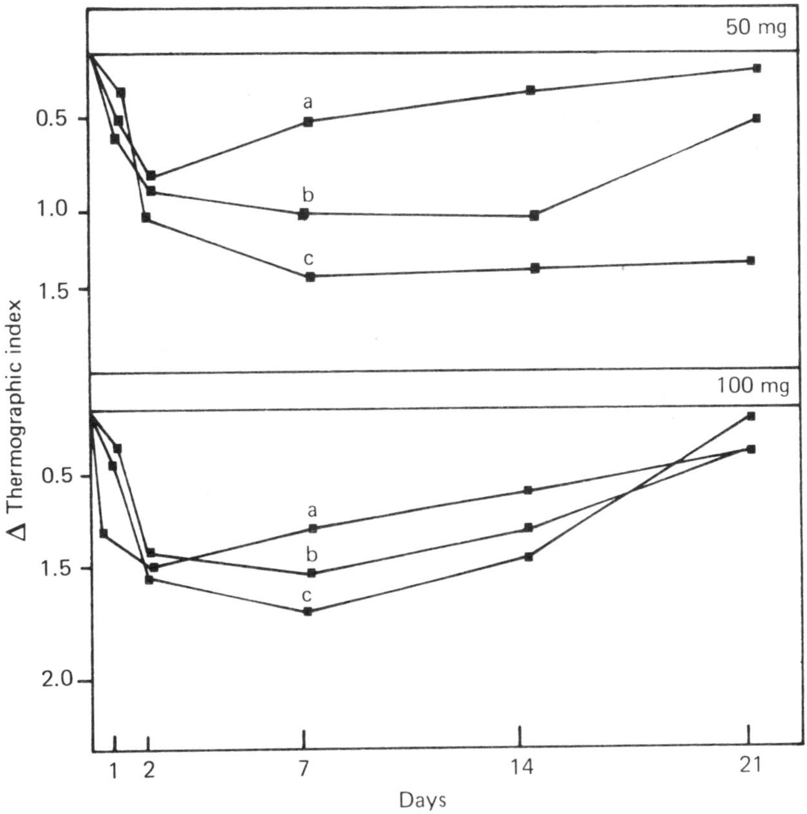

Figure 19.1 The mean fall in the thermographic index in the injected knee in the three groups of patients given each prednisolone analogue at the 50 or the 10 mg dose. Prednisolone acetate (a); prednisolone pivalate (b); and prednisolone tertiary butyl acetate (c). The difference between a and c is significant at 7 days ($p<0.05$), 14 days ($p<0.01$) and 21 days. (<0.001)

inflammatory polyarthritis, but also to quantify the differing effects of three steroid preparations of differing solubility. The data presented also confirm that the so-called insoluble compounds do indeed have a longer lasting effect in the injected joint.

ASSESSMENT OF ORALLY ADMINISTERED DRUGS

Since rheumatoid arthritis is a polyarticular disease it is clear that for the assessment of orally administered drugs the thermography of a single joint would not be representative. For these studies we have therefore used a compound joint index which is the mean of four separate joint areas. This usually

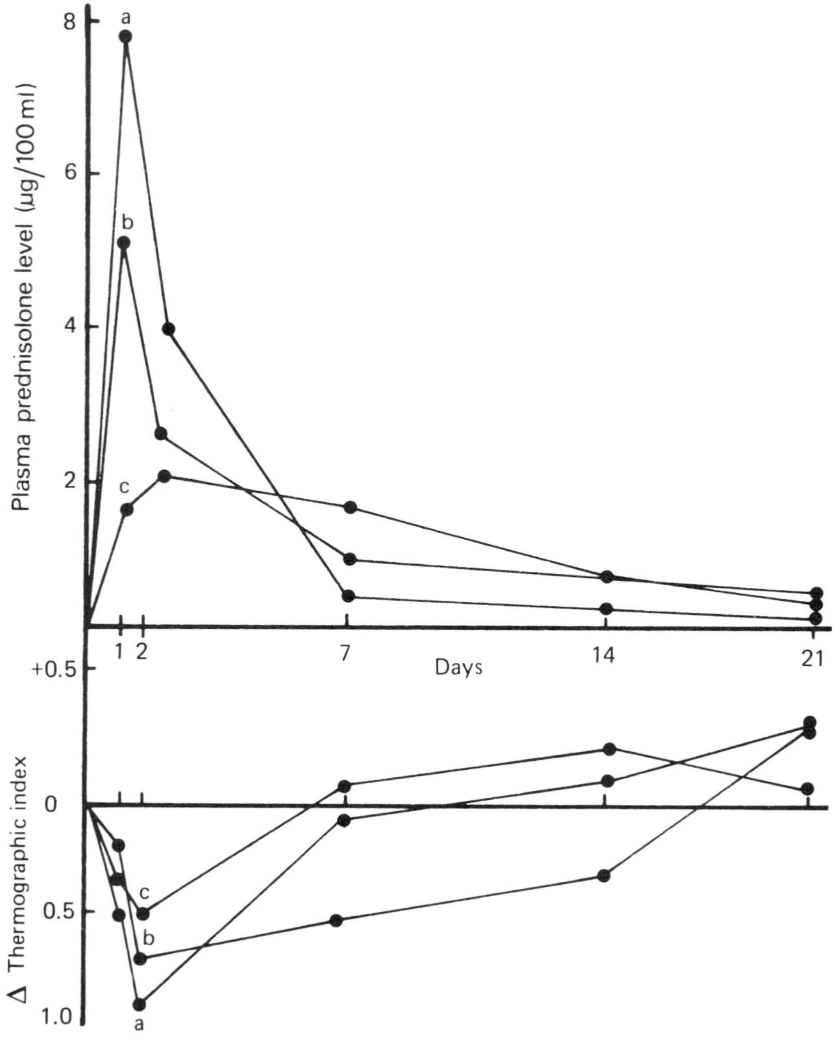

Figure 19.2 The plasma prednisolone levels after a single intra-articular injection of the three prednisolone analogues, each 100 mg. The plasma levels peak at 24 hours while the corresponding fall in the thermographic index in the uninjected contralateral knee is maximum at 48 hours. The maximum change in both measurements is seen with the soluble prednisolone acetate (a) and the minimum change with the least soluble prednisolone tertiary butyl acetate (c), results for prednisolone pivalate (b) lay in between

includes both hands and a pair of involved larger joints such as knees, ankles or elbows. The anti-inflammatory effect of an oral non-steroidal drug as shown by the thermographic index was found to be slow and cumulative over a period of 10 days to 2 weeks. Also it was necessary to allow a wash-out period for any previous anti-inflammatory drugs. We have therefore followed a standard methodology, with a one week wash-out period on paracetamol followed by a 2 week period on the chosen agent, for all our studies of non-steroidal drugs. To achieve reproducible quantification over this period the technique and the conditions of examination were also carefully standardized as previously described[1].

Data for six standard non-steroidal anti-inflammatory drugs (NSAIDs) and five similar compounds under development, or in the pre-marketing stage, are reported below. In addition to these 11 quick acting compounds the present report includes also some data on the effect of two slowly acting orally administered compounds on rheumatoid arthritis.

Table 19.1 The mean fall* in TI induced by each of six drugs. The total group and the responders within each group have been compared

	Total group 2 weeks NSAID			*Responders*	
Drug	*No.*	*Mean fall TI*	*Non-responders*	*No.*	*Mean fall TI*
Aspirin	10	0.53	2	8	0.86
Benorylate	10	0.42	3	7	0.72
Ibuprofen	10	0.54	2	8	0.73
Indomethacin	10	0.39	2	8	0.73
Ketoprofen	10	0.69	1	9	0.81
Naproxen	10	0.40	3	7	0.81
Total	60	0.51		47	0.78

* $p<0.025$

Effect of six standard NSAIDs

The drugs assessed were: aspirin, benorylate, ibuprofen, indomethacin, ketoprofen and naproxen. Results for 60 patients, 10 of whom received one of six compound for 2 weeks are summarized in Table 19.1. It can be seen that there was no significant difference between the fall in the compound thermographic index induced by any of these drugs. Further analysis of the data showed that in each case the mean value concealed a very wide range of individual responses. In each treatment group there were between one and three non-responders (Table 19.1) and, overall, out of 60 patients as many as 22% showed no measurable response to the drug for which they were selected. This is a surprisingly high figure but Huskisson *et al.*[5], using a very different method of assessment, found a similar wide variation in response and an inability to predict responders to an individual drug. A non-responder should be tried empirically on one drug after another until a suitable one is found.

Analysis of the responders only, again showed a remarkably similar fall in mean thermographic index between each group (Table 19.1). This was significantly higher than with the entire group ($p<0.025$) but still did not separate out the individual drugs in any way. Thus it is clear that the established non-steroidal anti-inflammatory drugs produced a very similar response to each other both in terms of the number of patients responding and of the degree of response in those who did well. This very small difference between the groups is at variance with the enormous difference in potency detected when one examines their ability to inhibit prostaglandin synthetase. In this system there is a 5000 fold difference between compounds. This wide discrepancy between the two indices may suggest that inhibition of prostaglandin synthetase is unrelated to the clinical effect of these drugs.

Finally we have analysed these 60 patients according to the height of their starting thermographic index, irrespective of the drug therapy they received. This was to detect whether the activity of the arthritis affected the response to a non-steroidal drug. It can be seen (Table 19.2) that there was no significant difference in the fall in thermographic index whatever the starting index.

Table 19.2 The fall in TI has been ranked according to the starting index in 60 patients, irrespective of which non-steroidal drug was used. The initial index is seen not to influence the change induced by the drug

		Mean fall	
TI	*No.*	*2 weeks NSAID*	*SD*
5.00–6.00	5	0.66	0.50
4.00–4.99	21	0.44	0.81
3.00–3.99	22	0.57	0.60
<3.00	12	0.47	0.86

Effect of five new NSAIDs

The first point which becomes obvious from the data summarized in Figure 19.3 is that compared with the fall in the compound thermographic index of patients receiving the six established NSAIDs, the response of patients receiving the five new NSAIDs was quite variable. Only one of the new drugs was found to be as active as the established group.

The lesser effect of the newer drugs could be related to lower intrinsic effectiveness or could be a dose-related effect. To examine this we tested two of these drugs at a number of dose levels. The first of these, fenclofenac, was initially introduced on the basis of animal experiments at a dose of 200–600 mg a day. Our results with that dose increasing over a period of several weeks in a few patients showed an almost straight line, which we regard as being more a tribute to the stability of our method than to the effectiveness of the drug. Once further trials established the safety of the drug, a second investigation was undertaken at 1200 mg a day. On this occasion there was some response seen in a few patients but the mean response was small and still significantly less than that seen in the established drug group ($p<0.05$). For this reason a further investigation at 1800 mg (over 3 times the original dose) was commenced. It is currently under way. A larger fall in the compound thermographic index is seen with the high dose but, in the incomplete group so far, this does not reach statistical significance.

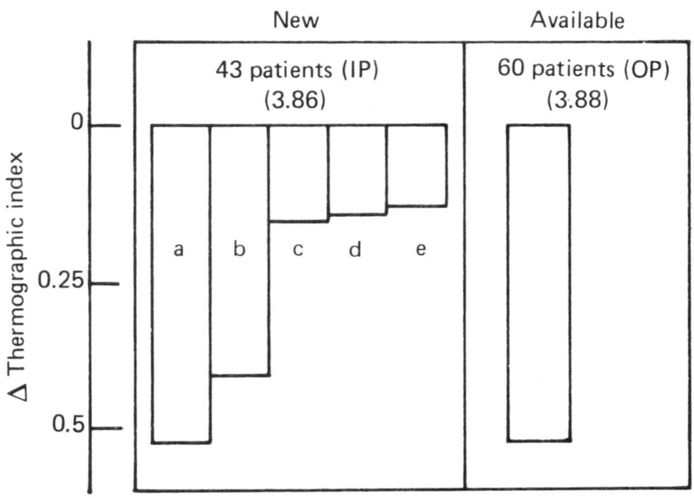

Figure 19.3 The mean fall in TI in five groups of patients each receiving one of 5 new non-steroidal anti-inflammatory drugs compared with that induced by a group of established agents. The mean starting index of the two groups before treatment was similar

The second compound investigated at several doses is azapropazone (Figure 19.3). It is now available on the UK market. Our initial studies at the suggested dose of 1200 mg indicated that it had an analgesic but only weak anti-inflammatory action. A further group of patients examined at 1800 mg showed a very wide scatter of response but the mean response was not significantly improved. A third group examined on a dose of 2400 mg per day showed a more impressive group response though still a wide scatter of individual responses. The differences between the mean thermographic index of patients receiving 1200 mg and 2400 mg in the case of responders only was highly significant ($p<0.005$).

The data suggest that quantitative thermography is capable of detecting a dose-response effect of anti-rheumatic drugs in humans, which is probably not possible with any other methodology at present.

Effect of slowly acting drugs

To study the effect of D-penicillamine and cyclophosphamide, assessment of the thermographic index was conducted over periods of 6 months to 1 year in different individuals. To assess the stability of the thermographic index in non-diseased joints over such long periods, repeated measurements were made on one of the technicians. The mean index for 22 measurements was 2.15 with a standard deviation of 0.21; data which clearly establish that the degree of fluctuation in the thermographic index despite widely varying ambient temperature is acceptably small in the absence of joint disease.

Penicillamine is widely accepted as a powerful anti-rheumatic agent similar in efficacy to gold but the necessary dosage has not been firmly fixed. Original studies showing its efficacy were performed at a fairly high dose and were attended with appreciable toxicity. For this reason lower doses have been advocated but as yet there is poor evidence for their efficacy. In our unit a study performed on varying doses of penicillamine for rheumatoid arthritis[6] showed that the group of patients on a high dose (1000 mg a day) had a more marked fall in thermographic index than those on the low dose (600 mg a day) at all periods up to one year. However, toxicity was also higher in the high dose group. When patients who developed side-effects were analysed separately, it was found that they had a more marked fall in thermographic index than those in whom no toxicity was observed. This suggests that the therapeutic ratio for penicillamine is quite low.

Another study has looked at the effect on two regimens of oral cyclophosphamide in RA[7]. The same total dose of cyclophosphamide was given either as 1 mg/kg on a daily basis or as 2 mg/kg daily for alternate weeks only. The improvement in the thermographic index was much greater with the intermittent dose than with the continuous low dose regimen. This methodology is being used to assess other cyclophosphamide regimens in an attempt to improve efficacy and reduce toxicity.

It is interesting to compare the results of long-acting drugs with those obtained with the non-steroidal drugs (Figure 19.4). Both the groups of drugs show a positive effect on inflammation quite different from the effect of a pure analgesic such as paracetamol which augments the thermographic index. The action of the non-steroidal drugs is much more immediate than that of the longer-acting drugs. Indeed the very slow initial response seen with both penicillamine and cyclophosphamide suggests that these drugs are acting in a different way from the non-steroidal drugs. There is also a difference in the total response obtained, it being greater with penicillamine and cyclophosphamide than with the non-steroidal drugs. However, if we examine the data in terms of a 'cure' of rheumatoid arthritis, it is clear that maximally

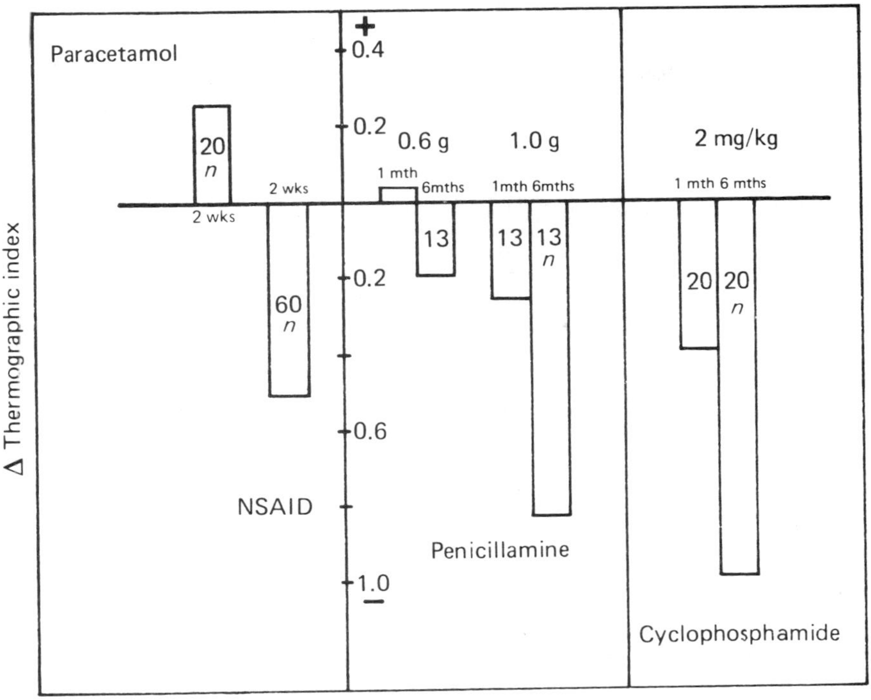

Figure 19.4 The mean change in the thermographic index induced by an analgesic (paracetamol) and established non-steroidal anti-inflammatory drugs over 2 weeks is compared with that found after administration of 2 longer acting agents, penicillamine and cyclophosphamide over 1 and 6 months. The numbers within each block refer to the number of patients in that group. The difference between the increase in the thermographic index on paracetamol and the fall on the non-steroidal agents is highly significant ($p = 0.0005$)

tolerated doses of neither group of drugs are capable of suppressing the thermographic index to anywhere near the normal range, considering that most of the groups started with an index above 4.00.

In conclusion quantitative thermography can show an effect of both intra-articularly and orally administered anti-rheumatic drugs. It provides a useful, harmless and objective method of assessing the anti-inflammatory effects of these drugs in individual patients and also in assessing the mean effects of new and established treatments on groups of patients.

ACKNOWLEDGEMENTS

I am grateful to my colleagues Dr R. C. Bucknall and Dr H. A. Bird who allowed me to include data from their current studies. I am glad to acknowledge the help of Mr Francis Ring whose skill and technical expertise made the whole investigation possible.

References

1. Bacon, P. A., Collins, A. J., Ring, E. F. J. and Cosh, J. A. (1976). Thermography in the assessment of inflammatory arthritis. *Clin. Rheum. Dis.*, **2,** No. 1., 51
2. Collings, A. J., Ring, E. F. J., Cosh, J. A. and Bacon, P. A. (1974). Quantitation of thermography in arthritis using multi isothermal analysis. 1. The thermographic index. *Ann. Rheum. Dis.*, **33,** No. 2., 113
3. Hollander, J. L., Brown, E. M., Jessar, R. A. and Brown, C. Y. (1951). Hydrocortisone and cortisone injected into arthritic joints. *J. Am. Med. Assoc.*, **147,** 1629
4. Eselinckx, W., Bacon, P. A., Demottaz, D. Ring, E. F. J. and Crook, D. (1977). *Brit. J. Clin. Pharmacol.* (in press)
5. Huskisson, E. C., Woolf, D. L., Balme, H. W., Scott, J. and Franklyn, S. (1976). Four new anti-inflammatory drugs: responses and variations. *Br. Med. J.*, **1,** 1048
6. Bucknall, R. C., Bacon, P. A. and Ring, E. F. J. (1977). (In preparation)
7. Bird, H. A., Bacon, P. A., Ring, E. F. J. and Hall, N. D. (1977). (In preparation)

20
Standardized Radiological Evaluation of Rheumatoid Arthritis in Therapeutic Trials

A. LARSEN and K. DALE

INTRODUCTION

The importance of radiological evaluation in therapeutic trials of rheumatoid arthritis (RA) is traditionally well recognized[1]. In fact the radiological approach appears to be the only practical method for the assessment of permanent destruction of the cartilage and bone in RA. Besides reviewing a number of published methods designed to assess the severity and progression of RA on the basis of radiological changes in the affected joints, the present paper introduces a new system which involves the use of standard reference radiographs for that purpose.

PREVIOUS SYSTEMS

The two most widely employed methods for the assessment of radiological changes in RA [2,3], though simple in format and easy to execute, are not sensitive enough to be useful in therapeutic trials. For instance, an English multicentre trial on D-penicillamine[4] involving the use of one of these methods[3] failed to reveal any noteworthy differences between the radiographs of hands and feet taken before and 12 months after commencement of therapy. All the patients had advanced erosive changes on entry to the trial, and so although it was possible that the disease was far too advanced to be significantly arrested it was also possible that the grading system used was too crude to detect small alterations in the severity of joint disease due to drug treatment.

Other systems that have been advocated for use in the assessment of the effects of drug treatment are reviewed below.

1. In the Empire Rheumatism Council trial on cortisone acetate[5], a classical example of a well planned assessment of drug treatment of RA, radiographs of hands and wrists taken before commencement of therapy were compared with those taken at the end of the trial. In all a total of 44 small joints, 8 in each wrist and 14 in the digits of each hand were routinely examined for four types of alterations, namely, joint space narrowing, surface erosion, periosteal reaction and articular subluxation; and the changes were graded as slight or marked.

Two methods for scoring the progression of disease were used. In the first, a joint scored one point when only slight deterioration had occurred, but two points either when there was marked deterioration in a particular feature present in the initial radiograph or when features not present in the initial radiograph were detectable in the final one. By this method the maximal score per patient was 88. The second scoring method was similar except that joints not affected initially scored an additional point if they became affected by the end of the trial. The maximum score per patient by the second method was 132.

2. In the trial on gold therapy[6], also by the Empire Rheumatism Council, the procedure employed for the evaluation of therapeutic effectiveness of cortisone acetate[5] was slightly modified. The initial radiographs of 20 finger joints (excluding the distal interphalangeal joints) were compared with radiographs of the same joints taken at the end of the trial for detection of additional narrowing of the joint space (1 point), enlargement of an old erosion (1 point) and the appearance of a new erosion (2 points). The maximal score per patient was 80. The wrist joints were assessed separately on a four grade scale with verbal definitions.

3. A significant departure from the need to compare the final radiograph with the initial one has been made possible since the introduction in 1971 by Sharp and colleagues[7] of an approach which allows the assessment of the severity as well as progression of joint disease through the examination of an individual radiograph.

In the method of Sharp *et al.*[7] osseous defects (erosions) and joint space narrowing are assessed separately. For assessment of osseous defects 29 areas of each hand and wrist are observed and the number of erosions for each area are counted. Individual erosions up to four are recorded and 5 points are assigned to an area with a greater number of erosions. A defect score (D) is the sum of points in both hands and wrists, i.e. 58 areas. A corrected defect score (Dc) is obtained by dividing the observed score D by the maximum possible D. Dc divided by the number of months from the onset of RA gives the ratio Dc/T(time) which provides a measure of the rate of progression of osseous changes in the individual radiograph.

For the evaluation of joint space narrowing (JSN) Sharp *et al.*[7] examined 27 joints of each hand and wrist, and assigned 1 point to each joint that showed narrowing on one side only, 2 points when it showed narrowing of the space to less than half of the original space, 3 points when it showed narrowing greater than half the original space and 4 points when the joint was ankylosed. The joint space narrowing score (JSN) as well as the corrected score for it, i.e. JSNc, and the rate of progression of JSN (JSNc/T) were determined in the same way as the corresponding indices for the osseous defects.

The method of Sharp *et al.* has been effectively employed in the evaluation of the effect of cyclophosphamide[8] and gold[9] on the joint disease in RA. However, despite offering important advantages over other methods, the scoring system of Sharp *et al.* is not without its limitations. Ankylosis valued as 4 points in the assessment of joint space narrowing may not be relevant since the loss of cartilage which actually accounts for joint space narrowing might not be related to the ossification process responsible for ankylosis. In addition, even complete loss of cartilage is not necessarily (or always) followed by bony ankylosis and the reverse is also true, i.e. that the joint space can remain well preserved despite bony ankylosis[10].

Other possible limitations of the method of Sharp *et al.* concern the assessment of osseous defects. Not only is the counting of erosions in an individual joint up to 4 seemingly arbitrary but it is also possible that the enlargement of an existing erosion rather than an increase in the number of erosions may be more relevant to the progression of R.A. As against this, the results of an important study[11] described below suggest that the progression of RA can be judged by enumeration of new erosions.

4. In the study of the effect of cyclophosphamide on RA conducted by the Cooperating Clinics Committee of ARA[11] radiographs of the hands taken at the beginning of a 32 week trial were compared with films prepared at completion. The initial and final radiographs were randomly marked X and Y before reading. Two observers enumerated the erosions in 18 joints of each hand recording whether the erosions remained constant or became more numerous in X or Y. One observer assessed radiographs without grading the severity of erosions, the other graded them using a 4 point scale as: questionable, minimal, moderate and maximal. This approach revealed no difference in the degree of worsening reported by the two observers examining the same set of radiographs of patients receiving a low dose of cyclophosphamide (up to 15 mg daily), and there was no disagreement between them as to the beneficial effect of a high dose (up to 150 mg daily).

Many other reports[12,13] do not however provide as detailed an account of the methods employed for the assessment of radiological changes as the few cited above.

NEWLY PROPOSED METHOD INVOLVING USE OF STANDARD RADIOGRAPHS

We suggest that radiological assessment for the evaluation of effect of drug treatment should routinely include radiographs of hands, wrists and feet, all taken before the commencement of therapy and preferably at 6 monthly intervals thereafter. The joints to be assessed should include all those depicted in Figure 20.1. They should be graded using the standard reference radiographs shown in Figure 20.2, 20.3 and 20.4 into the following six categories:

Grade 0: nominal appearance

Grade 1: presence of one or more of the following changes – soft tissue swelling, osteoporosis and only a slight degree of joint space narrowing.

Grades 2 to 5: presence of erosions and joint space narrowing in increasing severity as demonstrated by the standards.

The original negatives of the standard radiographs shown in Figure 20.2 to 20.4 are available on request from the authors and those wishing to have

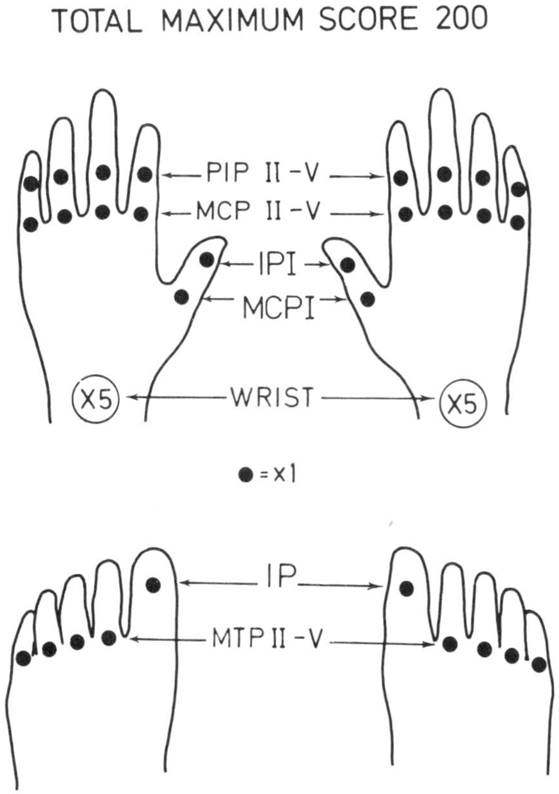

Figure 20.1 The joints depicted in the figure are graded using standard radiographs. The scores for the wrists are multiplied by five. The sum of the individual gradings gives the total score

further details concerning the interpretation of observations made using them are referred to published reports[14,15].

To make a general assessment of the severity of RA in the extremities we find it useful to determine a total score for the radiographed joints of the hands, wrists and forefeet. In calculating the total score the wrist, being a large joint, is

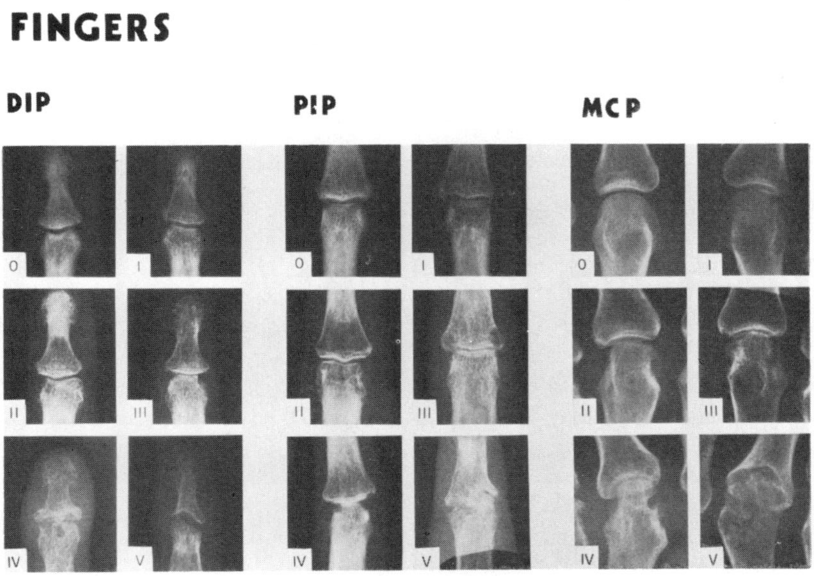

Figure 20.2 Standard radiographs for the finger joints. DIP joints are not considered in the present scoring system

weighted by multiplying its score by 5. Using this approach the total maximal score per patient is 200 as indicated in Figure 20.1.

Other types of analysis are also possible. For example the small joints may be assessed separately from the wrists. It is possible that the mean scores for the two sub-sets of joints so obtained might not prove sensitive enough for the detection of drug effect especially in the later stages of RA. This is why it may be more useful to record the scores for the presence of soft tissue swelling, osteoporosis, joint space narrowing and erosion in each individual joint and assess them separately for changes at the recommended intervals. Also it may prove useful to assess changes in the size of erosions in sequential radiographs joint by joint.

The radiographs should be interpreted without knowledge of the order in which they were taken and to minimize inter-observer differences it is suggested that having interpreted the radiographs independently the observers

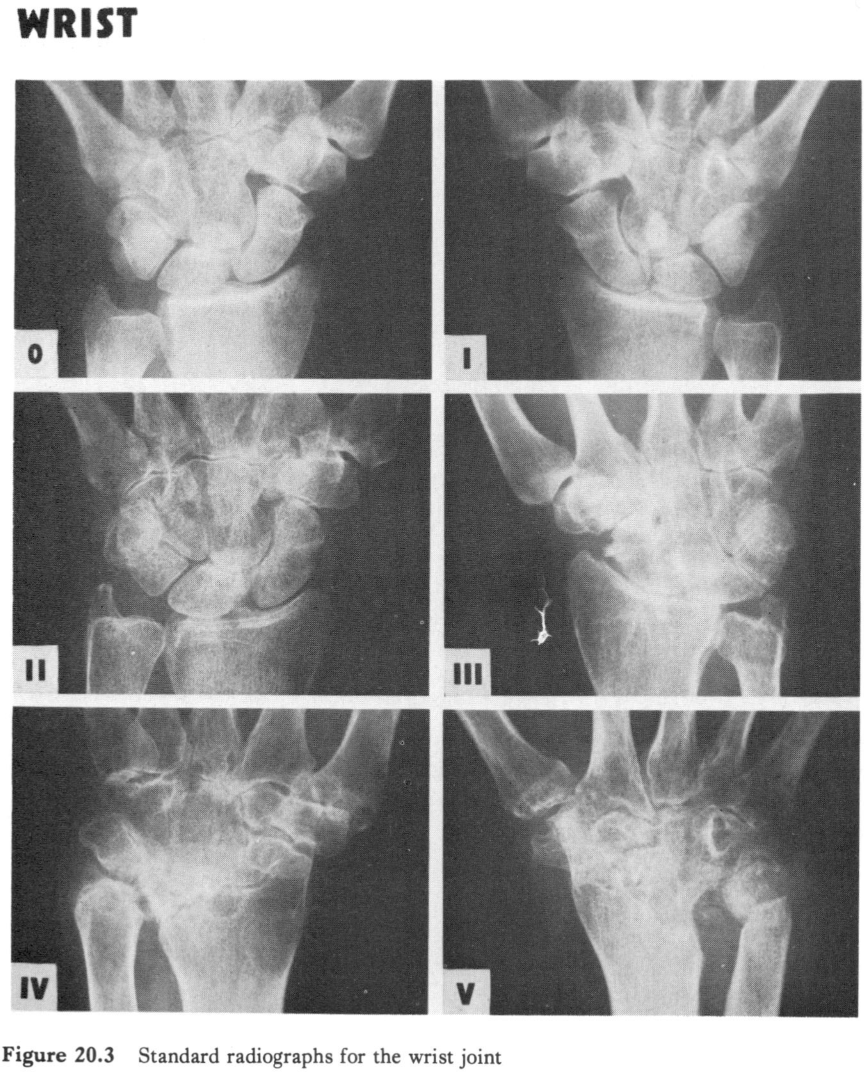

Figure 20.3 Standard radiographs for the wrist joint

agree upon any discrepancies by re-examination of the relevant radiographs.

The radiographs in therapeutic trials are usually taken by conventional technique which in our experience is rather similar in most countries. This is why the standard radiographs were selected from films made using standard equipment. Mammographic equipment or industrial films, though more advantageous than the conventional techniques were avoided mainly because they are readily available in only a few hospitals.

Finally in most previous therapeutic trials only the hands and wrists have been radiographed for the assessment of drug effect. Such an assessment overlooks the fact demonstrated by several studies[16–19] that the forefeet display even more severe radiological changes than the hands and wrists. One of these studies[18] also reported that the first diagnostic erosions were found most frequently in the metatarsophalangeal (MTP) joints. We have found[19] the MTP and wrist joints to be more frequently and severely affected than the metacarpophalangeal (MCP) and proximal interphalangeal (PIP) joints.

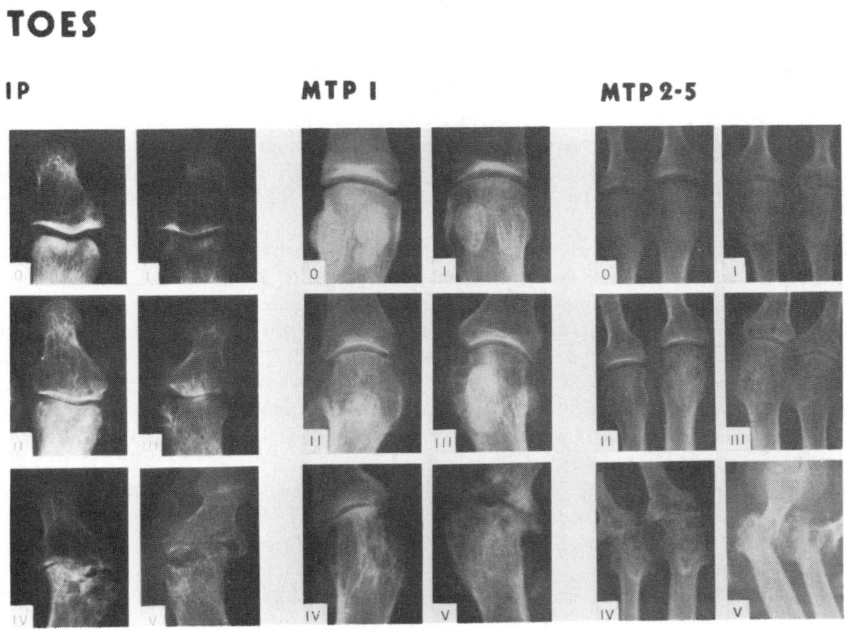

Figure 20.4 Standard radiographs for the toe joints. MTP 1 joints are not considered in the present scoring system

CONCLUDING REMARKS

Apart from emphasizing the need for routine assessment of joints of the forefeet, the newly proposed system recommends the use of standard radiographs.

References

1. Bollet, A. J. and Bunim, J. J. (1955). The importance of serial x-rays in the evaluation of treatment of rheumatoid arthritis. *Med. Clin. N. Am.*, **39**, 439

2. Steinbrocker, O., Traeger, C. H. and Batterman, R. C. (1949). Therapeutic criteria in rheumatoid arthritis. *J. Am. Med. Assoc.*, **140,** 659
3. Kellgren, J. H., Jefrey, M. R. and Ball, J. (1963). Atlas of standard radiographs of arthritis. In *The Epidemiology of Chronic Rheumatism,* Vol. II. (Oxford: Blackwell Scientific Publications)
4. Multicentre Trial Group (1973). Controlled trial of D-penicillamine in severe rheumatoid arthritis. *Lancet,* **i,** 7798
5. Empire Rheumatism Council (1955). Multi-centre controlled trial comparing cortisone acetate and acetyl salicyclic acid in the long-term treatment of rheumatoid arthritis. *Ann. Rheum. Dis.*, **14,** 353
6. Empire Rheumatism Council (1961). Gold therapy in rheumatoid arthritis. *Ann. Rheum. Dis.*, **20,** 315
7. Sharp, J. T., Lidsky, M. D., Collins, L. C. and Moreland, J. (1971). Methods of scoring the progression of radiological changes in rheumatoid arthritis. *Arthr. Rheum.*, **14,** 706
8. Lidsky, M., Sharp, J. and Billings, S. (1973). Double-blind study of cyclophosphamide in rheumatoid arthritis. *Arthr. Rheum.*, **16,** 148
9. Sigler, J. W., Bluhm, G. B., Duncan, H., Sharp, J. T., Ensign, D. C. and McRum, W. R. (1974). Gold salts in the treatment of rheumatoid arthritis. *Ann. Int. Med.,* **80,** 21
10. Ball, J. (1964). The articular pathology of rheumatoid arthritis. In M. Crater (ed.) *Radiological Aspects of Rheumatoid Arthritis* 25 (Amsterdam: Excerpta Medica Foundation, International Congress Series No. 61)
11. Cooperating Clinics Committee of the American Rheumatism Association (1970). A controlled trial of cyclophosphamide in rheumatoid arthritis. *N. Engl. J. Med.*, **283,** 884
12. Cooperating Clinics Committee of the American Rheumatism Association (1973). A controlled trial of gold salt therapy in rheumatoid arthritis. *Arthr. Rheum.*, **16,** 353
13. Hunter, T., Urowitz, M. B. Gordon, D. A., Smythe, H. A. and Ogryzlo, M. A. (1975). Azathioprine in rheumatoid arthritis. *Arthr. Rheum.*, **18,** 15
14. Larsen, A. and Dale, K. (1978). In D. C. Dumonde and M. W. Steward (eds.) *Laboratory Tests in the Rheumatic Diseases.* (Lancaster: MTP Press Limited) (in preparation). Standardized radiological evaluation of rheumatoid arthritis
15. Larsen, A., Dale, K. and Eek, M. (1977). Roentgenologic evaluation of rheumatoid arthritis and related conditions by standard reference films. *Acta Radiol. Diagnosis,* **18,** 481
16. Fletcher, D. E. and Rowley, K. A. (1952). The radiological features of rheumatoid arthritis. *Br. J. Radiol.*, **25,** 282
17. Thould, A. K. and Simon, G. (1966). Assessment of radiological changes in the hands and feet in rheumatoid arthritis. *Ann. Rheum. Dis.* **25,** 220
18. Brook, A. and Corbett, M (1977). Radiographic changes in early rheumatoid disease. *Ann. Rheum. Dis.* **36,** 71
19. Larsen, A. (1976). The value of individual joints for radiologic assessment of rheumatoid arthritis. *Scand. J. Rheumatol.*, **5,** 119

21
The Effects of Specific Drug Therapy on Neutrophil Chemotaxis in Rheumatoid Arthritis

A. G. MOWAT

INTRODUCTION

An important function of the neutrophil leukocyte is the phagocytosis and digestion of foreign and dead material. Although essentially a beneficial function, in patients with rheumatoid arthritis phagocytosis of immune complexes may lead to cell death and the release of lysosomal enzymes[1,2].

Neutrophil chemotaxis and phagocytosis are abnormal in patients with rheumatoid arthritis[3,4]. The impairment in chemotaxis can be attributed both to the prior ingestion of complexes and cellular metabolic changes[3,5].

No correlation between chemotaxis and measures of disease activity such as the erythrocyte sedimentation rate and the articular index has been found and to date no relationship between chemotaxis and standard non-steroidal, anti-inflammatory drug therapy has been noted. D-Penicillamine and gold salts are established drugs in the treatment of rheumatoid arthritis while the promising initial findings with the anti-helminthic drug levamisole[6,7] has led to further clinical studies. The drugs have a comparable clinical effect, both in quality and speed of onset, although the exact mode of action of the various drugs is unknown. Since changes in neutrophil function could produce changes in cellular and immunological reactions, the effect of these drugs upon neutrophil chemotaxis has been studied.

MATERIAL AND METHODS

Since earlier studies[8], have shown that neutrophil chemotaxis is not dependent upon the age and sex of the subject, nor, in patients with rheumatoid arthritis, the duration or severity of the disease or titre of rheumatoid factor in the serum, the subject groups were not matched for these factors.

For the tests with D-penicillamine neutrophils were obtained from 12 normal controls, from 19 patients with rheumatoid arthritis who had been treated with the drug ('Distamine' – Dista) for periods ranging from one day to four years with daily doses ranging from 250 mg to 2 g, and from 17 other patients with rheumatoid arthritis many of whom were about to commence D-penicillamine therapy.

For the tests with gold salts the neutrophils from 18 normal controls, from 8 patients who had failed to respond to gold therapy, from 12 patients who had had a clear clinical response to gold, and from 20 patients who had never received gold therapy, were employed.

For the tests with levamisole the neutrophils from 9 normal controls and 10 patients, untreated with the drug, were employed. Standard measurements of neutrophils untreated with the drug were also undertaken on 8 patients before and during the initial weeks of treatment with levamisole; the drug being given on the first three days of the week in a dose of 50 mg/day in week one increasing to 150 mg/day in the third and subsequent weeks.

Chemotaxis was measured by the method of Baum *et al.*[8] a mixture of casein and standard AB serum being used as an attractant, and the results expressed as an index. The results of drug treatment are expressed as a percentage of the index found for untreated cells tested at the same time. Pure D-penicillamine powder (Dista), sodium aurothiomalate ('Myocrisin' – May and Baker) and levamisole powder (Janssen) were dissolved or diluted in Hank's solution in concentrations of 1000, 100, 10 and 1 μg/ml (10^4 μg/ml added for levamisole) without significantly altering the pH of the solutions. These solutions were added to the upper, cellular non-attractant compartments of the Sykes-Moore tissue culture chambers and the chambers incubated for 3 hours at 37 °C. In a smaller number of cases the cells were pre-incubated with the drugs for 1 hour at 37 °C before being centrifuged onto the millepore filter and enclosed in the chambers without washing or addition of further drug.

RESULTS

D-Penicillamine

The results found after 3 h incubation with D-penicillamine are listed in Table 21.1. There was no alteration in the chemotactic index for any patient group at any drug concentration. A concentration of 100 μg/ml represents the approximate plasma concentration expected with a daily dose of 1 g of D-penicillamine.

The results found after pre-incubation for 1 h with D-penicillamine are listed in Table 21.2. These results are quite different to those in Table 21.1 and show significant ($p<0.01$) impairment in chemotaxis at both drug concentrations. The inter-group differences are not significant. Standard chemotactic tests in

Table 21.1 Neutrophil chemotaxis: effect of incubation at 37 °C for 3 h with D-penicillamine

Subjects (number)	*Basal*	*Chemotactic indices (Mean ± SE) % basal value*			
		D-penicillamine concentration (μg/ml)			
		10^3	10^2	10	1
Normal control (9)	551 ± 15	96 ± 10	97 ± 6	101 ± 9	103 ± 7
RA treated (15)	364 ± 12	104 ± 8	99 ± 7	104 ± 8	100 ± 8
RA untreated (13)	345 ± 18	101 ± 9	103 ± 5	103 ± 8	97 ± 9

Table 21.2 Neutrophil chemotaxis: effect of pre-incubation at 37 °C for 1 h with D-penicillamine

Subjects (number)	*Basal*	*Chemotactic indices (Mean ± SE) % basal value*	
		D-penicillamine concentration (μg/ml)	
		10^3	10^2
Normal control (4)	565	39 ± 5	62 ± 6
RA treated (5)	501	63 ± 15	85 ± 8
RA untreated (7)	432	39 ± 3	69 ± 5

patients before and during D-penicillamine therapy showed no immediate change but tended to improve as the activity of the rheumatoid disease was controlled.

Gold salts

The results found with gold are listed in Table 21.3. Normal controls had approximately dose-related impairment in chemotaxis while there were similar, but significantly less marked dose-related changes in the patients who had never received gold ($p<0.01$ at each concentration). The patients showing a clinical response to gold had a similar but less closely dose-related reduction in chemotaxis to that found in normal subjects. The reduction was significantly ($p<0.01$) less marked at drug concentrations of 1000 and 10 μg/ml but was not different ($p<0.5$ >0.2) at the other two drug concentrations. However, the reductions were significantly greater than those found with the neutrophils of patients who had never received gold therapy ($p<0.01$ at each concentration). Patients who failed to respond to gold therapy showed only a modest reduction in chemotaxis and this was not dose dependent.

Levamisole

The results summarized in Table 21.4 show that compared with changes found in normal subjects, levamisole (10^4 μg/ml) inhibited the neutrophils of rheumatoid patients to a significantly lesser extent ($p<0.01$). On the other hand, at concentrations between $10–10^{-3}$ μg/ml, it stimulated the chemotactic response of neutrophils of rheumatoid patients to a greater extent than that of the neutrophils of normal subjects. The stimulation of neutrophil chemotaxis was most noticeable in the range of therapeutic concentrations, namely 10–100 μg/ml.

Table 21.3 Neutrophil chemotaxis: effect of gold salts

Subjects (numbers)	*Chemotactic indices (Mean ± SE) % basal value*				
	Basal	*Gold concentration (μg/ml)*			
		10^3	10^2	10	1
Normal controls (18)	471 ± 22	39 ± 6	54 ± 6	59 ± 8	69 ± 8
RA untreated (20)	441 ± 32	68 ± 8	73 ± 7	77 ± 6	86 ± 5
RA gold response (12)	398 ± 46	47 ± 7	56 ± 6	70 ± 5	72 ± 7
RA no gold response (8)	323 ± 33	88 ± 13	88 ± 9	89 ± 9	85 ± 8

Table 21.4 Neutrophil chemotaxis: effect of levamisole

Subjects (numbers)	*Chemotactic indices (Mean ± SE) % basal value*					
	Basal	*Levamisole concentrations (μg/ml)*				
		10^4	10^3	10^2	10	1
Normals (9)	517 ± 35	28 ± 4	122 ± 15	118 ± 8	102 ± 8	89 ± 8
Rheumatoid arthritics (10)	409 ± 41	56 ± 5	166 ± 20	162 ± 24	122 ± 12	106 ± 6

The results of standard chemotactic tests in patients before and during the initial weeks of levamisole therapy, before any clinical benefit was apparent, are listed in Table 21.5. A marked improvement in the chemotactic index was found after two days treatment each week, i.e. on day 3, the value being similar for each patient each week despite an increasing drug dosage and representing a significant ($p<0.01$) improvement beyond the normal range not only for rheumatoid subjects but also for controls. By day 5, some 36 hours after the last dose of levamisole, the chemotactic index had shown a slight fall.

Table 21.5 Neutrophil chemotaxis. Eight patients treated with levamisole

		Mean chemotactic indices
Initial		430
Week 1	Day 2	818
	Day 5	783
Week 2	Day 2	876
	Day 5	722
Week 3	Day 2	865
	Day 5	735

DISCUSSION

Defective neutrophil chemotaxis *in vivo* may arise due to intrinsic defects in the leukocyte, either familial or acquired, and these have been demonstrated in a number of conditions including rheumatoid arthritis. A number of drugs have also been implicated in the causation of such defects. Defects may also arise due to familial or acquired abnormalities in the complement system while inhibitors against both the leukocytes or chemotactic factors have been described[9–11]. Thus it is possible to find either similar defects in several functions of one cell type or several cell lines similarly affected, for instance by a cell poison. Alternatively a specific defect may occur in only one cellular function with other cellular activities remaining unaffected. The standardized *in vitro* method used here eliminates a number of possible mechanisms. In particular, owing to the use of a standard AB serum instead of the individual patient's serum it eliminates mechanisms relating to complement system and its inhibitors, such as have been described for gold salts[12].

In the standard *in vitro* system D-penicillamine does not alter chemotaxis of neutrophil leukocytes. However, as noted by others,[13] pre-incubation of the neutrophils for one hour produces significant impairment in chemotaxis. It is suggested that the drug might produce a dose-dependent inhibition of the pro-esterase found in the cell membrane and which is essential for activation of chemotaxis[13]. The different results with different incubation methods could reflect changes in competition for activation of the pro-esterase, the effect of D-penicillamine being overcome in the presence of chemotactic complement components.

The changes noted in neutrophil chemotaxis in patients treated for some months with D-penicillamine are consistent with the finding that there is some improvement in the rheumatoid disease, although this improvement correlates more closely with a feeling of well-being than with changes in the erythrocyte sedimentation rate or articular index (Mowat, unpublished observations). Thus it cannot be concluded from these studies that D-penicillamine produces its clinical effect by a change in neutrophil chemotaxis.

However, gold salts do affect neutrophil chemotaxis, the percentage impairment being similar in normal controls and in those patients with rheumatoid arthritis who responded to gold therapy. Interestingly, the results in patients who had never received gold suggest that the group included both those who would and would not show a drug effect. The concentrations of sodium aurothiomalate were chosen in the knowledge that in treated patients serum, and probably synovial fluid, concentrations of gold rise to 1 and 10 μg/ml[14,15] while mean synovial tissue concentrations in patients on maintenance therapy could reach 20 μg/ml (range 1–76 μg/ml)[16]. A similar reduction in the phagocytic activity of human macrophages has also been demonstrated[17], and the changes shown to correlate with clinical improvement.

How gold salts produce these changes is unknown. Since they are known to inhibit a variety of enzymes they may simply alter the metabolism of neutrophils and other cell lines in a non-specific manner and this is reflected in comparable percentage impairment of neutrophil chemotaxis in both normal controls and successfully treated patients. It is perhaps of greater interest to speculate on why patients who did not respond to gold therapy showed only a minor impairment in chemotaxis. The results suggest that the metabolism of these rheumatoid neutrophils has been inherently altered and that the cells are no longer susceptible to the metabolic effects of gold salts. Although there is some scatter in the results, the findings suggest that changes in neutrophil chemotaxis in the presence of gold salts may allow selection of suitable cases for treatment with these drugs.

Levamisole, a potent anti-helminthic drug, appears to have immunostimulatory properties. In conventional animal models and skin tests the drug has no anti-inflammatory activity but stimulates cells, notably the macrophage, involved in immunological responses[18,19]. The drug stimulates *in vitro* chemotaxis in both patients and controls, and rapidly raises the chemotactic index to supra-normal values in treated patients. Others have reported similar *in vitro* results in controls[20]. It has been suggested that levamisole increases intra-cellular levels of cyclic 3,5–guanosine monophosphate thereby sustaining microtubular assembly and enhancing cell motility[20].

It is postulated that in patients with rheumatoid arthritis phagocytosis by neutrophils of the immune complexes in the synovial fluid and perhaps in the serum and other fluids, lead to cell death and the release of lysosomal enzymes. Chemotaxis is an essential preliminary to phagocytosis. It is simpler to imagine that the impaired chemotaxis produced by gold salts leads to a reduction in the rate of destruction of immune complexes and the subsequent release of inflammatory enzymes, than it is to imagine that the increased neutrophil activity induced by levamisole can be beneficial. However, it is possible that when in the longer term, the sustained attempts by the neutrophils to remove immune complexes become successful a comparable clinical improvement may also result. Sequential examination of joint fluids could provide the answer.

The test system described here identifies distinct differences in drugs with a similar clinical effect. The extension of such tests, particularly to macrophage studies, may help in the assessment of new agents and in the selection of patients for treatment.

SUMMARY

The effect of therapeutic concentrations of D-penicillamine, sodium aurothiomalate and levamisole on *in vitro* neutrophil chemotaxis was studied. D-Penicillamine produced no changes. Sodium aurothiomalate produced dose-related reductions in chemotaxis in normal subjects and in patients who had a good clinical response to gold therapy, while patients who had failed to respond to gold showed a minimal, non-dose dependent reduction. Levamisole produced dose-dependent stimulation of chemotaxis, a greater effect being found with the patients' cells.

Neutrophil chemotaxis improved to normal values in most patients responding to several months of D-penicillamine treatment but showed an immediate and marked stimulation in patients treated with levamisole.

ACKNOWLEDGEMENTS

The author wishes to acknowledge the expert technical assistance of P. Brooks, Esq. He is grateful to Dr Fisher of the Oxford Regional Blood Transfusion Service for the provision of fresh AB serum, to Dr W. H. Lyle of Dista for D-penicillamine powder and to Dr J. G. Adams of Janssen for levamisole powder. The author wishes to express his thanks to Mrs S. Strudwick for typing the manuscript.

References

1. Hollander, J. L., McCarty, D. L. Astorga, G. and Castro-Murillo, E. (1965). Studies on the pathogenesis of rheumatoid joint inflammation. 1. The 'R.A.' cell and a working hypothesis. *Ann. Int. Med.*, **62,** 271
2. Rosenthal, M., Graf, U. and Muller, W. (1976). Nachweis und Vorkommen von immunkomplexen bei rheumatischen erkrankungen. *Schweiz. Med. Wochenschr.*, **106,** 1116
3. Mowat, A. G. and Baum, J. (1971). Chemotaxis of polymorphonuclear leukocytes from patients with rheumatoid arthritis. *J. Clin. Invest.*, **50,** 2541
4. Turner, R. A., Schumacher, H. R. and Myers, A. R. (1973). Phagocytic function of polymorphonuclear leukocytes in rheumatic disease. *J. Clin. Invest.*, **52,** 1632
5. Roberts-Thomson, P. J., Hazleman, B. L., Barnett, I. G., MacLennan, I. C. M. and Mowat, A. G. (1976). Factors relating to circulating immune complexes in rheumatoid arthritis. *Ann. Rheum. Dis.*, **35,** 314
6. Schuermans, Y. (1975). Levamisole in rheumatoid arthritis. *Lancet*, **i,** 111
7. Huskisson, E. C., Dieppe, P. A., Scott, J., Trapnell, J., Balme, H. W. and Willoughby, D. A. (1976). Immunostimulant therapy with levamisole for rheumatoid arthritis. *Lancet*, **i,** 393

8. Baum, J., Mowat, A. G. and Kirk, J. (1971). A simplified method for the measurement of chemotaxis of polymorphonuclear leucocytes from human blood. *J. Lab. Clin. Med.*, **77,** 501
9. Ward, P. A. (1972). Insubstantial leukotaxis. *J. Lab. Clin. Med.*, **79,** 873
10. Keller, H. U., Hess, M. W. and Cottier, H. (1975). Physiology of chemotaxis and random motility. *Semin. Haemat.*, **12,** 47
11. Miller, M. E. (1975). Pathology of chemotaxis and random motility. *Semin. Haemat.*, **12,** 59
12. Schultz, D. R., Volanakis, J. E., Arnold, P. I., Gottlieb, N. L., Sakai, K. and Stroud, R. M. (1974). Inactivation of C1 in rheumatoid synovial fluid, purified C1 and C1 esterase, by gold compounds. *Clin. Exper. Immunol.*, **17,** 395
13. Chwalinska-Sadowska, H. and Baum, J. (1976). The effect of D-penicillamine on polymorphonuclear leukocyte function. *J. Clin. Invest.*, **58,** 871
14. Billings, R., Grahame, R., Marks, V., Wood, P. J. and Taylor, A. (1975). Blood and urine gold levels during chrysotherapy for rheumatoid arthritis. *Rheum. Rehab.*, **14,** 13
15. Lorber, A., Simon, T. M., Leeb, J. and Carroll, P. E. (1975). Chrysotherapy: pharmacological and clinical correlates. *J. Rheumat.*, **4,** 401
16. Grahame, R., Billings, R., Laurence, N., Marks, V. and Wood, P. J. (1974). Tissue gold levels after chrysotherapy. *Ann. Rheum. Dis.*, **33,** 536
17. Jessop, J. D., Vernon-Roberts, B. and Harris, J. (1973). Effects of gold salts and prednisolone on inflammatory cells. *Ann. Rheum. Dis.*, **32,** 294
18. Editorial (1975). Levamisole. *Lancet,* **i,** 151
19. Trabert, U., Rosenthal, M. and Muller, W. (1976). The effect of levamisole on adjuvant arthritis in the rat. *J. Rheumat.*, **3,** 166
20. Anderson, R., Glover, A., Koornhof, H. J. and Rabson, A. R. (1976). *In vitro* stimulation of neutrophil motiligy by levamisole: Maintenance of cGMP levels in chemotactically stimulated levamisole-treated neutrophils. *J. Immunol.*, **117,** 428

Discussion VI

Standardization in Clinical Measurement (Chapter 16)

E. V. BARNETT: Do we have insight into systems, measurements, or identification procedures that would tend to select more homogeneous populations for drug studies and allow the distinction of potential responders from non-responders? Are there any techniques?

W. WATSON BUCHANAN: There clearly must be techniques. What one would require to do would be to take patients and to treat a group of patients who are representative as far as possible of the general population of rheumatoid arthritis. They would have to be treated with two drugs: (a) and (b). One would then need to identify the patients who appeared to respond to drug (a) and those who did not respond, and the other patients who appeared to respond to drug (b) and those who did not respond. One would then have to wait until they threw out yet another exacerbation and treat them again with the two drugs, and then one would wait again and do a crossover to prove that there were subgroups of patients who are responding to one drug and not another.

The other problem is that some of the patients will have side effects from a drug, and they would be the dropouts. With some drugs, e.g. aspirin, that would be quite high. It is worth doing, and we shall be trying to do it with the compliance studies that I mentioned.

E. V. BARNETT: Is it possible that since there are correlates with activity of disease, joint counts, grip strength and latex titre and sedimentation rate, and staging of articular erosion, that a realistic hypothesis for greater homogeneity might be to identify patients not only in terms of whether or not they have arthritis, but statistically to group them in bands of latex titre, sedimentation rates, immune complex levels, etc.?

W. WATSON BUCHANAN: They would be important variables in determining whether they were responding to one or other drug regimen. They would have to be looked at. But I do not know whether it is the case. Dr Huskisson has examined the distribution of responders and non-responders, but his data show a normal distribution curve. It is exactly what one would expect of a homogenous group: 2.5% will be highly responsive to one drug and 2.5% will be highly responsive to another.

J. WEBB: Is Professor Buchanan proposing at this stage that the pain index is the only measurement that needs to be taken?

Secondly, has he ever done one of these studies including a narcotic analgesic.

W. WATSON BUCHANAN: I am not suggesting that only one method be used. Clearly we should use all the methods. I am pointing out the fact that the most relevant method is measurement of the patient's pain – and that is easy. Pain is easily measured. One measures it in terms of its relief. But of course with short-term trials on a small number of patients one might include all the other measurements that are available.

We haven't done a study including the narcotic analgesics, such as morphine. But others have done it. There has been a study with pethidine, and pethidine does not relieve pain in rheumatoid arthritis. Aspirin does, but pethidine does not. We have done it with Fortral (pentazocine) and it does not work in rheumatoid arthritis, whether it is given alone, or whether it is given in association with a non-steroidal anti-inflammatory drug. Similarly with paracetamol. Yet the interesting point is that 40% of the patients we see are being prescribed paracetamol.

M. F. CUTHBERT: I should like to give some quantitative information to support Professor Buchanan's remarks on gold. I also have a question about his mortality or his morbidity figures related to rheumatic drugs.

In the 10-year period, 1964–1974, we had 102 reports of adverse reactions associated with the use of gold reported to the Committee on Safety of Medicines. Of these, 32 were fatal. There were 41 reports affecting the haemopoietic system, of which 22 were fatal, and 11 of gastrointestinal bleeding, two of which were fatal. Of all the major anti-rheumatic drugs that we have analysed, gold carries the highest mortality in terms of those reported to us. Most of the blood dysplasias were thromocytopenia or aplastic anaemia.

I have done a quick tally of the figure that Professor Buchanan showed quoting Professor Goodwood's paper. Of the 40 000 reports received in the 10-year period – that is adverse reactions to all drugs – some 5000 reports, were associated with the use of major anti-rheumatic drugs. Out of those 5000 there were 709 deaths, but I have no comparable figure with me for the number of deaths relating to my total figure of 40 000. I would therefore like Professor Buchanan to clarify whether the figures he quoted were for deaths or for reported adverse reactions.

W. WATSON BUCHANAN: Deaths – which is the ultimate in adverse reaction. These were deaths. The important thing is not the numerator, but the denominator, in these adverse reactions. With phenylbutazone, for example, one will give 80 000 prescriptions before one sees the first haemopoietic disorder.

M. WEATHERALL: A word of caution on the reporting of adverse reactions. The criterion by which the particular drug concerned is held responsible is not always completely clear. Most patients are treated with more than one drug, and often with two or more toxic drugs at the same time. The actual cause of the adverse reaction is not always proven to what one might call the scientific standard of acceptability.

M. F. CUTHBERT: This will come out in my own paper. It is abundantly clear that many drugs are associated with adverse reaction, but it is quite another matter to establish the cause – effect relationships.

M. K. JASANI: Would Professor Buchanan look at the future and outline what in his view should be the type of developments for assessment of severity of disease in patients with or without drug treatment.

W. WATSON BUCHANAN: There is no doubt that if this is to be done a unit will be needed that can measure the blood levels of the drugs, that can do clinical pharmacology, and that can assess the response of patients. It will need a clinical unit, preferably with the laboratories by the side.

It will require a system where patients can be quickly tested against placebo. The first step is to test the drug against placebo in varying doses, to see whether it works. Having done that, one should do short-term trials comparing it with other standard drugs. Then one should perhaps use Peter Lee's method, and then go on to long-term one year follow-ups, compliance studies.

J. G. HAWKES: A word in support of gold. In the Empire Rheumatism Council Study surely the gold was administered only for a short period and up to a total of 1 g? As one of the shop-floor workers, I actually have to treat patients, and I find gold is a very effective agent, particularly when used as a maintenance dose of around 20 mg, or 50 mg each 4 weeks, month, or thereabouts. I would not want the symposium to run away with the idea that gold is the most dangerous drug in the pharmacopoeia, or that its effectiveness is practically zero.

W. WATSON BUCHANAN: I have looked at all of these trials, not only with gold, but at the American Rheumatism Association trial of cyclophosphamide. If only the mean differences are taken, none of them can be judged as very dramatic drugs.

Of course they work. If they are given to the milder cases they will work and they will appear to have a greater therapeutic benefit than if they are given to severe cases. We happen, unfortunately, to have given them to severe cases. They are the second-line drugs.

It still behoves us to appreciate that we are dealing with potentially very toxic compounds.

M. K. JASANI: Is Professor Buchanan prepared to amplify his remarks with respect to the type of measurements which could be evolved in the future?

W. WATSON BUCHANAN: We are limited by the fact that inflammation has only five cardinal features, and we have to relate our measurements to these features. At the moment it would appear that the most sensitive measure is the patient's response, and that is unfortunate. The technitium uptakes and other laboratory measures are the least sensitive. They are more objective, but unfortunately they are least sensitive.

A. T. A. DOBLE: Professor Buchanan might be giving the impression that pain is perhaps the most important thing to change when treating rheumatoid patients. The correlate of that is that perhaps the drug companies should try to develop analgesics rather than anti-inflammatory agents.

How good is the tie up between pain relief and anti-rheumatic effect?

W. WATSON BUCHANAN: It is not good at all. I showed a patient's hand. That patient had received every drug that we are able to prescribe, over long periods. The histology of synovium from that patient is used as our standard teaching slide. None of these drugs has a really marked effect on the disease process. That is my view. They have an effect, but they are reducing the effect from *there* to *there* when they still have to get from *there* to zero.

A QUESTIONER: One comment. Should we not be trying to develop a method with regard to joint swelling which measures joint volume rather than joint circumference.

If we measure joint circumference, we are measuring one parameter of the joint and we are missing – possibly – the soft tissue swelling which occurs on either side of an affected joint, which may be shrunk down by effective therapy. If we measure the circumference we may miss that completely.

I have two questions. Regarding the trials of ibuprofen, Professor Buchanan mentioned (to me) that only 12 of these were properly controlled. Can he confirm whether each of the twelve used either only in-patients or only outpatients in the trial?

Could he comment, too, on what his feelings are about the visual analogue scale for measuring pain. It is something that I have used quite a lot. I am quite impressed, but I should like to know what the professor thinks.

W. WATSON BUCHANAN: We have used the visual analogue scale, and it works. It shows changes between effective drugs and placebo. One cannot do comparisons with other scales of pain. One cannot find out how they correlate, because the patient's response is immediately conditioned to the next method. If he is asked what is his pain on an adjectival scale and he says 'moderate' and he is then given a line to point out where his pain is, he will tend to pick the mid-point. In other words, one conditions the response, so one cannot really do comparisons with different methods. But we have used the visual analogue scale, and it works. Of course it works.

On the point about ibuprofen let me say at once that it is not a criticism of the drug. It is a criticism of the clinicians who are doing the trials. The same was true with William O'Brien's paper in 1969 on indomethacin. He found exactly the same result when he looked at the trials of indomethacin. I would suggest that O'Brien's article on indomethacin trials should be a standard paper for every student.

Of the 12 ibuprofen trials, one was done on an in-patient basis and the others were done on an out-patient basis. Most of the poor trials were done in countries where English is not spoken. The word 'control' does not seem to exist in other languages.

E.V. BARNETT: Different measurements are useful for different purposes. Changes in inflammation mobility may be an excellent end-point change for a drug on pre-marketing trial, for public health measures, if viewed from the standpoint of the re-employability of the individual may be a much better criterion than pain relief or joint count. Indeed, bed rest is not an employable result, even though it reduces joint counts and may well be anti-inflammatory.

Multivariate Analysis of Laboratory Tests (Chapter 17)

W. WATSON BUCHANAN: One of the problems in a disease like rheumatoid arthritis when trying to do multivariate analysis is time. At any one point in time, the variables may not correlate as well as at another. For instance, it is well-known amongst clinicians – or at least it is taught to medical students – that anaemia correlates well with the severity of the disease. If this is assessed at a point in time in rheumatoid arthritis, however, it may correlate only weakly with the articular index, ESR, perhaps serum albumin, but nothing else.

E. V. BARNETT: Along those lines, the changes over the time and the rate of change, which may include final data and initial data, would be missed by looking at just final data, just initial data, or even the combination. The degree of slope may reflect both better than the combination.

M. K. JASANI: With respect to the many parameters that he measured, does Professor Barnett have any system whereby he could delete or add other discriminant functions to the analysis?

E. V. BARNETT: Agreed. If one sees that the slopes are parallel in a highly consistent fashion between two test systems, then obviously one of the measurements is redundant from the cost–benefit analysis standpoints, especially when the patient has to pay for it. That is one spin-off of looking at all the measurements. If they are seen to correlate with each other and with the third variable to be measured, e.g. renal function, but do not completely correlate with each other, then there is a greater potential for the tests in combination to be of greater utility than singly.

M. K. JASANI: I like Professor Barnett's approach. It is obviously comprehensive and one could do longitudinal studies with probably greater interpretative value.

I should like to take the opporunity of expanding on the comment in his presentation with respect to the discriminative power of certain biochemical measurements such as acid phosphatase and β-glucuronidase in the skin graft model (*J. Physiol.*, **219,** 525; 1971). I might then expand also on the implications to the clinical situation (*Clin. Rheum. Dis.*, **2**(1) pp 273; 1976).

After quite a long investigation of that problem we feel that the enzymes measured, as Professor Barnett rightly inferred, may not have a direct role in the mediation of inflammation. Nevertheless, they may be reflecting some cellular event which, if we knew and we were able to identify, could be integrated into the type of matrix that he outlined in order to have a specific probe with respect to what a drug is doing to that particular cell type.

E. V. BARNETT: The results of test systems applied at different times to patients with disease on therapy and remission may at first seem to contradict the hypothesis, and the experimental data. For instance, in immune complex disease there is activation of the complement system, hypocomplementaemia, and a relationship with antigen and antibody. Yet, when these variables are measured, there are patients with active disease who have no evidence of circulating complexes, and there are patients with circulating complexes but no evidence of renal disease. This may indeed negate the hypothesis. But it is also possible that the elements involved in the pathogenesis of renal disease tend to be consumed in the kidney in some patients, whereas in other patients the surveillance mechanisms such as the reticulo-endothelial cells in liver and spleen, clear the elements and then protect target organs from punishment.

D. ALARCON-SEGOVIA: For the record I should like to contest the notion that patients with SLE that have gone into remission resemble mixed connective tissue disease. This seemed to be the case superficially at the beginning, when we looked into the question, but on looking back at their sera that we had had stored for years we found that they had an ENA, anti-ENA, or the anti-RNP antibody for a long time, and that altogether they did seem to have a different disease. We also had patients who had been diagnosed as mixed connective tissue disease to begin with, and without the intervention of treatment.

To consider that a mixed connective tissue disease could be in some of the instances artificially induced disease would not be warranted by our data.

Patients with mixed connective tissue disease are more likely to go into remission than patients with SLE. I might therefore suggest that what Professor Barnett is seeing is patients with mixed connective tissue disease to begin with who went into remission because of that.

E. V. BARNETT: This sort of discussion and controversy illustrates the entire problem in diagnosis and definition of rheumatic diseases. What Dr Alarcon-Segovia has said may be entirely correct. It is possible that the 47 patients, all of whom had biopsy evidence of diffuse proliferative or membrano-proliferative glomerulonephritis, may have been by unknown selection factors nearly all good responders and mixed connective tissue disease cases. However by the usual criteria these patients would have been classified as classical lupus, if they were read blindly.

Nonetheless, it may well be true that mixed connective tissue in addition is a definable entity, and not attributable to therapy. I did not state that that was not the case.

W. WATSON BUCHANAN: To come back to Professor Barnett's first slide. He presented a group with a very clearly-defined sub-group in clinical rheumatology: those patients with an associated HLA B-27 gene. It is often said by clinicians that patients with ankylosing spondylitis respond particularly well to phenylbutazone. Indeed, in a standard textbook of rheumatology published in the US, this statement is still made. It could be that the response might be genetically determined, and one wonders whether it might be worth looking at that, particularly as Professor Barnett's group have so clearly defined the problem.

E. V. BARNETT: That is a very good question. Since we also will have patients with criteria of ankylosing spondylitis who are B-27 negative, we could find out whether their therapeutic responses are indeed different.

Isotope Analysis of Joint Inflammation (Chapter 18)
Thermography in the Assessment of Rheumatic Inflammation (Chapter 19)

G. P. LEWIS: I welcome hearing about some scientific objective approaches from clinicians. I have been becoming depressed over the past week or two, even more so today, probably reaching a height with Professor Buchanan's paper when it looked as if we should have to bring back the clinicians from the Dark Ages. I am therefore very pleased to see such nice scientific experiments adapted to the clinic.

One specific point. Dr Dick mentioned that he measured xenon-133 coming from the dog joint in femoral vein blood and lymph. Has he measured lymph separately? In rabbits, Dr C. S. Bach and I have looked at the anatomy of the lymphatic system and there we could not actually trace any lymphatics from the joint itself – and this would be useful information.

W. CARSON DICK: I am well aware of the work of Professor Lewis and Dr C. S. Bach. We have looked for the presence of ^{133}Xe in the lymphatics in great detail. However, like Professor Lewis we could not find a really big change, I think because there was such a low flow rate.

G. P. LEWIS: Was radioactivity detected?

W. CARSON DICK: Yes, but not enough to quantify it reliably. In other words we had the same difficulty as you.

G. P. LEWIS: It might be a significant factor if a joint does not have a lymph drainage.

W. WATSON BUCHANAN: All the joints have a lymph drainage. If a very large particle is put into a joint, it will be cleared by the lymphatics.

G. P. LEWIS: Might I have a reference?

W. WATSON BUCHANAN: 'Buchanan' – 1977.

J. R. VANE: Dr Dick hinted that he had, in his xenon clearance tests, an animal model for inflammation. Which model has he chosen as the one most relevant to the human situation?

W. CARSON DICK: The work we did was with the veterinary college. It is a model of osteoarthrosis (OA) in the long term, but of an inflammatory synovitis in the short term. It is a simple model. One simply cuts the cruciate ligament and lets the animal run about, and it will gradually develop OA.

J. R. VANE: I was also interested in Dr Bacon's suggestion that inhibition of PG synthetase has no relevance to the mode of action of the aspirin-like drugs. Was he extrapolating from *in vitro* data? Were your results on rheumatoid synovia obtained *in vitro*?

P. A. BACON: These were *in vitro* data, but we have looked in the *in vivo* situation. We have looked in synovium from patients treated with different drugs too, and there is a very large difference in the action of some of these drugs.

J. R. VANE: I am sure that there is a large difference *in vivo*. To go from direct cells *in vitro* through all the barriers that a drug has to pass before it reaches the rheumatoid synovium *in vivo* is a considerable step, and there are all sorts of things, absorbtion, plasma protein binding, selective uptake that might interfere with, or reduce, the correlations that one sees.

P. A. BACON: I accept that. It is just that as a simple clinician that very big difference suggests to me that it is not very relevant.

J. R. VANE: What then is relevant? What is the mode of action of aspirin-like drugs?

P. A. BACON: That is really for the pharmacologists.

A. A. J. GOLDBERG: If one examines Dr Bacon's responders in the fenclofenac group, it looks as though there was a dose-related response curve, as with azapropazone. Does the fall in the responders on the fenclofenac correlate with the fall seen on standard drugs?

P. A. BACON: We are still completing the high-dose group and I would not like to answer that question until it is completed. With both of those, taking the responders only, there seems to be quite a similarity.

M. K. JASANI: My first comment concerns the possible establishment of a middle ground in the comments made by various persons on lymphatic drainage. Even if it is accepted that the normal joint has a lymphatic drainage, it should be remembered that in the rheumatoid synovium, or the rheumatoid joint, there is an element of lymphatic blockage due to fibrin. Here I am not simply extrapolating from the experimental model that I described, but basing it on the fact that the osmolality of persistent synovial effusions is that of a plasma transudate rather than that of an exudate (*see Arthr. Rheum.* **8**, 29; 1965), implying that there is retention of fluid.

Dr Bacon is it possible that with your methodology you are testing, in the clinic, the vasoconstrictive ability of some of the drugs. Is there any way you could visualize that would enable you to distinguish whether the lowering of the thermographic index is due to an effect against arteriolar dilatation or venous congestion?

P. A. BACON: We have not even tried to look at that. It might be interesting to do so, but perhaps in an animal model rather than the human situation.

E. V. BARNETT: I would like to put forward a possible alternative interpretation for Dr Bacon's data concerning the lack of suppression of PG synthetase in the rheumatoid synovium. It is that although all the active drugs suppress inflammation and also suppress PG synthetase, an increased potency of suppression of PG synthetase does not result in increased potency of anti-inflammation. Therefore, the next step would be to find mechanisms for anti-inflammation other than PG synthetase.

P. A. BACON: The problem has been very little looked at in the clinical situation.

S. ORLOFF: I have a comment on Dr Jasani's remark. When one measures infra-red emission, one measures something that is not emitted from 1 mm, or 0.5 mm, or so. Therefore, whatever we measure is just the response of the superficial blood flow to what is happening deeper down. There is a gradient there, and the question that arises is whether the drugs are as specific as we might think.

Dr Bacon showed various non-responders. Were these the same patients for all the drugs, or were they different patients? Is a non-responder to aspirin a non-responder to phenylbutazone, and so on?

P. A. BACON: That is not necessarily true. We have not formally tested it and patients are not going sequentially from one drug to another. There are certainly some patients who have not responded to one and have responded to another, but we have not done what Professor Buchanan suggested this morning – that is to come back to the same patients during their next flare-up and to look at it then. A comment on the blood flow. The figure of 0.5 cm is often quoted, yet very little work has been done on it. We have also looked at Paget's disease where it seems that most of the blood flow is in the underlying bone. We have not yet done enough to reach a good conclusion, but it looks as though measurements are often of things deeper than 0.5 cm.

S. ORLOFF: Physically the infra-red is absorbed. If there is an absorbtion, it cannot be emitted.

P. A. BACON: The absorbtion has not been looked at in any great detail in human tissues. It depends a lot on the type of tissue; whether it is adipose tissue, or what.

J. R. VANE: I have a comment on Professor Barnett's suggestions. He has said that if some drugs are too potent then they may not show up as being more active in the clinic. In this case the dose could easily be reduced, thereby reducing the potency. This is what Dr Bacon is doing when he compares indomethacin with aspirin. I presume that he uses a much higher dose of aspirin than of indomethacin. He then already has a fairly large factor in the dosage which has to be considered.

Another point. I do not know about the methodology, but aspirin acetylates the PG synthetizing system, the cyclo-oxygenase. If a piece of tissue is taken out of the body and the PG synthetase activity is measured, it will not recover from an aspirin effect *in vivo* whereas if it is kept in a solution whilst it is being prepared, and so, it may well wash out the indomethacin. I do not whether that could have happened in the experiments.

P. A. BACON: It is a possible partial explanation. I would agree.

W. CARSON DICK: This debate is becoming polarized and lost, but there is no doubt on whether or not PG synthetase mechanisms are of importance. That is not the point. Our quarrel is with the phrase 'the mode of action'. Our feeling is that if we become too preoccupied with one system alone, without looking at all the others that are inter-related, then we shall never find what I consider to be the biological effects of these drugs.

Standardization of Radiological Criteria (Chapter 20)

W. WATSON BUCHANAN: By taking the whole of the wrist, Dr Larsen is making things difficult for himself. With all these carpal joints it is a very difficult area to assess. Why not localize, for instance simply to the styloid of the ulnar head, which is frequently involved, which one can easily see and count the number of erosions. Why not limit the number of joints looked at in hands? Why not take the second and third metacarpal joint which is frequently involved, and perhaps maybe only two or three of the metatarsal heads? The films then could be read more quickly, and perhaps, conceivably, the accuracy could be increased.

A. LARSEN: Professor Buchanan is right about the wrist. We do not really know how to get it into the scoring system since usually the whole wrist is involved in rheumatoid arthritis and not only the ulnar head. Still it may be a good idea to take just the ulnar head as a reference point for the whole wrist joint.

As regards the finger and toe joints, all of them should be included because they are very often affected in random order. Although it is true that the second and third metacarpals are frequently affected, they are not invariably the first to be affected.

W. WATSON BUCHANAN: To include juxta-articular-osteoporosis also seems to make it difficult. The observer error in that is tremendous.

A. LARSEN: Why more difficult? It is very reliable. We have studied the reliability of reading osteoporosis and have had 80 per cent agreement. The old papers say that it is not reliable, but if we follow the patient from the beginning and compare the left and right sides, we can always see the osteoporosis.

W. WATSON BUCHANAN: Are all the films read blind?

A. LARSEN: Yes.

E. V. BARNETT: In a patient who has other criteria of polyarthritis, latex positivity and high ESR, the metatarsal heads may be the most sensitive radiographic abnormality. However, from other data they may be the least specific in distinguishing rheumatoid arthritis patients from osteoarthritic patients because there are several traumatic and degenerative processes that mimic the destructive process in metatarsal heads. It may be inappropriate to use the metatarsal heads for case-finding or distinguishing patients – including patients by that criterion alone in a drug study.

A. LARSEN: It may be true that they have more unspecific changes but it is not a good feature of drug studies to exclude feet and we stand by our opinion that they should be included. It is a matter of opinion.

A. G. MOWAT: One can become very confused by putting together erosion and joint damage with osteoporosis. Looking at erosions and progressive joint damage, there is not much evidence that any of the anti-rheumatic drugs do much to slow that, let alone reverse it, whereas in osteoporosis I would suggest that much depends on the return of function in the joint, particularly in regard to the hand. It has been shown post-synovectomy, and we have recently shown by following patients on penicillamine, that a dramatic improvement in osteoporosis can be shown even where the erosions and joint damage continue to deteriorate. If the patient's pain from inflamed joints is reduced by drug therapy, the patient will use the hand more and the muscle action will improve the osteoporosis.

A. LARSEN: That is probably right. We have had considerable problems in selecting criteria. It may be true that only erosion is enough in follow-up studies – but we presented the method to get opinions before we use it.

Standardization of Immunological Laboratory Tests (Chapter 21)

D. C. DUMONDE: How variable is the difference between the chemotactic index in rheumatoid and non-rheumatoid individuals from one set of patients to another? I noticed, for example, that on the penicillamine slides there was very little difference between the normals and the rheumatoid patients, whereas on the other two there was quite a marked difference.

A. G. MOWAT: In general terms they are separate groups. With a large group of rheumatoid patients and a large group of controls there is very little overlap, but there is a small number of patients who fell within the same range.

D. C. DUMONDE: Can subsests be identified according to extent of chemotactic index reduction? i.e. seropositive versus seronegative, peripheral versus axial, vasculitic versus non-vasculitic, etc.

A. G. MOWAT: I have tried all the clinical parameters and have failed to correlate individual measurements with any group of chemotactic indices. I cannot separate off a sub-group in that way.

D. C. DUMONDE: Have only two chemotactic stimuli been used?

A. G. MOWAT: I have studied only the casein-induced complement-mediated chemotaxis. I have not used *E. coli* or anything else as a chemotactic stimulus.

D. C. DUMONDE: It is not clear what was done with the serum nor whether it was present in both the upper and the lower compartments.

A. G. MOWAT: In the lower alone. There was no serum in the top.

D. C. DUMONDE: Is this a standard AB serum?

A. G. MOWAT: Yes. From a single donor. Stored and then used continuously.

D. C. DUMONDE: Heat inactivated?

A. G. MOWAT: No.

D. C. DUMONDE: Frozen fresh at −70 °C?

A. G. MOWAT: Yes.

D. C. DUMONDE: What concentration?

A. G. MOWAT: A standard aliquot of frozen serum.

D. C. DUMONDE: A 100% serum in the lower compartment?

A. G. MOWAT: Yes.

D. C. DUMONDE: And when the casein is in there, is the serum in there as well?

A. G. MOWAT: Yes.

D. C. DUMONDE: What strength casein?

A. G. MOWAT: I am not certain, but it is 5 mg/ml.

D. C. DUMONDE: So there can be two stimuli with the casein, i.e. the serum and the casein, and one stimulus only, i.e. the serum. does this identify subsets?

A. G. MOWAT: No.

R. R. A. COOMBS: Is it possibly not an advantage to the rheumatoid patient to have a reduced chemotactic index?

A. G. MOWAT: It could be argued either way. I have an answer to why both these drugs work. It is bad news to go around gobbling up immune complexes, and it might be a good idea to have a reduced ability so to do. One could argue that gold, by suppressing it further, was actually to the patient's benefit, but I suppose it could equally well be argued that in the long term it would be a good idea to clear the body of those immune complexes, and therefore that is perhaps how levamisole works. It is perhaps how neither drug works.

R. R. A. COOMBS: What does Dr Mowat think is actually going on?

A. G. MOWAT: I do not know. This is an interesting observation at the moment but I do not really know how to take it any further. One can come out with pat answers as to why one drug should work and another drug not, but the three drugs, which as clinicians we tend to lump together, clearly are doing quite different things in this test system. Whether that really has any relevance, I do not know, but it is an observation that I want to extend to the macrophage which might have more relevance, particularly in a long-term chronic inflammatory situation, and see what happens.

P. A. BACON: I was surprised that no effect was found with the non-steroidal drugs. When Alan Brown in my own department looked at leukocyte motility and at electrophoretic mobility he found an effect of non-steroidal drugs and of penicillamine. Has random migration without a chemotactic stimulus been looked at, as well as directional chemotaxis?

A. G. MOWAT: I have looked at random migration and this particular chamber method is not very good at measuring random migration. It will do it, but the number of cells and its sensitivity is much less than it is with chemotaxis. My impression is that the non-steroidal drugs do not work. I know Brown's results and I am a little worried by some of those results in terms of the drug concentrations used, but I cannot really answer that question.

GENERAL DISCUSSION

W. WATSON BUCHANAN: A word of caution. It has been suggested that there are patients who respond and patients who do not respond. This is not proven. Response to a treatment is determined by a number of factors, including the height and the weight of the patient, the dose of the drug and the natural history of the disease. There is at present no evidence to indicate that there are subsets of patients who are responding and others who are not responding. There may well be, but it remains to be proven.

D. M. BURLEY: Perhaps we use the drugs that we do use the wrong way round. Practitioners seem to treat the mild cases with drugs like paracetamol or small doses of other non-steroidal anti-inflammatory agents, and the severe cases with prednisolone, gold and cyclophosphamide which then do not seem to do any good. Would it be more logical to apply the more active drugs, gold and prednisolone, in the early and mild cases. No one treates pneumonia with paracetamol, switching to penicillin when it gets a lot worse.

W. WATSON BUCHANAN: Nor does one use chloramphenicol to treat pneumonia! We are discussing drugs with a high degree of toxicity. Cyclophosphamide causes baldness and gives haemorrhagic cystitis. Gold knocks off patients with aplastic anaemia. The list is horrendous. Dr Burley is proposing to use a sledge-hammer to kill a fly crawling up a window.

D. M. BURLEY: Rheumatoid arthritis is quite a severe condition, and it often gets bad. We should be doing our best to knock it on the head right from the outset.

W. WATSON BUCHANAN: But that might break the window.

D. M. BURLEY: It might.

W. WATSON BUCHANAN: Rheumatoid arthritis is not necessarily a severe disease. The natural history of the disease in patients referred to hospitals has been well worked out. Perhaps 25 per cent seen after 10 years are doing quite well, taking the odd aspirin, keeping their jobs – sedentary occupation, light occupation. A further 25% will be taking their aspirin regularly, and they will be functioning reasonably well. Only half do badly, and the problem is that there is great difficulty in predicting into which group the patient will fit.

E. V. BARNETT: Which is the exact point of the session. The hypothesis is very viable that all the measurements enumerated, radiographic criteria, serological criteria, immune complexes, chemotaxis, may identify the subset of patients who have a rapidly progressing disease and would justify earlier intervention with the toxic drugs. It may further identify the responders as compared with the non-responders, although I would agree with Professor Buchanan that as yet we have not accomplished the documentation. This increase of data strongly suggests that we should be looking at these variables to indeed predict those patients would justify the strongest, most toxic and potentially most therapeutic programmes.

W. CARSON DICK: One answer to Dr Burley. All over the world individual physicians have energetically treated rheumatoid arthritis with toxic drugs in terms of giving patients early gold in one centre, cyclophosphamide in another. When one travels round one sees the results. They may be very enthusiastic in the early stages of the treatment, but there is not that much difference in the patient groups, and there is nobody who would claim that any of their treatments radically alters the course of the disease at the moment.

The answer to Dr Burley is that it has been done.

M. K. JASANI: I would like, however, to point out that what still requires to be done in rheumatoid arthritis is to establish whether a short course of cyclophosphamide and high doses of prednisolone together could alter the natural history of the joint disease as has been shown by Professor Soothill to be the case in the nephrotic syndrome of childhood (see *Lancet*, **ii**, 479; 1970; *Lancet*, **i**, 55; 1975).

We need to know the point in time when we should intervene in rheumatoid arthritis. I can see no difficulty in the basic concept that something of the sort should apply to RA as much as to renal disease that is mediated by immunological mechanisms.

W. WATSON BUCHANAN: My argument would be this. In renal disease the end-result is death. It is an entirely different situation from a disease that is essentially benign.

M. K. JASANI: It is no longer death with transplants and renal dialysis available.

W. WATSON BUCHANAN: But the natural history of renal disease —

M. K. JASANI: And the natural history of rheumatoid arthritis is to be seized up.

W. WATSON BUCHANAN: Living death!

M. K. JASANI: Exactly.

C. SCHNEIDER: A question to Dr Bacon. Is there yet any evidence that thermography is of use in the early diagnosis of rheumatoid arthritis?

P. A. BACON: It is not of much use as a diagnostic criterion. One can show evidence of inflammation before there are fixed changes on the x-ray, for instance, but these can also be detected clinically. Non-involved joints can be picked up, but these can also be detected clinically. I would not have thought that it had very much use as a diagnostic tool.

Professor Buchanan has said that the end-result of rheumatoid arthritis is not death, yet long term follow-up for 15 years, as has been done in Bath shows quite a significant excess mortality in the rheumatoid group, a lot of which can be related to the rheumatoid disease itself. If we had good evidence that treating with gold or with penicillamine at the beginning really produced long-term suppression of the disease, we should be doing exactly what Dr Burley suggests. We do not have that evidence.

W. WATSON BUCHANAN: I accept that rheumatoid patients do not live as long as normal subjects, but I should also point out that our observations indicate that there is a very high iatrogenic death rate which has not been looked at by other people, and it is the drugs which are proposed for the early cases that are the very drugs that cause the exitus.

J. G. HAWKES: I have to support gold on a maintenance dosage basis, that is for a prolonged period, when carefully monitored, patients can do very well.

There is another point. Rather than prescribing penicillamine, another useful drug that I have not heard mentioned as yet, but that would seem to arrest rather than to suppress the disease, would be Plaquenil (hydroxychloroquine). I use it and other drugs belonging to the group quite frequently. I know that there is a risk of eye effects, but the reports are few and far between, and provided the patient is closely monitored, with ophthalmological checks every three months, they do very well. I have many patients for whom I have prescribed that drug early on, and who would otherwise – by the criteria I use – have gone on to develop very severe rheumatoid arthritis.

I know that this is a clinical impression, but I should like comments about the role the drug fulfills, when it should be prescribed, and what its action is.

W. WATSON BUCHANAN: Chloroquine has innumerable effects. It is a very interesting drug. As to side effects, it is again a question of the denominator. One would need to treat between 1000 and 2000 patients for a whole year before picking up one's first case of irreversible blindness.

Secondly, gold. Aplastic anaemia, agranulocytosis and thrombocytopaenia come on like lightening. There is no way in which that side effect can be predicted, and again a lot of patients will have to be treated before the first fatality ensues.

M. K. JASANI: Going back to the point about severe toxic reactions encountered in people receiving these rather toxic drugs, is it not true that the people that Professor Buchanan has encountered have been treated randomly before they came to his attention, and in view of that would there not be a difference if there was a pre-planned programme of introducing certain restricted regimens of toxic treatment with very good rationales?

I am again drawing the analogy with respect to glomerular nephritis and some of the other conditions, where there is no necessity to prolong the treatment once there is clinical improvement, and there are long-term remissions.

Perhaps the failure to take a decision on this point will delay the better care of rheumatoid patients.

W. WATSON BUCHANAN: It is possible, but I very much doubt whether the physician has very much effect on the incidence of side effects. It is the drug that causes the side effects, and whether it is prescribed by the general practitioner or by the hospital consultant is unlikely to make a significant difference. But I may be wrong.

W. CARSON DICK: I hate to point out that the session is not addressed to the treatment of rheumatoid arthritis, and if we get lost in that discussion we shall get nowhere.

M. F. CUTHBERT: Before we move off that topic might I ask one question for clarification, and also to show that the drug regulatory authority in the UK is interested in efficacy as well as in the toxicity of drugs.

Mention has been made of the possibility that chloroquine may alter the course of rheumatoid arthritis. A similar claim has also been made for alclofenac. Professor Buchanan has not replied to the question of whether chloroquine does alter the course of the disease. Would he, or anybody else, comment on that statement in relation to the two particular compounds to which I referred, and for which the claim has been made.

W. WATSON BUCHANAN: These drugs have an effect but they do not alter the course of the disease to any clinically significant degree.

E. V. BARNETT: It is a controversial subject. In several studies, Plaquenil (hydroxychloroquine) as compared with gold responses induced remissions and was correlated with decreased erosions on x-ray. The toxicity of hydroxychloroquine may be minimal. In a recent study in the United States, 100 patients on no more than two tablets per day of hydroxychloroquine for up to ten years did not show one single case of irreversible ophthalmological damage. That data, coupled with the patients being monitored prior to initiation of therapy and every six months, makes Plaquenil a viable candidate in the armamentarium.

Dr Dick has pointed out that we are not necessarily discussing the therapy of rheumatoid arthritis, but the entire purpose of the symposium is to evaluate current therapy and mechanisms for improving that therapy.

I would again give my biased viewpoint, to compare with Professor Buchanan's, that I am very optimistic about the use of currently available drugs. In my practice, and in our group practice at UCLA, in patients who come in with polyarthritis, most respond and have minimal progression of erosion for long periods of time on acidic non-steroidal anti-inflammatory drugs. When there is evidence of seropositivity and peripheral erosions, the two most important criteria for classical or definite RA, an inexorably progressive and crippling outcome can be confidently predicted in a majority of the patients if left untreated. For such patients the administration of hydroxychloroquine or gold therapy – which are not investigational drugs in the US is fully justified. The non-responders to that group, those who either do not respond or cannot continue drugs because of toxicity, amount to a very small fraction of the initial numbers, and they are candidates for investigative protocols, and we have all of them going at one time and another, and concurrently. That includes azothioprine, cyclophosphamide, penicillamine, etc. I happen to be highly biased to the use of azothioprine and very biased against the use of corticosteroids, and with the bias I have very few patients who have come to me, to us, in stage 1 or 2 who have progressed over 15 years to stage 4.

I would say that with the appropriate selection of patients, even with the current armamentarium, it is possible to greatly alter what appears to be the natural crippling course of rheumatoid arthritis.

G. P. LEWIS: It is clear now where non-steroidal anti-inflammatory drugs and the new loose group of delayed action drugs fit into therapy. What about steroid therapy? Is that now altogether out of fashion, and if not, where does it fit in?

W. CARSON DICK: I did not wish to get into a discussion on therapy because every member of the symposium has his own bias. Any one of us can produce evidence over fifteen years to show that most of the patients do well, whether it be azothioprine or what. The first and major variable is the patient. The second is not the drug, but it is the clinician. The wee bit at the top may be the drug. But it has not been clearly shown in any acceptable scientific sense.

To answer the next point. We have thrown corticosteroids out – I must put this carefully – in an emotional sense. We have flung away from them because we are all desperately trying to teach against the misuse and abuse of corticosteroids. Dr Jasani may be correct that we should re-evaluate the therapeutic ratio of corticosteroids (*Clin. Rheum. Dis.*, **1**, (2): 359; 1975), but we are frightened that the minute we say that in public, everybody will prescribe them for seronegative early disease, and we shall end up with iatrogenesis. There lies the difficulty.

W. WATSON BUCHANAN: Perhaps we might go back to the evaluation, the methods of evaluating. For the assessment of heat in a joint by thermography. Dr Bacon, what is the cost of the instrument to measure it and what are the requirements? Does it require a room at stable temperature? How difficult is it to do? Could he also slot thermography into the league table that Dr Dick showed. Where would it fit into that league table?

P. A. BACON: With regard to the first part of the question, unless the technique is carefully standardized, the results are meaningless, and therefore there has to be a standard room temperature, a special room, and probably one technician who will devote his time to it. So there is some expense there, and the machinery is expensive, with cameras costing around £20 000. I suspect that like most things, as the apparatus is used more its cost would become cheaper.

In regard to the second part of the question, I can only guess where thermography might fit into the league table since we have not done the sort of multivariate analysis that others have done. It is a guess, but I should imagine that it would come in the same sort of place as radioactive technitium (^{99m}Tc).

W. CARSON DICK: Dr Bacon knows better than that. It is not really a guess, and we are not comparing one against the other. It is not Celtic versus Rangers. Each is measuring a different aspect of the inflammatory and disease process, and instead of arguing one against the other we should be using them together to see what is happening.

There is already a paper, an early one, on that. I would suggest that that is what we should all be doing, and not comparing or contrasting one against the other.

P. A. BACON: I would absolutely agree. The problem is that unless we actually compare our methods with each other, someone else will be doing a different methodology for technitium and a different methodology for thermography. We want a transfer: Celtic and Rangers combined.

M. K. JASANI: Corticosteroids have been mentioned, and for the sake of the record I should like to clarify the situation.

Although I remain firmly committed to their use investigatively in experimental systems, I do not advocate any of the currently available steroidal drugs for *long-term* rheumatoid therapy.

T. J. WILLIAMS: Coming back to the cost of thermography, has anybody tried a simple ultraviolet probe coupled directly to a printout? Much of the cost of the machine is to get a very nice picture, and then the cost is doubled for the computer to get a number again. Has it been tried with a fixed area probe, which I imagine would be about one-twentieth of the cost.

P. A. BACON: I agree. The problem is that the small area of the probe does not necessarily correlate with the integration of the whole area from something the size of a knee joint. It works very well for small finger joints or for animal arthritic studies, and we have used it, but there is no reason why it should not be extended and why one should not go straight for the integration. I quite agree that the pretty pictures are totally irrelevant.

P. H. EVANS: Professor Buchanan made a comment in relation to Dr Barnett's paper on the difficulty of making correlations between various parameters at a fixed point in time. If the time phase was shifted, he moved from telepathy to precognition, what sort of correlation can be achieved by such phase shifts?

Secondly, can some factor be included in the correlation which includes the length of time by which a particular parameter has been measured?

W. WATSON BUCHANAN: We have tried to do it. The problem is that the disease is so variable that one would need so many assessments. One would require to measure the area under the undulating curve. It is the total amount of whatever factor is being measured under the curve that will correlate with whatever it is that one wants to correlate with. That is the difficulty. We cannot get slopes. We have tried it all. It is not possible to do it in a disease like rheumatoid arthritis.

This morning has been interesting because it shows that the clinician is at one end of the spectrum and the scientific worker is at the other end. They are looking at the same problem with somewhat different viewpoints. It is slightly irritating to the clinician to see doses of drugs which he would have to prescribe in tons to a patient being used in an experimental animal far distant from man. At the same time it is irritating to the scientific worker to see the clinician having to use clinical methodology which he would really not deign to use.

But hopefully meetings such as this will bring the two together, and perhaps, who knows, we may even meet in the middle.

Section: VII
Progress and Pitfalls in the Clinical Evaluation of Anti-Rheumatic Drugs

Chairman: J. Seldrup

22
A Statistician's View of Clinical Trials of Anti-Rheumatic Drugs

J. SELDRUP

"... It is impossible to calculate accurately events that are determined by chance"
Thucydides (ca. 400 BC)

INTRODUCTION

It happened not so long ago when the χ^2 tests played the t tests in the final of the FS Cup. (Incidentally, in case you have forgotten, or you do not know, the FS Cup is the False Statistics Cup played annually by teams from all over the land.) The t tests had had a fairly normal run, beating the Wilcoxon tests, who were very highly ranked in the semi-final; but then they are quite powerful tests and they had been very efficient on the night. The χ^2 tests had struggled in their semi-final to beat the Exact Probability tests, mainly by not allowing them the same degrees of freedom, in fact they did not allow them any degree of freedom at all. Everybody was waiting for the big match to start. Weeks and weeks had been spent on preparations and now they wanted it finished as quickly as possible, so that the reports could be written and published.

Both teams were dressed in the same coating. It was a double-blind match. The null hypothesis was stated and they were away. It had always been obvious that it was not going to be a fair trial of strength, with two teams being so markedly different in their distributional approach. Had there not been a preponderance of dichotomous data throughout Phase I of the trial, the χ^2 tests may not have been ahead. After Phase II, however, chance changed the picture and following the next cross-over p was equal to 20% in favour of the t tests.

As the teams go out at the confidence interval, without having arrived at a statistically significant result, we will take a break and examine seriously certain aspects of a clinical trial as seen by a statistician. Although the title includes the words 'clinical trial of anti-rheumatic drugs', much of the comment is of a general nature, applicable to clinical trials en masse. The views expressed may well be coloured by my background in the pharmaceutical industry, but I should stress that they are not necessarily those of my employer.

A REVIEW OF ANTI-RHEUMATIC DRUG TRIALS

Recently a paper was published in the *British Medical Journal*[1] highlighting statistical deficiencies in publications of medical work. Does this also apply to work published by rheumatologists? To shed some light on this question, a review was done of the 1976 issues of an international journal, which shall be nameless. Six papers reported on clinical trials of anti-rheumatic drugs. One paper was from Romania, one paper was from the USA and one paper was from Canada. Of the remaining three papers, two were from the UK and one had authors from the USA and Columbia. One of the authors of the Canadian paper was a statistician, and statistically, perhaps, this was the most acceptable of the papers. The USA paper acknowledged the statistical expertise, but the other four papers had no reference to or acknowledgement of statistical advice.

The most startling shortcoming in the papers reviewed was the omission of any explanation of the statistical techniques used. Twenty-two times in the text a p value was given. In at least two papers the phrases 'statistically significant' and 'statistically comparable' were used without explanation. In four papers the tables included p-values, but no reference to the kind of test used, although one column was headed ominously 'F' — but neither Fisher's exact probability test nor (Fisher's) variance ratio test seemed applicable.

The paper with the statistical co-author is the only one which explains the statistics. The null-hypothesis that there is a 50–50 chance of clinical trial reports explaining their statistics is rejected. Using a binomial test $p = 0.109$ and it is concluded that a much smaller percentage of such trials are up to standard. Although I sometimes suspect that the only two tests known to the medical world are the χ^2 test and the t test; surely we are not just to choose at random which of the two tests holds the key to the magic p-value.

To round off this critical look at publications of anti-rheumatic drug trials, one trial did not report the type, i.e. randomness of allocation of treatment. Indeed the same report did not mention anything about blindness of the study. Two trials were in osteoarthritis: one was a one-by-one week cross-over study of two drugs in 55 patients, the other was a six week between patient study of 195 patients. Of the four trials in rheumatoid arthritis, three were cross-overs: a two-by-two week cross-over in 23 patients, a three-by-three week cross-over in 36 patients and a six-by-six week cross-over in 40 patients. The last study was a between patient study of 32 patients for two years. Two of the trials were positive in the sense that two drugs were shown to be different on several parameters, differences which were statistically significant, usually at the 5% level. The other four trials were negative.

It is always a very worthwhile exercise afterwards to examine why a trial proved positive or negative. No attempt is being made to exhaust the numerous possibilities. However, a few comments seem pertinent. First of all it should always be remembered that '. . . it is impossible to calculate accurately events that are determined by chance'. Events in clinical trials are not solely, hopefully, determined by chance, but chance plays a part in any piece of research: there is always the possibility of being wrong, even if the outcome is statistically significant with $p < 0.05$. Secondly, the concepts of clinical and statistical significance should be considered. Clinical significance is often used to describe the clinical importance of a trial result which may or may not have the magic '$p < 0.05$' attached to it, whilst statistical significance is often synonymous with $p < 0.05$, bringing the statistician or statistics into disrepute if the result is not meaningful clinically. I do not particularly subscribe to the distinction although I admit that the two concepts may be useful. I submit that if clinical and statistical significance are not one and the same thing, the wrong null hypothesis has been tested. If statistics was only done by qualified statisticians, as medicine seems to be only for medics, maybe other than 5% p-values would now be acceptable. If I read an elementary text book on surgery, I wonder how many of you would let me replace your right hip. However, I accept that we, as statisticians, often seem more than willing to teach research workers how to do χ^2 tests and Student t tests, when what we should do is to teach the concepts of statistics, so that we have a common ground and can communicate to the mutual benefit of both professions. Today research teams are multi-disciplinary and I for my part spend a fair amount of time in trying to understand the clinical implications of any piece of work I get involved with, before it gets off the ground. Who knows, one day we may be able to abandon the 'NS' (not significant) and give the actual p-values in our reports and let other people get a chance to judge the significance of our results. In this respect, it was very refreshing to read recently in the editorial of the *British Journal of Clinical Pharmacology*[2] an appreciation of the statistical assistance provided for the medical department of a pharmaceutical company.

To come back to our anti-rheumatic drug trials, I would like to suggest that anybody who considers doing a cross-over trial, should stop and think again. This trial design, where each patient acts as his own control through being administered more than one of the trial drugs, is often heralded as the ideal design. This may well be so, but unfortunately that does not necessarily make it a practical proposition. I am getting more and more convinced that this design should be used less and less in clinical trials, including trials of anti-rheumatic drugs for the simple reason that neither patient nor disease is ever again, after the first drug is administered, in a situation comparable to the start of the trial.

Trials should always be of a sensible length on a sensible number of patients. I am confident that if this principle had always been followed, the medical literature would have been the better for it. The easiest thing in the world is to 'show' that two drugs are comparable by treating too few patients for too short a period. And we should not be allowed to get away with it, Dr Editors. On the other hand, we should not be pushed, i.e. not be given any alternative, into doing exactly that kind of trial, Mr Authorities. I have just had the opportunity of forming a group of statisticians in the pharmaceutical industry, and one of our aims is to promote professional standards in statistics in matters pertinent to the pharmaceutical industry.

I believe we have more to give than just doing your *t* tests and looking up the statistical tables. I am concerned as a statistician about the trials we do: the number of trials and the reasons for doing them. It seems to me that the bodies which govern what can and cannot be done in terms of clinical research should take a fresh look at themselves and their regulations. I am not offering any solutions, but maybe we should be encouraged to spend much more time and effort in studying what happens to man when he is fed a chemical substance, and have less faith in the necessity to provide almost standard evidence in species inferior to him.

I have spent a long time being critical, but then I often see my role as the devil's advocate. To try to win you over to my side, however, I will change the tactic and spend the rest of the time on discussing some recent research in the methodology and analysis of clinical trials.

RECENT RESEARCH IN CLINICAL TRIAL METHODOLOGY

About four years ago, I was involved with designing a clinical trial of superficial thrombophlebitis[3] in which a marketed compound was compared with a placebo. No stratification factors were used, i.e. it was not thought necessary to attempt to achieve treatment balance for any prognostic factors. After the trial, which lasted about a year, and in which some 54 patients were treated, we regretted this decision. When we compared the two treatment groups, we discovered that on almost all parameters the active group was more severe than the placebo making a meaningful comparison of effect of the treatment impossible. We are currently repeating that trial. An examination of the first trial suggested that all severity measures were highly correlated and the problem of imbalanced treatment groups would be avoided by stratifying for 'length of indurated vein'. The second trial uses a 'balanced block' allocation scheme, whereby for each of four patients in each stratum, two patients will be allocated treatment A and two treatment B, but in a random order. A simulation study by Pocock and Simon[4] suggested that this procedure is highly effective in achieving treatment balance. However, the study also suggested that as the number of prognostic factors, for which treatment balance is desirable, increase, so this procedure tends to be no better than purely random assignment.

A possible alternative procedure has been suggested by Taves (1974)[5] who called it minimization. This procedure was given a more formal theoretical description in the afore-mentioned paper by Pocock and Simon[4]. The object of this treatment assignment procedure is to minimize over any number of levels of prognostic factors the imbalance of treatments.

It is best described by considering a practical example. Suppose we want to compare drugs A and B in the treatment of rheumatic conditions. Five centres are to participate. They will admit only rheumatoid and osteoarthritic patients and let us consider that initial severity may be an important factor in determining the outcome of the trial. We will therefore consider mild, moderate and severe cases appropriately defined. In other words, we have described a trial with three stratification factors:

(1) Centre (at 5 levels)
(2) Type of disease (at 2 levels) and
(3) Severity (at 3 levels)

Let us assume that we have already allocated treatment to 30 patients, 15 are on treatment A and 15 on treatment B. Table 22.1 gives the details of the calculations necessary to decide the treatment for the next patient, patient 31.

Table 22.1 Example of treatment allocation following the minimization procedure

	Centre					*Disease*		*Severity*			*Sum*
	1	2	3	4	5	R	O	*Mild*	*Mod*	*Sev*	
A	2	3	1	6	3	10	5	2	8	5	
B	3	1	3	4	4	9	6	3	6	6	
Patient 31	0	0	1	0	0	1	0	0	0	1	
A + 31			2			11				6	
B			3			9				6	
|A + 31 – B|			1			2				0	3
B + 31			4			10				7	
A			1			10				5	
|B + 31 – A|			3			0				2	5

Allocate treatment A to patient 31

A number of variations on this scheme are possible, one obvious one is to give weights to the levels of the various factors. It may, for example, be considered most desirable to achieve balance of treatments between centres in which case centres would be given higher weights than type of disease and severity. One draw-back may be the amount of administration which would have to be done centrally, although this would be counter-balanced by the number of randomization lists which would be required for the 'balanced block' allocation scheme. In the example above, suppose we wanted 10 patients from each centre. Then to cater for the possibility that all patients fall into any of the six possible groups created by 2 levels of disease and 3 levels of severity, we would have to provide for each centre 6 randomization lists, each with 10 patients or 30 lists all together. This could mean packing and labelling trial materials for 300 patients. Simulation studies performed by Pocock and Simon[4] suggest that even with several factors, this new method would achieve more balanced trials than traditional methods.

From a method of treatment allocation, I want to turn to a method of analysis which has not been given much attention in the literature in the hope that some academic statisticians may dig it out and study it in more detail, because unfortunately not much is known about its theoretical properties. However it seems to be eminently suited to a lot of data, not least of which are collected in trials of anti-rheumatic compounds. The type of data to consider is categorical data that is to say, for example, pain rated 0 = absent, 1 = mild, 2 = moderate, 3 = severe, or tenderness rated likewise. To demonstrate the technique, consider again the situation with two drugs A and B to compare. Suppose 30 patients on each drug have been assessed on the 0–3 pain scale before and after treatment. For each of the treatments we can now devise a so-called transition probability matrix, as illustrated in Table 22.2.

Table 22.2 Transition probability matrices for the comparison between treatment A and treatment B

Before treatment A	*After treatment A*				*Before treatment B*	*After treatment B*			
	0	1	2	3		0	1	2	3
0	0	1	0	0	0	0	0	0	0
1	3	9	0	0	1	5	4	1	0
2	1	2	10	2	2	8	5	4	0
3	0	0	0	2	3	3	0	0	0

Test statistic LR = 23.243; $p = 0.026$

The number in each cell, numbered i for row and j for column, represents the number of patients who before treatment had a pain score of i and after treatment the pain score had changed to j. It is obvious that the difference between A and B lies in the transition of pain scores corresponding to the two treatments. I shall not go into any more detail about the statistical test, but refer any interested parties to a paper in the Royal Statistical Society, series C by Hilton[6].

Finally, I want to return to the trial discussed above of two drugs in superficial thrombophlebitis in which we were unable to reach any firm conclusion of the relative effectiveness of the two treatments, because the two treatment groups of patients had different characteristics, in so far as one group was more severe than the other. Sometimes this problem is dealt with in the literature by covariance analysis (see, for example, Fisher[7]), i.e. by adjusting the effects of treatment according to the difference in initial severity. However, I remain firmly convinced that this use of covariance analysis has no place in the clinical trial, but is only a mathematical manipulation of the data which cannot meaningfully be interpreted. As an illustration I did a covariance analysis of the pain scores rated on a 0–100 scale, adjusting the change in pain by the initial pain level. The result is shown in Table 22.3.

Table 22.3 Analysis of covariance

Treatment	*Initial mean pain*	*Mean response*	*Adjusted mean response*
T	54.6	43.8	38.1
P	41.7	26.5	31.9
t test or variance ratio test (F) for difference between T and P:		$t(43) = 2.331$ $p = 0.025$	$F(1,42) = 1.376$ $p = 0.247$

It will be seen that the hypothesis of equality of the adjusted cell means could not be rejected ($p = 0.247$). However, I maintain this is a purely artificial result and has nothing to do with what would have happened if the severity of pain had been similar before the start of the trial.

CONCLUSION

Rather than giving you a more or less traditional account of statistical methodology in clinical trials, the concepts of which many of you may be more or less familiar with, I have tried to point out some of the more common deficiencies in the reporting of statistics in trials of anti-rheumatic drugs. I have dealt with a relatively new concept in the allocation of treatments to patients and drawn your attention to an alternative method of analysing categorical data, often dealt with by the χ^2 technique. I have warned you against accepting the conclusions of a covariance analysis, where response have been adjusted according to initial state.

Before I go, I suppose I had better give you the result of the FS Cup Final. You may recall that the t tests were leading the χ^2 tests at the end of Phase III. When the final whistle was blown at the end of Phase IV, the match was declared a draw, despite the type 1 error declared after Phase II. When the trial was restarted a week later (to avoid any carry-over effects), it was decided to have no cross-overs and no adjustments could be made for injuries. The match again ended in a draw and after five successive draws the match was finally decided by the toss of a coin, the finest demonstration of the simplest and most basic concept in statistics: chance.

SUMMARY

This paper contains a critical view of six international publications of trials of anti-rheumatic drugs seen through the eyes of a statistician. Further, it presents some recent research concerning the allocation of treatment to patients, pointing out that this new 'minimization' procedure will often be superior to more traditional methods of treatment allocation in achieving balanced treatment groups, i.e. balanced in respect of chosen prognostic factors. A method of analysis of categorical data is promoted, which is eminently suited to the before/after treatment analysis of symptoms rated on, say, 0–3 scales. Finally, the use of analysis of covariance in the analysis of clinical trials is discussed.

References

1. Gore, S. M., Jones, I. G. and Rytter, E. C. (1977). Misuse of statistical methods: critical assessment of articles in BMJ from January to March 1976. *Br. Med. J.*, **1**, 85
2. Kendall, M. J. (1977). A year in Industry. *Br. J. Clin. Pharmacol.*, **4**, 3
3. Archer, D. S. and Fowler, P. D. (1977). Comparison of oxyphenbutazone and placebo in the treatment of superficial thrombophlebitis: An object lesson in clinical trial design. *The Practitioner*
4. Pocock, S. J. and Simon, R. (1975). Sequential treatment assignment with balancing for prognostic factors in the controlled clinical trial. *Biometrics*, **31**, 103
5. Taves, D. R. (1974). Minimisation: A new method of assigning patients to treatment and control groups. *Clin. Pharmacol. Ther.*, **15**, 443
6. Hilton, G. (1971). An algorithm for detecting differences between transition probability matrices. *Appl. Stat.*, **20**, 80
7. Fisher, R. A. (1970). *Statistical Methods for Research Workers*. 14th Ed. 272p (Edinburgh: Oliver and Boyd)

23
Prescribing of Anti-Rheumatic Drugs in General Practice

A. W. PATTERSON

INTRODUCTION

The aims of this symposium state that 'now is the time to assess both the usefulness of laboratory methods and standardization in disease assessment' and that the symposium 'should facilitate the recognition of more effective anti-rheumatic drugs'. New medical knowledge must be disseminated throughout the medical profession and particularly to general medical practice, the situation of which by its nature, is peripheral to the mainstream of medical research. With the development of continuing education in medicine and increasing interest in what has become known as medical audit, it is important that facilities be improved, not only for the successful dissemination of new knowledge but also for the assessment of its application and effectiveness. In short, operational research is required to supplement fundamental research.

It has been said that 'medical audit will be practicable only when we know what we do and what we should be doing'[1]. More recently certain rheumatologists have expressed the view that 'although a great deal of effort and thought has been expended in devising monitoring systems for recording toxicity of drugs, trials of their therapeutic efficacy, reducing prescribing errors, and utilizing the choice of drug therapy to assess quality of patient care there remains a relative paucity of information on how drugs are being used by physicians in practice'[2]. In pursuit of information on how drugs for rheumatoid arthritis were being prescribed the same workers collected information on general practice prescribing and expressed dissatisfaction therewith[3]. A correspondent of the Lancet has also fulminated on the uncertain rationale for anti-inflammatory drug therapy[4] in osteoarthritis and in February of this year, with regard to general practice prescribing, a Lancet review stated that 'Doctors need education and guidance in the prescribing of drugs and medicines'[5]. The problem of what to do about it remains substantially unresolved at present. This paper presents information on what some 650 prescribers in general practice did in the application of drug therapy for rheumatoid conditions and offers suggestions for monitoring whether prescribing habits change over time, in which direction they change, and how they could be influenced.

SOURCES OF INFORMATION

The best source of information on which drug therapy general practitioners prescribe, and for what reason, would be their own records. Even if such records were well kept, however, it would be an undertaking of considerable magnitude. Something less satisfactory has often to be accepted if any progress is to be made.

Much information, albeit of a general nature, can be derived from the prescriptions written by general medical practitioners within the National Health Service (NHS) in Britain. The collection and processing of these data has been, until very recently, almost entirely cost-orientated and of little use in the clinical setting. There has been no adequate feedback to prescribers and the data tend to be too retrospective. New approaches are, however, being investigated at present by the Department of Health and Social Security (DHSS).

Data resources, even though imperfect, may yet yield much valuable information and on this premise a large scale longitudinal study of a cohort of prescribers has been sponsored by the DHSS. It is referred to as the Sociology of Prescribing Project[6]. There are two main components to the study. First, at the Medical Sociology Research Centre, University College of Swansea in Wales, sociologists, in collaboration with a medical researcher, try to assess the influence on prescribing of medical education, information resources used, practice characteristics etc. This work is based on contact with prescribers by questionnaire and, in some cases, interviews and is supported by analysis of prescription data supplied for the purpose by the Unit for Research into Drug Usage, Department of Pharmacy, Heriot-Watt University.

Secondly, the Heriot-Watt Research Unit also analyses the prescriptions written by members of the GP cohort but from a more medico-pharmaceutical point of view. One objective is to observe prescribing patterns and changes in such patterns in drug usage over time. It is the latter work that has provided the data on which the present paper on anti-rheumatic drug usage is based. Any other therapeutic category, or categories taken in conjunction, can be similarly scrutinized.

DESIGN OF THE STUDY

The design of the part of the cohort study relevant to this paper is as follows. The Department of Health and Social Security process the prescribing data for one month per annum, excluding August, for each general medical practitioner

(GP) in the National Health Service (the PD2 analysis) and thereafter the prescriptions may be released to an approved research group. In this way the prescription bundles of some 650 GPs for one month per annum have been made available for study over several recent years through the good offices of the Prescription Pricing Authority. The prescriptions are read, interpreted and the data encoded for computer input by trained coders under the supervision of research pharmacists with substantial computer expertise. After undergoing various validation procedures the data are matched with 'fixed information' such as therapeutic class etc. and archived to magnetic tape. The data may then be retrieved by appropriate programmes for a variety of purposes.

Some of the work currently in progress is designed to observe changes in prescibing patterns over time through the comparison of 'prescribing years' one with another and to account for such changes. This approach can be applied to any selected therapeutic group or groups of drugs as a series of sub-studies. This paper refers to the first two stages of a sub-study on drugs presumed to have been prescribed for the treatment of rheumatic and related disorders. Inevitably work of this nature is retropsective but at least it has the merit of giving a base-line of prescribing information uninfluenced by artificial changes due to awareness of the sub-study.

Composition of the Cohort

The cohort of 650 general practitioners whose prescribing data has contributed to this study derives from an originally larger cohort of 859 doctors who entered general practice in England and Wales as principals between 2 July 1969 and 1 July 1970. Further details of this cohort are available in Supplement No. 1, Vol. 26, December 1976 entitled 'Prescribing in General Practice', published by the Journal of the Royal College of General Practitioners[6].

VOLUME OF DATA AND ITS ANALYSIS

Preparations of drugs specified for rheumatic diseases and gout constitute some 3% of all items prescribed in the National Health Service in Britain. In order, therefore, to derive facts and figures of sufficient magnitude to be meaningful a very large volume of NHS prescriptions requires to be scanned.

The data deriving from the PD2 analysis (p. 326) consists of one month's prescriptions per doctor per PD2 year (Sept. to July, August omitted). This 'prescribing year' was the basis for the longitudinal study from which the data for this paper were derived. The main 'prescribing year' involved was 1973–74, but data from the first three months of the following year (1974–75) has also been scrutinized to assess trends. Included are also the preliminary data of a smaller scale study of the prescribing habits in Scotland during the first three months of 1975.

The data for 1973–74 consisted of 656 534 prescribed items, of which 22 396 were for items specified in the DHSS therapeutic classification[7] (old category 65) for rheumatic diseases and gout. The data for the first three months of 1974–75 consisted of 206 196 prescribed items, of which 7162 items were for preparations specified for rheumatic diseases and gout.

On further analysis of the 1973–74 data, to assess concomitant prescribing, it was found that the 22 396 items generated 21 300 pairs of drugs, that is, the drugs specified or recommended for rheumatic diseases appeared on a prescription form with one or more other items. For example, three drugs on one prescription form generate three pairs and so on. These other items belonged to many other therapeutic categories but concomitant prescribing of additional anti-rheumatic drugs and of analgesics, glucocorticoids and antacids have particular significance in the drug-therapy of rheumatic and related disorders.

In the absence of information on the therapeutic intent when prescribing drugs, evidence of use must be presumptive. To overcome this difficulty, drugs were usually allocated to a therapeutic classification based on their customary or most frequent therapeutic application. Drugs with a specific or narrow usage spectrum are relatively easy to classify but drugs capable of more than one application presented considerable difficulty.

THE MORBIDITY SPECTRUM IN ASSOCIATION WITH RHEUMATIC DISEASES AND GOUT

It has been stated that 'rheumatic diseases are second only to respiratory infections as a cause of medical consultation in this country'[8]. Additionally though, patients with rheumatic or arthritic conditions present a variety of medical problems as is only too clearly implied by results of PD2 analysis summarized in Table 23.1.

Table 23.1 shows the rank order of drugs in other therapeutic categories prescribed together with preparations specified for rheumatic disease and gout. The data reveal that apart from the expectedly high frequency for the prescription of anti-pyretic and analgesic drugs, patients with rheumatic disease and gout were frequently prescribed diuretics, hypnotics, anti-hypertensives, preparations acting on the heart and anti-depressives, in that order. It is possible that whereas the preponderance of prescriptions for preparations active on the cardiovascular system reflect the age and sex spectrum of the patient sample (see Table 23.2), that of the prescriptions for anti-depressives may reflect the prevalence of depression in chronically disabled patients with rheumatoid arthritis[9]. Further speculations on the possible significance of the prescription of drugs from many other therapeutic categories in the sample of patients studied is left to the particular interests of the reader.

AGE/SEX DISTRIBUTION OF PATIENTS

Table 23.2 illustrates another problem of prescription analysis. The way in

Table 23.1 Drugs of other therapeutic categories prescribed concomitantly with anti-rheumatics of therapeutic group 65 (DHSS old therapeutic classification)

Rank order	*Number of items*	*Percent n = 22 396*	*Therapeutic classification*
1	2690	12.01	anti-pyretic analgesics
2	1873	8.36	diuretics
3	1795	8.01	tranquillizers
4	1026	4.58	barbiturates (unadmixed or if principal ingredient)
5	935	4.17	hypnotics (non-barbiturate)
6	848	3.78	local anaesthetics and counter-irritants
7	822	3.67	anti-hypertensives
8	774	3.45	preparations acting on the heart
9	599	2.67	corticosteroid preparations acting on the skin
10	590	2.63	anti-depressants
11	581	2.59	expectorants and cough suppressants
12	565	2.52	preparations specified for rheumatic diseases and gout
13	560	2.50	iron and other erythropoietic preparations
14	539	2.40	vasodilators
15	514	2.29	antacids

Items in other therapeutic groups were of lower frequency

Table 23.2 Age/sex distribution of patients receiving anti-rheumatic drugs of therapeutic class 65 (DHSS old classification)

Age (yrs)	*Male*	*Female*	*Sex?*	*Age/sex?*	*Age totals*	*Percent n = 22 396*
0–16	55	72	20		147	0.66
16–64	5236					
16–59		7059				
16–64			1075		13370	59.70
65+	2022					
60+		5039				
60/65+			487		7528	33.61
Age/sex				1351		6.03
Sex totals	7293	12170	1582	1351	22396	
Percent	32.56	54.34	7.06	6.03		100.00

which a prescription is written may leave data coders with inadequate information and this could give rise to categories of 'unknown'. Information on age and sex would also be difficult to obtain were it not for the supplementary information available on the back of prescription forms regarding exemption from prescription charges. A further problem arises with prescriptions from areas of high immigrant population. Coders would not normally know the sex of Chandrakant Singh for example just from the forename while John or Rosemary leaves little doubt if legibly written. National Health Service prescriptions only permit a very broad age classification as Table 23.2 indicates. An interesting feature of Table 23.2 is the relatively high proportion of males to females in the 16 to 60 or 64 category. The figure for females would, of course, have been higher had it been possible to include females of age 60–64. As they stand the figures in the age category are not strictly comparable. The total percentage of all males to all females representing about 60 males per 100 females, is higher however than the sex incidence of about 40 males per 100 females sometimes quoted for rheumatic diseases and gout[8].

PRESCRIBING RELEVANT TO RHEUMATIC AND RELATED THERAPY

As explained above, the drugs and formulations principally intended or specified for rheumatic diseases and gout were placed in therapeutic class 65 (old classification) by the DHSS for prescribing analysis purposes. A considerable number of drugs used in rheumatic therapy, however, particularly those used as adjuncts to the principal therapeutic agent, e.g. immunosuppressives, are used for other purposes. Thus many drugs in the therapy of rheumatic, arthritic and related disorders cross the boundaries of several therapeutic categories. This renders logical analysis difficult in the absence of any indication of the therapeutic intent of the prescriber.

As a compromise to what would otherwise be sheer guesswork the drugs prescribed concomitantly with established anti-rheumatic drugs can in some cases be presumed to be associated with the treatment of the rheumatic or related condition. If this approach is adopted further analysis is feasible.

Detailed results of PD2 analysis for 1973–74 revealed as shown in Table 23.3 that the 22 396 prescriptions for preparations specified for rheumatic diseases and gout could be sub-classified under 15 different sub-groups. Further inspection of the data (not included in the report) revealed that the 15 groups embraced a total of 74 different formulations and preparations, and even these were found to represent only a relatively small range of individual drugs contained in analgesic formulations or other combination products currently recommended for the treatment of rheumatic diseases. For instance, the bulk of the analgesics, salicylates and corticosteroids are excluded from Table 23.3. Realizing their limitations, the DHSS has revised its therapeutic classification and this will be discussed below under salicylate therapy.

Data from the first three months of the succeeding year 1974–75 showed remarkable stability in the drug usage pattern represented in Table 23.3. They showed in addition a trend towards an increased interest in the propionic acid derivatives ketoprofen, fenoprofen and naproxen.

Even more interestingly, the results of a small-scale study based on 15 880 items of all categories prescribed in Scotland during January 1975 also showed an overall pattern for the prescribing of anti-rheumatic drugs such as that contained in Table 23.3. Minor exceptions included the fact that of the two major anti-inflammatory drugs of Table 23.3, the rank order for indomethacin was higher than that for phenylbutazone. However, the reversal did not constitute a significant deviation in prescribing habits because fluctuations in figures that are already fairly close together as in Table 23.3 can be inevitable. The Scottish data confirmed the trend towards ketoprofen, fenoprofen and naproxen.

Table 23.3 Preparations specified for rheumatic diseases and gout therapeutic group 65 (DHSS old classification) 'Prescribing Year' 1973–74

		Frequency
Uricosuric agents		736
Gold		49
Anti-inflammatories		20345
Flufenamic acid	35	
Indomethacin	6060	
Oxphenbutazone	1245	
Phenylbutazone	7307	
Propionic acid derivs.	5698	
Corticosteroids (Prednisone)		290
Analgesics		954
Alclofenac	172	
Aspirin variants	41	
Dextropropoxyphene	75	
Pentazocine	666	
Others		22
Total		22396

The uricosuric agents include allopurinol, probenecid, ethebenecid and sulphinpyrazone. For convenience colchicine is also included here. The propionic acid derivatives include fenoprofen, ibuprofen, ketoprofen and naproxen

It would however be unwise to read too much into figures from small scale studies and only the follow through of the larger scale studies can confirm or refute a continuing trend. In view of recent comment regarding the addictive tendencies of dextropropoxyphene[10], increased future interest in the use of alternative analgesics should be screened for in the data for 1976–77.

Anti-rheumatics and concomitant prescribing

It is common for anti-rheumatic drugs to be prescribed together[11]. The data presented in Table 23.4 further confirm this point. They show that not only was one type of anti-rheumatic drug concomitantly prescribed with another type but also that corticotrophin was prescribed together with glucocorticoids. Of drugs not exhibiting an anti-rheumatic effect, the analgesics featured most prominently and antacids, iron preparations and anti-depressants to about the same extent.

While the concomitant prescription of antacids may be related to the problem of dyspepsia and other gastro-intestinal disturbances attendant upon the use of many anti-rheumatic drugs, that of iron preparations to patients with rheumatoid arthritis may be related to the underlying joint disease. Leaving aside for the present the detailed examination of the therapeutic combinations of antacids and anti-rheumatics, it is pertinent to note that despite a

Table 23.4 Concomitant prescribing with (22396) anti-rheumatics of therapeutic group 65 (DHSS old classification)

Anti-rheumatics, other	565
Glucocorticoids + corticotrophin	382
Immunosuppressives	7
Analgesics	2719
Antacids	514
Iron	560
Anti-depressants	590

recommendation for the use of parenteral iron for the treatment of anaemia of rheumatoid arthritis[12], of 560 prescriptions for iron only 5 were for parenteral iron.

Although the data for concomitant prescription of tranquillizers (Table 23.3) and anti-depressants (Table 23.4) are of considerable interest in view of the reported association between depression and rheumatic diseases[9], detailed analyses of the figures reveals some interesting facts. For instance the combined total for the two categories, i.e. 2385 prescriptions (Tables 23.3 and 23.4), amounts to only 5.46% of the 43 696 drugs involved and is not much more than half of what the entire patient population receives nationally (approx. 9%). The anti-depressants alone constitute 1.35% in this study compared with around 2.4% nationally. Is it therefore possible that sufferers from rheumatoid type disorders sustain their problems better than the population at large in some ways?

COMBINATIONS OF NON-STEROIDAL ANTI-INFLAMMATORY DRUGS

In Table 23.5, of the 96 prescriptions for two indomethacin preparations, 77 were for 100 mg suppositories. The popularity of combining the newer propionic acid derivatives with the longer established anti-inflammatory drugs is obvious. It is also clear that the prescribers of indomethacin and of phenylbutazone consider that combination with other anti-inflammatory drugs is desirable in a number of cases. Some rheumatologists tend to discourage such combination therapy[13].

Table 23.5 Combined therapy of major non-steroidal anti-inflammatory drugs one with another (314 combinations)

	Indomethacin	*Phenylbutazone*	*Oxyphenbutazone*	*Propionic acid derivatives*	*Prednisone and Phenylbutazone*
Indomethacin	*96	43	7	118	
Phenylbutazone				28	
Oxyphenbutazone				7	
Propionic acid derivatives				12	3

* 77 of the 96 were for 100 mg suppositories

COMBINED STEROIDAL AND NON-STEROIDAL ANTI-INFLAMMATORY THERAPY

The prescription of glucocorticoids, if unassociated with anti-rheumatic drugs, does not reveal even presumptive evidence of therapeutic intent. For this reason assessment of involvement of steroids has been confined to those prescribed concomitantly with non-steroidal anti-inflammatory agents. Table 23.6 shows the range and frequency with which the glucocorticoids were prescribed together with non-steroidal anti-inflammatory agents and represents 2.98% of the 20 316 non-steroidal agents screened for this table. This form of analysis cannot, of course, give any information on glucocorticoids prescribed on an NHS script alone or with drugs not categorized as anti-rheumatics since evidence of therapeutic intent is too problematical in that case. Since the percentage of patients being treated with this combined therapy is relatively small (2.71%) it may be reasonable to assume that an orthodox approach is being adopted here, that is the type of third-line treatment suggested in *Prescribers' Journal*[14] in which the addition of small doses of corticosteroids are used to supplement other anti-inflammatory and analgesic therapy.

Table 23.6 Glucocorticosteroids prescribed with other non-steroidal anti-inflammatory drugs

	Total	*Indomethacin*	*Phenylbutazone*	*Oxyphenbutazone*	*Propionic acid derivatives*	*Other*	*Most popular strength of Glucocorticoid*
Prednisone	526	111	303	3	99	10	1.25 mg and 5 mg
Prednisolone	12	3	1	0	7	1	5 mg
Methylprednisolone	31	16	8	0	6	1	4 mg
Betamethasone	18	5	3	1	8	1	0.5 mg
Dexamethasone	2	2	0	0	0	0	0.5 mg
Paramethasone	2	1	0	0	0	1	2 mg
Triamcinolone	8	2	2	1	3	0	4 mg
Corticotrophin	7	4	0	0	2	1	40 IU
Totals	606	144	317	5	125	15	

A further possible refinement here would be to find the daily dosage of each pair of drugs. A disadvantage is that the data available for such dosage calculations is frequently vitiated by lack of dosage detail on the original prescriptions.

On the face of it, however, the above figures may indicate a situation more satisfactory than that reported in a study of general practitioner prescribing[3], contemporary with this data, in which it was stated that 'about one-third of the patients had been prescribed oral corticosteroids', a point concerning which the rheumatologists reporting the study were most unhappy.

GOLD, PENICILLAMINE, IMMUNOSUPPRESSIVES

Gold has been used for fifty years for rheumatoid therapy while penicillamine has been introduced for this application relatively recently[15] as have the immunosuppressive agents. Rheumatologists recommend the use of this group of drugs by those with experience in this field since close supervision of the patient is considered to be mandatory. It is not surprising therefore to find that the use of these agents, as shown by this study (see Table 23.7), is very limited. It can, however, be expected that the use of penicillamine will increase since the data-base for the present study refers to 1973–74 when trials of penicillamine largely began. The immunosuppressive antimetabolite azathioprine is also of interest in this connection and comparative trials with penicillamine have been carried out recently[16].

Again, in this study, presumptive evidence of therapeutic intent has to be based on concomitant prescription with anti-inflammatory or uricosuric agents. From the small figures it seems probable that these agents were being regarded with caution by the prescribers who generated these data. It is interesting that three of the five immunosuppressive agents were prescribed with allopurinol (Table 23.7), concurrent therapy with which allows reduction in dosage of an-

Table 23.7 Gold, penicillamine and immunosuppressives prescribed alone or with other items

	Totals	*Allopurinol*	*Gold*	*Indomethacin*	*Phenylbutazone*	*Propionic acid DVS*	*Prednisone*	*Analgesic*	*Antacids*
Gold	•49		3	3	1		2	6	3
Penicillamine	5			2	1	2			
Azathioprine	2			2					
Chlorambucil	1	1							
Busulphan	1	1							
Cyclophosphamide	1	1							

• Of the 49 gold only 18 were coupled with other items

tipurines such as azathioprine[17]. In the case of the antineoplastic agents such as chlorambucil, busulphan and cyclophosphamide featured in Table 23.7, it is possible that allopurinol was prescribed for the treatment of hyperuricaemia associated with malignancy.

Of the 49 prescriptions for gold injections recorded (see Table 23.7), 18 were coupled with other items ranging from indomethacin through to prednisone and antacids. The three prescriptions which showed that gold was prescribed concomitantly with gold bore two different strengths of gold injection and in all likelihood represented attempts to administer a dosage intermediate between the commercially available strengths. The prescriptions for antacids were probably related to problems arising from the use of drugs other than gold.

The data of Table 23.7 shows also that the use of penicillamine was associated in all 5 instances with the prescription of one or other of the major anti-inflammatory drugs.

URICOSURIC AND OTHER AGENTS USED FOR GOUT

The classification of therapeutic agents on whatever basis results in anomalies from time to time. For example, the use of the anti-inflammatory agents indomethacin and phenylbutazone in the treatment of gout is largely concealed in this type of analysis except when used concurrently with recognized or established uricosuric agents as illustrated in Table 23.8. This again highlights the shortcomings of prescribing analysis in the absence of declared therapeutic intent. A consequence is that the incidence of gout relative to other rheumatic type disorders cannot be satisfactorily arrived at by this means.

Table 23.8 Uricosuric and other agents for gout prescribed alone and with other items

	Frequency (total usage)	*Combined therapy usage*	*Uricosuric agents*	*Prednisone*	*Major anti-inflam-matories*	*Analgesics*	*Antacids*
Allopurinol	560	133	18	2	71	36	6
Ethebenecid	4	1	0	0	1	0	0
Probenecid	102	16	3	2	7	3	1
Sulphinpyrazone	13	3	1	0	1	1	0
Colchicine	57	22	12	0	5	5	0
Totals	736	175	34	4	85	45	7

The incidence of concurrent prescribing with major anti-inflammatories is indicative of the place of such agents in the treatment of gout

ANTACIDS PRESCRIBED CONCOMITANTLY WITH ANTI-RHEUMATIC DRUGS

The data summarized in Table 23.9 show that in 2.29% of all prescriptions issued in the 1973–74 survey, antacids were prescribed concurrently with anti-rheumatic drugs. In up to 20% of the 514 prescriptions the antacids were used in association with indomethacin or phenylbutazone, whereas the corresponding figure for the group of propionic acid derivatives (fenoprofen, ibuprofen, ketoprofen and naproxen) was 40%.

The antacids prescribed included aluminium and magnesium salts in a wide variety of formulations some of which had added antispasmodics or sedatives. Approximately 25% of the antacids were tablets or mixtures of the British

National Formulary (BNF). In all there were 39 different preparations prescribed of which 6 were BNF. When looked at overall as in Table 23.1, the concurrent use of antacids ranked fifteenth which suggests that dyspepsia and other gastro-intestinal disorders associated with the use of anti-inflammatory drugs might not be the most pressing of the additional medical problems of rheumatic patients.

Some time ago the *Prescribers' Journal* (1974, **14,** 48) carried an article entitled 'Anti-Rheumatic Analgesics and the Stomach' which reviewed the four drugs, relatively new at that time, alclofenac, naproxen, ketoprofen and fenoprofen. The article ended in the statement that 'whatever the reports of initial trials may be it is at least several months after general release before the true incidence of side effects becomes apparent in the use of any new anti-rheumatic drug'. The data shown in Table 23.9 is of special interest in the light

Table 23.9 Antacids prescribed concomitantly with anti-rheumatic drugs

	Frequency		*Frequency*	*Per cent*
Anti-rheumatic drugs	22396	Antacids	514	2.29
Indomethacin	6060		116	1.91
Phenylbutazone	7307		78	1.07
Oxyphenbutazone	1245		16	1.28
Propionic acid DVS.	5698		176	3.09

of the above statements and also in view of more recent observations of the clinical effects of propionic acid derivatives[18]. Although the figures derived as these have been can in no sense take the place of properly controlled clinical trials, the experience of a group of general practitioners handling large numbers of patients is no doubt of some value particularly when those conducting clinical trials find it difficult to ascertain the frequency of gastro-intestinal complications[18]. It will be interesting to follow this through subsequent 'prescribing years' of this cohort study.

ANALGESICS AND SALICYLATES

The assessment of analgesic therapy concurrent with other anti-rheumatics is rendered difficult by the fact that the therapeutic classification in use in this study (DHSS old classification) places certain analgesic formulations recommended for rheumatic and arthritic therapy in the same therapeutic group as the major anti-inflammatory agents and not in the antipyretic or addictive analgesic groups. In addition there are certain combined analgesic/anti-inflammatory formulations available and these are quite naturally placed with the major anti-inflammatory drugs in group 65 of the old DHSS classification.

Analysis of data as shown in Table 23.10 was an attempt to discover the spectrum of combined use of analgesic and major anti-inflammatory drugs. A complete breakdown has not been attempted but it is interesting to note that analgesics were concurrently prescribed in 13.6% of all prescriptions for indomethacin, in 13.4% of those for the propionic acid derivatives, in 9.8% of those for phenylbutazone and in 4.4% of all the prescriptions for oxyphenbutazone. If, however, the available fixed combination formulations of analgesic plus phenylbutazone or oxyphenbutazone are included in the calculation the

Table 23.10 Analgesics (anti-pyretic and other) prescribed with anti-inflammatory agents

	Totals	*Indomethacin*	*Phenylbutazone*	*Oxyphenbutazone*	*Propionic acid derivatives*	*Others*
Aspirin and variants	274	136	65	4	69	
Paracetamol and variants	922	299	287	24	312	
Benorylate	66	27	4	1	34	
Dextropropoxyphene and variants	738	240	239	18	241	
Pentazocine	110	40	30	3	37	
Ethoheptazine and variants	109	40	43	2	24	
Dihydrocodeine	95	36	31	2	26	
Mefenamic acid	48	8	21	1	18	
Other	357					357
Total	2719	826	720	55	761	357

Table 23.11 Soluble forms of aspirin modal dose calculation attempted on 1402 items

Daily dosage (No. of 300 mg Tablets) – Top line
Frequency of occurrence – Bottom line

1	2	3	4	5	6	8	9	10	12	16	18	Other	Total
20	39	140	167	11	293	244	7	79	6	5	1	1	1013

Ten tablets of 300 mg = 3 g

percentages of combination therapy change to 15.4% for phenylbutazone and 22.1% for oxyphenbutazone. Even so these figures are perhaps not as high as might be expected for this form of combined therapy and the question of salicylate therapy is left unanswered.

One of the drawbacks of classifying drugs into therapeutic groups for prescribing analysis arises from the fact that some drugs may have more than one therapeutic application. For this reason, and even when prescribed concomitantly with other anti-rheumatic drugs, it is difficult to arrive at a satisfactory assessment of salicylate therapy in rheumatic conditions. Table 23.10 gives an indication of aspirin alone or in various combinations prescribed concurrently with the major non-steroidal anti-inflammatory agents, but this can give no real guide as to the entire spectrum of salicylates used for rheumatic treatment.

Table 23.11 illustrates an attempt to reach some concensus by examining the modal dosage of the most frequently prescribed soluble aspirin preparations. Of one group of 1402 such preparations extracted from 656 534 prescribed items it was possible to calculate a daily dose in only 1013 cases. If 3 g per day is taken as the minimum effective dose of aspirin for rheumatoid treatment[3] then only 92 prescriptions for soluble aspirin could be regarded as possible salicylate controlled therapy. The modal dose investigation was not pursued further on this occasion.

If, however, the more recent DHSS therapeutic classification (Revised November 1975) is used to analyse the data for aspirin and aspirin based preparations in the 1973–74 study the results summarized in Table 23.12 were obtained. It will be observed that the apparent salicylate based therapy is substantially increased by comparison with the figures for concomitant prescribing of aspirin and non-steroidal anti-inflammatory drugs. This approach would give a figure of approximately 11% for therapy involving salicylate as such but can give no guide as to whether the therapy is merely an adjunct to other therapy or whether it is being used as initial or first-line treatment. Modal dose calculations might be of some assistance here.

Table 23.12 Apparent salicylate based anti-rheumatic therapy*†

	Frequency
Aspirin in soluble and effervescent forms	1514
Aspirin, enteric coated	283
Aspirin as principal ingredient in admixture or combination	1066
Mix. sod. sal. BNF	88
Total	2951

* Based on DHSS revised Therapeutic Classification (Revised November 1975) Included in Class 061 ... Preparations prescribed for rheumatism ... Anti-inflammatory drugs other than steroids.
† Abstracted from 656534 prescribed items *'Prescribing Year'* 1973–74

The three approaches used above clearly emphasize the difficulty of using presumptive evidence of therapeutic intent based on 'therapeutic codes'. Too much depends on therapeutic classification decisions and on incomplete data. False conclusions may therefore be reached all too readily and engender speculations on the value of this kind of study. Something better is required in order to make 'operational research' more effective.

MORE ADEQUATE METHODS OF OPERATIONAL RESEARCH

Probably the best type of operational research into the prescribing habits and therapeutic intent of general practitioners is the sort of study mounted by a university department of rheumatology or clinic with the collaboration of a sufficient number of general practitioners in its own area. This opens up the possibilities of follow-up in the context of continued postgraduate education. An example of this type of study was reported recently[3].

The author has experience of conducting the data processing for another type of study which could prove very fruitful for studies of prescribing and morbidity in general, or for selected sub-studies such as rheumatic treatment. Participating prescribers were supplied with pads of NHS prescriptions interleaved with a yellow copy form of special design. These prescription 'sets' were printed on NCR paper requiring no carbon, only a ballpoint pen. Instructions on procedure were printed on a stiff card insert flexibly bound to the prescription pad. This card insert was placed below a prescription 'set' before writing the prescription to avoid copy carrying through several layers. The prescription was written and given to the patient as usual and the 'indication' or reason for prescribing the drug(s) immediately written on to the yellow copy. The 'indication' was later coded using the OXMIS problem coding system.

It is probably best to have this coding carried out centrally in order to avoid ambiguities. A patient identification code was generated after the fashion of Hogben and Cross[19] and written into a box provided on the yellow copy prescription. This code consisted of date of birth plus letters from a forename initial and part of the surname. A sex indication can be added with advantage. The top of the copy script was then guillotined off to remove the name and address of the patient and so preserve confidentially. Thus a partially coded but anonymous copy script reached the data processing centre where coding of the drugs was carried out and data processing put in hand. Data capture at this level of detail opens up almost unlimited possibilities for studies of prescribing and morbidity and if conducted in association with appropriate departments of a medical school great things could be achieved. Much of the travail and many of the difficulties of prescribing analysis discussed earlier in the present review would vanish in that event.

ACKNOWLEDGEMENTS

The author is grateful to the Department of Health and Social Security for support and facilities and for the collaboration in study of the cohort of prescribers by the Medical Sociology Research Centre, University College of Swansea. Thanks are also due to the Prescription Pricing Authority for the collection and despatch of the necessary prescriptions.

Acknowledgement is made of the assistance given in analysing the data by Mrs A. Cameron and Dr G. L. Geddes of the Research Unit staff.

References

1. Acheson, H. W. K. (1974). Medical audit. *Br. Med. J.*, **1,** 453
2. Mason, D. I. R., Brooks, P. M., Lee, P., Kennedy, A. C. and Buchanan, W. W. (1975). In-patient prescribing in a rheumatic diseases centre. *Health Bull.*, **33,** 74
3. Lee, P., Ahola, S. J., Grennan, D., Brooks, P. and Buchanan, W. W. (1974). Observations on drug prescribing in rheumatic arthritis. *Br. Med. J.*, **1,** 424
4. Mckenzie, L S., Horsburgh, B. A., Ghosh, P. and Taylor, T. K. F. (1976). Osteoarthrosis: uncertain rationale for anti-inflammatory drug therapy. *Lancet*, **i,** 908
5. Review article (1977). General Practice Prescribing. *Lancet*, **i,** 463
6. Medical Sociology Research Centre, University College of Swansea, Wales (1976). Prescribing in general practice. *J. R. Coll. Gen. Practitioners*, Supplement No 1, Vol 26, 4604
7. Prescription analysis, therapeutic classification, Revised November 1975, Department of Health and Social Security.
8. Office of Health and Economics (A.B.P.I.) (1973). *Rheumatism and Arthritis in Britain*, Studies on current health problems. Paper No. 45
9. Zaphiropoulos, G. and Burry, H. C. (1974). Depression in rheumatoid diseases. *Ann. Rheum. Dis.*, **33,** 132
10. Review article (1977). Dangers of dextropropoxyphene. *Br. Med. J.*, **1,** 668
11. Cosh, J. A. (1974). Anti-inflammatory drugs in rheumatic diseases. *Practitioner*, **213,** 519
12. Mowat, A. G. (1975). Anaemia in rheumatoid arthritis. *Prescribers' J.*, **15,** 64
13. Review Article (1976). Antirheumatic drugs: plenty is not enough. *Br. Med. J.*, **1,** 59
14. Taylor, R. T. (1975). Corticosteroids and corticotrophins in rheumatology and collagen diseases. *Prescribers' J.*, **15,** 64
15. Mowat, A. G. (1976). Rheumatology. *Practitioner*, **217,** 549
16. Berry, H., Liyanage, S. P., Durance, R. A., Barnes, C. G., Berger, C. A. and Evans, S. (1976). Azathioprine and penicillamine in treatment of rheumatoid arthritis: a controlled trial. *Br. Med. J.*, **1,** 1052
17. Lessot, M. H. (1973). Immunosuppressive Drugs and their Adverse Effects. *Prescribers' J.*, **13,** 144
18. Huskisson, E. C., Woolf, D. L., Balme, H. W., Scott, J. and Franklyn, S. (1976). Four new anti-inflammatory drugs: responses and variations. *Br. Med. J.*, **1,** 1048
19. Hogben L. and Cross, K. W. (1948). The statistical specificity of a code personnel cypher sequence. *Br. J. Social Med.*, **2,** 149

24
Evaluation and Reporting of Toxicity of Anti-Rheumatic Drugs

M. F. CUTHBERT

INTRODUCTION

The Medicines Act (1968) was implemented in September 1971 and exercises control over the manufacturing, importation, sale and supply, labelling and advertising of medicines. A Medicines Commission has been established to give general advice on the various aspects of the enforcement of the Act. It also functions as an appeal body in respect of the activities of a number of expert advisory committees. In the context of this chapter the most relevant of these expert committees are the Committee of Safety of Medicines which has replaced the Committee on Safety of Drugs, and the Committee on the Review of Medicines. The Committee on Safety of Medicines is served by a number of expert sub-committees and advises on the issuing of licences and certificates. The Licensing Authority issues Clinical Trial Certificates, valid for 2 years, for drugs approved by the Committee on Safety of Medicines; and Product Licences, valid for 5 years, for drugs similarly approved for marketing.

LICENSING AND REVIEW OF ANTI-RHEUMATIC DRUGS

Before a clinical trial can be conducted on a new anti-rheumatic drug in the United Kingdom, the supplier must hold a valid Clinical Trial Certificate (CTC); this implies that the drug is considered to be of adequate quality and safe in respect of the proposed clinical trials. An application for a CTC must include a detailed protocol and up to three centres are usually nominated.

Similarly an anti-rheumatic drug may be marketed in the United Kingdom only if the promoter holds a Product Licence issued by the Licencing Authority. Since 1971, Product Licences have been granted for new products only after their safety, quality and efficacy have been assessed on the advice of the Committee on Safety of Medicines (CSM).

Approximately 36 000 products were on the market before 1971 and some 1000 of these made claims for use in rheumatic disease; licences for these products were granted automatically, mostly without any detailed assessment. The Licensing Authority have become increasingly aware that the standards applied since 1971 have not been applied to anti-rheumatic and other drugs marketed before that date and for this reason *all* marketed drugs, including all anti-rheumatic drugs, are now being reviewed by the Committee on the Review of Medicines (CRM) using criteria similar to those applied to new products. It is expected that this task will be completed within the time limit allowed by the EEC directives.

Products have been allocated to therapeutic categories according to their medical claims and priority has been given to those which include drugs which are widely prescribed or sold to the public for non-fatal diseases and which give rise to a relatively high proportion of reported adverse reactions. On this basis the anti-rheumatic drugs are the first category to be reviewed and an expert sub-committee under the chairmanship of Dr F. Dudley Hart was established in February 1976 to provide advice to CRM on the quality, safety and efficacy of individual drug substances. Utilizing all available sources of information, general recommendations are being made on the appropriate claims, dosage, method of sale, contraindications, warnings, labelling and advertising; after consultation with the Pharmaceutical Industry and other interested organizations, these recommendations are then applied to individual products.

A most important source of information in the evaluation of anti-rheumatic drugs are the reports of adverse reactions which are sent on a voluntary and confidential basis to the CSM. Since most serious adverse reactions are rare events they are unlikely to be detected in animal toxicity tests and may also be undetected in early clinical trials. The problem is essentially one of numbers since relatively small numbers of both animals and patients are exposed to a new drug before it is released on to the market. Marketing may therefore be the first adequate safety trial.

Eighty to one hundred reports are received weekly and some 60 000 reports have been entered into the Adverse Reactions Register since it was initiated in 1964. It must be emphasized that all reports are treated in the strictest confidence and the identity of the patient or reporting doctor is not revealed without the written permission of the latter. The information is stored by computer after evaluation by the medical staff of the section. Problems signalled by this system may lead to immediate action or initiation of special studies involving follow-up by a team of 80 part-time medical officers who can interview doctors in any part of the country. After consultation with the pharmaceutical industry and presentation of the problem to the Committee on Safety of Medicines through their Adverse Reactions Sub-Committee, action may be taken voluntarily by the manufacturer, or the Committee may decide to issue a letter in the medical journals or to send an individual letter to every doctor (and possibly dentist and pharmacist) in the country, or to publish a statement in the Adverse Reaction Series. This may be accompanied by the publication of a scientific paper in the case of a detailed study. Occasionally, this action will result in a variation to the Product Licence for the drug concerned or, rarely, to withdrawal.

Since the reporting of reactions by the practising doctor is voluntary, the most serious limitation of the system is under-reporting, since only a proportion of those adverse reactions which actually occur are reported. An indication of drug usage is often valuable in assessing the importance of a problem and prescribing statistics from a sample of prescriptions in general practice are available and overall both sources of information are invaluable in the review of anti-rheumatic drugs in widespread clinical use.

ADVERSE REACTIONS TO NON-STEROIDAL ANTI-RHEUMATIC DRUGS

Signals can only be derived from small numbers of reports when the adverse reaction is serious, of high incidence, unusual or related in some precise way to drug administration. With few exceptions, the adverse reaction potential of an anti-rheumatic drug can only be assessed when it has been in use for some time. However, a simple tabulation of computer data can be most useful in establishing the adverse reaction profile and in drawing attention to particular problems. This can be particularly valuable if the profile of a new anti-rheumatic drug is compared with that of an established remedy.

It must be emphasized, however, that the recording of a drug-associated adverse reaction does not necessarily imply a cause-effect relationship nor is a drug being received concomitantly excluded as a possible causative factor. Thus, if three drugs are being given simultaneously to a patient and three adverse reactions are reported, this will result in nine adverse reaction 'events' being entered into the computer.

Phenylbutazone

Analysis shows that adverse reactions involving the blood predominate with gastrointestinal effects in second place in the fatal reactions. A total of 1276 reports were received in the period June 1964 to January 1973. Of these, 398 (204 fatal) were blood disorders which included 163 reports of aplastic anaemia (121 fatal); 59 were reports of thrombocytopenia (18 fatal); and 95 were reports of agranulocytosis, leucopenia or pancytopenia (44 fatal). Haemorrhage from the gastrointestinal tract was recorded in 104 cases (27 fatal). Comparison with prescribing statistics showed that approximately 40 reports and 9 deaths are associated with each million prescriptions for phenylbutazone.

Oxyphenbutazone

This shows an almost identical profile, perhaps because it is a known metabolite of phenylbutazone. Of a total of 421 reports received during the same period, 157 (74 fatal) were of blood disorders which included 63 reports of aplastic anaemia (40 fatal); 38 reports of thrombocytopenia (14 fatal); and 36 reports of agranulocytosis or pancytopenia (15 fatal). Haemorrhage from the gastrointestinal tract was recorded in 16 cases (5 fatal). Despite the smaller number of reports, the incidence of both reports and deaths are almost exactly double that associated with phenylbutazone (80 reports, 18 deaths per million prescriptions). No explanation for this finding is as yet forthcoming.

Indomethacin

This in contrast, is commonly associated with adverse gastrointestinal effects with blood disorders taking a second place in the fatal reactions. Of a total of 1261 reports received between June 1964 and January 1973, haemorrhage from the gastrointestinal tract was recorded in 121 cases (25 fatal). Blood disorders figured in 157 reports (25 fatal) which included 35 reports of thrombocytopenia (5 fatal); 21 reports of agranulocytosis or leucopenia (3 fatal); and 17 cases of aplastic anaemia (no fatalities). An interesting feature of indomethacin is the high incidence of non-fatal reports involving the central nervous system (total 397), mainly of headache, giddiness, vertigo, confusion, and abnormalities of vision. Overall, a total of 60 reports and 6 deaths are associated with each million prescriptions.

Aspirin

Aspirin shows a similar profile to that of indomethacin. Of a total of 787 reports (1964 to 1973), gastrointestinal haemorrhage was recorded in 128 cases (64 fatal) while blood disorders figured in 95 reports (17 fatal), the latter included thrombocytopenia, 26 reports (2 fatal); aplastic anaemia, 13 reports (7 fatal); and agranulocytosis or pancytopenia in 10 reports (2 fatal). Reporting here is certainly very incomplete because of vast over-the-counter sales, but it is worth drawing attention to the number of adverse reactions affecting the kidney. This is largely due to cases of analgesic nephropathy (53 reports, 26 fatal) associated with the use of combined preparations containing aspirin, phenacetin and codeine.

Ibuprofen

This is an anti-rheumatic drug, which though closely related to ibufenac, has not been associated with hepatic toxicity. It was introduced in the UK in 1969 and presents a profile similar to that of indomethacin. Of a total of 388 reports received up to January 1974, gastrointestinal haemorrhage was recorded in 37 reports (6 fatal) while blood disorders figured in 34 reports (5 fatal), the latter included thrombocytopenia, 9 reports (1 fatal) and agranulocytosis or pancytopenia, 6 reports (2 fatal). Again, minor adverse reactions involving the central nervous system were relatively frequently recorded (89 reports) among which 18 reports were of visual disturbances. Approximately 40 reports and 4 deaths are associated with each million prescriptions.

Alclofenac

This was marketed in the UK in June 1971. Its use has been associated with a high incidence of skin reactions (294 of a total of 412 reports), some of which have been severe. The Committee published a letter in the medical journals in December 1973 drawing attention to this hazard. Other adverse reactions have been reported rarely and only 5 reports of associated gastrointestinal haemorrhage (1 fatal) had been received up to January 1974.

Naproxen

Naproxen was marketed in the UK in September 1973 with the suggestion that its gastrointestinal tolerance might be better than with some other non-steroidal anti-inflammatory drugs. However, the pattern of gastrointestinal side-effects associated with its use, which include 52 reports of gastrointestinal haemorrhage and 5 deaths, is similar to that of other non-steroidal anti-inflammatory drugs.

CORRELATION WITH ANIMAL TOXICITY TESTS

All non-steroidal anti-inflammatory drugs produce ulceration of the gastrointestinal tract, particularly in the dog. This property appears, on present evidence, to be related to efficacy and to be predictive in terms of human toxicity.

Regarding the haemopoietic system, which is of prime importance in the toxic effects of many potent anti-rheumatic drugs, toxic effect in animals are usually secondary only to the gastrointestinal pathology. Rarely, if ever, can an indication of the possible hazard of aplastic anaemia or bone-marrow suppression in man be derived from animal studies or even from clinical trials involving several hundred patients[1]. Similarly, evidence of liver toxicity is rarely seen in animal studies when this may be an important target organ in man. Perhaps the best example of this is the experience with ibufenac. The potential of this drug to cause fatal cholestatic jaundice, only became evident when it had been released for general use.

Animal toxicity tests may be useful in predicting the stimulation or depression of the central nervous system, and the renal, cardiovascular, endocrine and neuro-muscular effects of anti-rheumatic drugs; but many common adverse reactions, e.g. those affecting the skin, and some serious adverse reactions affecting haemopoietic and hepatic functions cannot usually be predicted by such studies.

CONCLUSIONS

With few exceptions adverse reactions can *only* be detected when an anti-rheumatic drug has been in extensive clinical use. Examples which illustrate this point are ibufenac, naproxen, phenylbutazone and oxyphenbutazone. Animal toxicity tests and early clinical trials are of limited value in this respect.

Analysis of crude adverse reactions data and prescribing statistics are useful in drawing attention to particular areas of concern, particularly when data on recently introduced drugs is compared with that on established anti-rheumatic drugs.

The objective of the review, at present in progress in the United Kingdom, is to ensure that *all* anti-rheumatic drugs on the market are of adequate quality and are safe and effective in relation to their clinical indications or claims, irrespective of whether these are prescribed by doctors or are available to the general public without prescription.

ACKNOWLEDGEMENTS

Much of the data quoted in this paper has been previously published in the journal *Current Medical Research and Opinion* and in the book *Current Approaches in Toxicology*[2,3] and I wish to acknowledge this fact and to thank the editors in this respect.

References

1. Inman W. H. W. (1977). Study of fatal bone marrow depression with special reference to phenylbutazone and oxyphenbutazone. *Br. Med. J.* **1,** 1500
2. Cuthbert, M. F. (1974). Adverse reactions to non-steroidal anti-rheumatic drugs. *Cur. Med. Res. and Opinion,* **2,** 600
3. Cuthbert, M. F. (1977). Adverse reactions to anti-rheumatic drugs: some correlations with animal toxicity studies. In B. Ballantyne (ed.) *Current Approaches in Toxicology,* pp. 279–288. (Bristol: John Wright and Sons Ltd.)

25
The Quest for Anti-Rheumatic Drugs

J. R. VANE

INTRODUCTION

When he organized this symposium, Dr Jasani very cleverly guaranteed that at least one member of the audience would attend every single paper by asking me to try to sum up the two days' discussion. In view of the clinical fusillades which were fired yesterday across the gulf between clinician and scientist I must immediately declare my interest.

First, I am a pharmacologist, interested in the mode of action of drugs. Secondly, for the last 3½ years, I have been Director of Research and Development for a fairly large multi-national British-based pharmaceutical company, interested in the discovery of new drugs — hopefully, profitable new drugs! Thirdly, I intend to fire a few shots back!

Let us just for a few minutes discuss the problem as a general one, not specific for arthritis. Profitable new drugs have arisen from four broad approaches which are generally known as (a) 'empirical' or random, (b) molecular manipulation, or the examination of structures related to compounds of known activity, (c) extraction and/or modifications of natural substances and (d) 'rational' (or based on fundamental research), as exemplified by designing chemicals to interfere with enzymes known to be vital for the life of the invading organism but not of the host.

In fact, all these approaches are highly rational, although the one given that designation is the most pleasing scientifically. The boundaries between them are not always clear and when there is an overlay of serendipity, ingenuity (especially in the development of relevant tests) and inspired opportunism, all have their place in industrial research.

Empirical

This approach can only be regarded as 'random screening' up to the point that activity is found. Thereafter, the accumulated wisdom of the chemist rapidly develops the best structural modifications. In my opinion, there is still the need to encourage the development of high through-put screens (such as measurement of an anti-enzyme activity in a test tube) which allow rapid assessment of very small quantities of new (or old) chemicals.

Molecular manipulation

Random screening can be eliminated when structures are already known which have the desired activity. Chemists then study related structures to increase activity, reduce side effects, change features such as absorbability by mouth and even to discover new activities.

Extraction and/or modification of natural substances

The search in recent years for exploitable and extractable biological activity (usually of high molecular weight) has not led to immediate rewards, although we in Wellcome have been in the forefront of this type of research. There is great interest in the immunostimulant properties of *Corynebacterium parvum* and a recent revival of interest in interferon. We are now growing both in our Biological division in the UK. The interferon is produced by lymphoblastoid cells in culture and, over the next few years, we are likely to see a product of greater and greater purity. But, like vaccines, this type of biological product has a standard of crudity which is completely unacceptable when we deal with smaller molecules. Strengths in immunology and immunochemistry are vital to take this whole area on to a different scientific and chemical plane in the 1980s.

Rational

As we learn more about the workings of different cells and of the structure of the molecules in cells with which drugs react, so we shall be better able to design drugs. In this field, George Hitchings was a pioneer. He searched methodically and vigorously for 'exploitable information' and created within the Company an unparalleled data base of fundamental knowledge within a particular area. This is a long-term strategy; results come slowly, but new drugs which arise are likely to be fundamental breakthroughs of substantial scientific and commercial value. For George Hitchings, and Wellcome, the policy led to trimethoprim, allopurinol, azathioprine and several other new drugs.

Could we now turn to the quest for new anti-rheumatic drugs, the present ones being described as 'steroids' or 'non-steroids'. The non-steroids have recently been subdivided again, after our discovery that aspirin-like drugs inhibit prostaglandin synthetase. Although this knowledge of enzyme inhibition tells us the basic mode of action and gives us more fundamental knowledge — or even a new test system, to know that aspirin and indomethacin inhibit prostaglandin synthetase does not change their clinical efficacy. They are just the same drugs today as they were ten years ago.

How then, do we discover new anti-inflammatory drugs? In listening to questioning of the relevance of animal models yesterday, it began to appear relatively simple. We just take our new chemical entities, make sure that they are not too toxic and then ship them into the clinic, without any knowledge of efficacy. If this is what you want, Dr Dick, I could send you several hundred compounds a year to test in your patients! But I cannot believe it is – there has to be some preliminary sorting mechanism and that has to be based on a test system that the pharmacologist designs as being relevant to inflammation.

The successful ones in the past have been acute models and have produced the present-day plethora of aspirin-like drugs, or prostaglandin synthetase inhibitors. The well-used acute models such as the various carrageenan oedema tests correlate well with tests against prostaglandin synthetase in the test tube.

It was suggested yesterday that we do not need new aspirin-like drugs, for they only relieve the signs and symptoms without affecting the underlying course of the disease. This is to some extent acceptable, but until we have effective, non-toxic drugs that *do* affect the underlying disease process, we shall continue to need aspirin-like drugs. Division of patients by Drs Dick and Buchanan into sub-groups who respond differently to different aspirin-like drugs also suggests a new aspect of drug design which needs to be explored. As Dr Dick has suggested, the pharmacologist should go to his clinic to try to distinguish the differences between the sub-groups. One possibility is that different patients have prostaglandin synthetases which are more or less susceptible to a particular inhibitor. The first thing I would do would be to test the patients urine for prostaglandin metabolites, in order to measure the daily prostaglandin turnover. This would allow the patients to be titrated to a low level of prostaglandin metabolism with different drugs individually. But to say to the industry that there is no need to devote resources to finding yet another aspirin is to beg the question. The industry is market-orientated and generally provides what the clinician is seen to be using. As long as clinicians prescribe world-wide several hundred million pounds worth of the various aspirin-like drugs each year, the industry will continue to look for *better* aspirin-like drugs for them to prescribe!

Our own approach has been a fundamental one, and that is to study the role of prostaglandins in inflammation and to learn as much as possible about the pathways involved (see Figure 2.1 in Dr Moncada's paper).

I'm sorry to talk about pathways rather than patients, but we shall only come to new types of drugs through new methods or new knowledge. Unless we trample up and down these pathways, there will be no drugs arising from the new knowledge!

As Salvador Moncada told you yesterday, aspirin-like drugs interfere with the cyclo-oxygenase, so inhibiting production of PGE_2, $PGF_{2\alpha}$, thromboxanes, endoperoxides and prostacyclin. In inflammation, the culprits seem to be PGE_2 and possibly thromboxane A_2. As Dr Moncada also mentioned yesterday, we believe that more selective anti-inflammatory substances will arise from more selective enzyme inhibitors or from prostaglandin antagonists.

But what can we learn from the steroids? They are regarded clinically as more efficacious than aspirin, and a steroid without side effects could be an improvement on present-day therapy. There is increasing evidence that steroids affect the prostaglandin cascade – Piper and Lewis suggesting that they do so by preventing release of PGs, whereas others, including ourselves, favour an effect on phospholipase A_2: the enzyme which liberates arachidonic acid.

So the difference between steroids and aspirin may lie in the HPETE pathway, or in an event further back. Should we be searching for phospholipase A_2 inhibitors? Such an enzyme activity, incidentally, is claimed for mepacrine. Another difference is that steroids have an effect in two chronic types of inflammation – asthma and arthritis, whereas aspirin-like drugs have no general beneficial effect in asthma. What does this tell us? Perhaps one of the several mediators other than PGs is more important in asthma, such as SRS–A, than in arthritis. Or again, perhaps it is associated with the HETE pathway.

Let us now move away from the prostaglandin system, accompanied, perhaps, by an approving skirl of the bagpipes. How do we look for better non-aspirin-like drugs?

I am convinced that the real breakthrough will come from a fundamental understanding of the disease process itself. We already know that there are many mediators involved and I have in no way intended to imply that prostaglandins are the most important. They have only been highlighted because of the link with aspirin. A multitude of mediators may well be involved, including amines, peptides, prostaglandins, enzymes, lymphokines, complement and so on. There are two implications from this statement. First, a multitude of tests are possible, each designed around a single system. Secondly, and perhaps more importantly, a multitude of drugs may be necessary to attack the disease process. Perhaps we shall eventually reach the stage where the rheumatoid patient is titrated to find out which mediators are most important in his or her particular case and then we make up a cocktail of 10–20 drugs, each one to help one facet. I wonder how the Committee on Safety of Machines would react to such rational therapy?

During the meeting, we heard of several interesting new observations upon which a search for noval anti-rheumatic drugs might be based. The work of G. P. Lewis and his colleagues at CIBA on homograft rejection has the merit of providing information on a fundamental process and the possibility of becoming a useful screen – perhaps highlighting the role of the immune lymphocyte. The idea of developing a drug to prevent the immune response could also carry hazards! The study of vascular permeability which Lewis and Williams are now carrying out at my old home, The Royal College of Surgeons of England, is also of great fundamental importance and will surely lead to a better understanding of vascular damage in general.

Studies of the interactions between the effects of mediators, as initiated by my own group and Morley and Williams will also eventually help in the understanding of the overall picture. The work of Perper, again of a basic nature, also suggests a different type of screen which will select drugs which prevent migration of cells. In this context, I was excited by the results presented by Dumonde, who studied the penetration of lymphocytes into cultures of vascular endothelium. This could also be extended, presumably, to other white cells and could also be a valuable tool. Incidentally, we now know that healthy vascular endothelium mainly generates prostacyclin and not PGE_2.

A. J. Lewis showed some interesting results using a modification of the erythema test and compared topical and systemic drugs. This is essentially a model which detects PG synthetase inhibitors, although Lewis found effects with gold and D-penicillamine. But how much more interesting would a drug be which also prevented the scab formation!

Returning to the homograft model, the work of Bach suggested that a measurement of the fibrin deposits and monocytes could be a useful model and, remarkably, a clinician admitted that the histology was similar to human rheumatoid arthritis!

The work of Coombs on serum sickness in rabbits could well lead to another model, based on deposition of immune complexes. At this stage, it is difficult to predict how such a model would compare in its relevance (and in its convenience as a working screen) to the standard methods of adjuvant arthritis.

Another variation was discussed by Blackham, who specifically injected antigen into one knee joint of Old English rabbits in order to try to produce a relevant model. This also detected prolonged dosage with gold, but not D-penicillamine. He concluded that the spectrum of activity of known drugs in this model was similar to their spectrum of activity in the clinic — surely a sign of relevance! Even so, there were clinical doubts about the relevance of the test, expressed so forcefully as to make one wonder whether the attitude was essentially nihilistic or whether any constructive suggestions were going to arise.

Goldlust described the use of reversed passive Arthus as a potential model. Interestingly, it did not respond to the usual doses of indomethacin or aspirin but selectively picked up colchicine, a drug better known for its activity in gout than in arthritis. Could it be that he has a test for gout — I wonder how the test responds to allopurinol?

There was a strong implication during the 2 days that the pharmacologist should design tests which show the activity of gold, D-penicillamine and perhaps levamisole. I agree — but you must realize that this is an empirical approach. Prolonged dosage in animals may not be obligatory; for instance, the effects of anti-depressants take some weeks to become evident in man, but they were discovered using acute models in animals.

Is there anything I can say in way of a summary? Certainly as a pharmacologist, I shall continue to have faith in animal analogues of human disease, and as our fundamental research tells us more about the disease process, so the animal models will undoubtedly change. At the present time, those based on deposition of immune complexes seem to be the most relevant. As a research director, I shall continue to devote resources to the quest for new anti-rheumatic drugs, both through fundamental research and through screens. Dr Dick has kindly invited me to attend one of his ward rounds. I'm sure that will be a vivid and exhilarating experience. Perhaps Dr Dick would also like to visit our laboratories — and when he comes, I hope he brings some ideas on relevant animal models with him!

Discussion VII

A Statistician's View of Clinical Trials of Anti-Rheumatic Drugs (Chapter 22)

W. WATSON BUCHANAN: I was interested in what Mr Seldup had to say, particularly his criticisms of adjusting for initial pain rating which is exactly what we did. I would be very happy for him to experiment with his statistical methods in our unit in Glasgow. We shall arrange to do different methods of trials for him, and try out the different methods.

It would be interesting to know how Mr Seldrup determines the number of patients who should be put into a trial, and over what period of time should the drugs be tried out. The clinician seems to make a guess, according to his expectations. We think a week or two weeks on a drug that is affective in 18 patients compared against placebo will give a meaningful result.

J. SELDRUP: I have no constructive suggestions on the length of the trial. I must rely on the clinicians to tell me that over *X* weeks or days they are likely, if the compound is any good, to see a change in the condition.

With regard to numbers of patients, before involving oneself in a clinical investigation, one should always set out to determine how many patients are necessary to show an effect which would be meaningful clinically. I would need to come to the clinician to ask what is clinically meaningul in terms of change in a patient, and with a few other statistics from the clinician we could certainly decide how many patients need to be studied. That would not necessarily mean a successful trial, but it would mean that if there was something there to find, it would most certainly be found.

M. F. CUTHBERT: Could Mr Seldrup expand on his rooted objection to the double-blind crossover study that I have regarded to be quite a good method.

J. SELDRUP: Double-blind studies are necessary in most trials. However, there may be trials where double-blind is not required – bio-availability studies, for example.

With respect to the crossover trial, in all textbooks it is the thing to do because one cuts down on variations, one compares compounds within the same patient. What is not always recognized is the change brought about by the first treatment, so that when the patient starts the second treatment, the effect of that second treatment may not be in any way comparable to the first.

One may argue that there is a wash-out period in the middle, but even with a wash-out period, however long it is, the patient will never return to the level at which he started the first trial. That makes a comparison very doubtful – or the relevance of a comparison doubtful.

M. F. CUTHBERT: Even though another group may be starting on the other treatment and crossing over in the opposite direction. Does that help?

J. SELDRUP: Ideally one would hope that if one compared A to B and B to A, the response to A when it comes first is the same as the response to A when it comes second, and the same for B. In my experience that is rarely the case.

W. CARSON DICK: In fact one cannot step into the same river twice.

J. SELDRUP: Yes, that is my personal opinion.

W. CARSON DICK: We would agree.

One point for clarification. The criticism of Peter Lee's data on initial pain rating is not on the data (see *Br. Med. J.*, **2**, 685; 1973), but on the handling of it by co-variance analysis. We showed that the major influence on the result of a simple study was the severity of the initial pain of the patient, and we re-analysed it taking that into account. The criticism was surely of the method of re-analysing it?

J. SELDRUP: The paper was written before any data were presented at the Symposium and no criticism of any particular person is intended. It is that second step that I am against. I accept that sometimes in clinical trials there are two groups that are not comparable initially, but one should forget about it and do it again and try and amend it.

W. WATSON BUCHANAN: It would be very interesting to give Mr Seldrup the data which was reported in the *Q.J.Med.*, (**42,** 387; 1973) in which I showed the mean differences between the groups. In the statistical analysis of that paper, the order in which the drugs were given was taken into account, and there was quite a clear difference between those on effective therapy and those on placebo, irrespective of whether the placebo came in week 1 or week 6 of the study. Is the criticism of the double blind crossover trial justified when it does something, it works, it gives the answer. When something works, why should one be so worried about it?

J. SELDRUP: I am worried because of my own experience in doing crossover trials. I think I have still to do one where with two treatments the response of a treatment is the same irrespective of whether it is given first or given second. It may be a fault in our methodology, but there it is.

W. WATSON BUCHANAN: One other question. Drug A was compared with Drug B but there was no placebo in that design. How does one know, in that particular trial, that Drug A = Drug B = Zero?

J. SELDRUP: I was careful not to say what Drug A and Drug B were, so Drug A could be placebo.

W. WATSON BUCHANAN: Would a placebo always be included?

J. SELDRUP: Generally yes. There might be occasions where one would be justified in not doing a placebo-controlled trial.

Prescribing of Anti-Rheumatic Drugs in General Practice (Chapter 23)

W. CARSON DICK: Is there any comparable control group in the studies on concomitant prescribing. I am thinking of diabetics, or asthmatics who are of roughly the same age group and who might also be taking a major drug concomitant with other drugs.

A. W. PATTERSON: The studies are only beginning and are nowhere near complete. We have in mind to look at as many of the problems as possible and to compare one group of patients with another, and so on.

A. G. MOWAT: The data that are being put together are fascinating and it is important for clinicians that we know that the right drugs are being prescribed in the right instances, etc, and that we get some sort of feedback, particularly in hospital departments, which must be giving the lead in prescribing. The next stage of the plan, to use copy prescriptions as they are already doing in the Oxford Study, is admirable, but there are some instances where even that falls down. If I could pick out two from the data that we have been given.

One is as regards the concomitant prescription of antacids with anti-rheumatic drugs. The higher prescription was with propionic acids. One might conclude from that that the propionic acids are more ulcerogenic, cause more dyspepsia, and therefore need more antacids with them. The other way around is that propionic acids are being prescribed because the patient has tendencies to dyspepsia in any case and needs an antacid as an adjunct drug. A copy prescription would answer that question, or go some way to answering it.

A. W. PATTERSON: Yes.

A. G. MOWAT: The second point that I would pick out would be on anti-depressants and tranquillizers. From the data that we have been shown – and I would tend to agree with it as a clinician – rheumatoid patients are a lot more depressed than the general population; whether they are less or not I do not know. But one reason for not prescribing the drugs may be because the doctor thinks that the patients are taking enough tablets anyway, and that information will not come back out of copy prescriptions.

A. W. PATTERSON: No.

There are decided shortcomings in this type of analysis, as I am sure Dr Mowat has noticed and appreciates. The next move is to do something better, and we hope that it can be done.

W. WATSON BUCHANAN: I take issue with Dr Mowat. Patients with rheumatoid arthritis are frequently depressed, but both he and I fail to recognize the depression because we both work in hospital settings. When a patient comes up as an outpatient, it is a social outing, and the patient does not appear depressed. But when questioned, at least 50 or 60 per cent are severely depressed. We have studied this (*Ann. rheum. Dis.*, **33,** 132; 1974).

They are not depressed because of pain, but they become depressed when they lose function, when they become dependent on others. Most general practitioners know that their patients are depressed, and they know not to give anti-depressants because they do not work. The study has a vast amount of information.

The findings on aspirin are very interesting. The general teaching is that at least 3 g of aspirin per day to achieve an anti-inflammatory effect, yet the great majority of patients being prescribed aspirin were getting less than an adequate dosage.

We really require more information as to what conditions a doctor in terms of his prescribing habits. What influences him? I suspect strongly that his prescribing habits are built into his psyche. Recently we did an educational exercise. We took residents as they came – they come to us for four weeks – and we gave them a one-hour talk on how to prescribe drugs to the patients. These are very good residents. We compared their prescribing habits after the exercise with those of the residents who had not been instructed, and there was no difference. The same number of patients got two or three drugs.

Evaluation and Reporting of Toxicity of Anti-Rheumatic Drugs (Chapter 24)

W. WATSON BUCHANAN: Since Dr Cuthbert is on the Committee for Safety of Medicines, he might answer a simple question.

He has made a statement that the commonest cause of aplastic anaemia resulting from therapy is pheynlbutazone and oxyphenbutazone. We have been told that this occurs in 1/80 000 prescriptions. Is this not the rheumatologist's chloramphenicol? Chloramphenicol was quite acceptable as a drug. It caused aplastic anaemia in 1/30 000 prescriptions, but there were no alternative antibiotics. Today we have alternative anti-inflammatory drugs. Is there any reason why we should not now remove phenylbutazone and oxyphenbutazone?

M. F. CUTHBERT: It is not definitely a cause. In the data that I presented, I said the drugs most often associated with aplastic anaemia are oxyphenbutazone and phenylbutazone. But one must be very careful – until we have the data – not to say that the aplastic anaemia is caused by the drug.

Secondly, I cannot answer the question. That is for my peers to consider and pontificate upon.

It is true to say that many rheumatologists would not be happy to see oxyphenbutazone and phenylbutazone removed from the market. I am not a rheumatologist, but I should have thought that these are useful, if toxic, drugs. Perhaps, expressing a personal view, one should have reservations about their use in trivial indications.

W. CARSON DICK: Dr Cuthbert has already said that reactions are idiosyncratic. One should perhaps add that they occur in particular groups of patients, although we do not know that yet. Perhaps it is the patient who should be flagged, and not the drug. Having documented an idiosyncratic reaction in one patient, is there no way in which we can put a red flag on to that patient and follow him thereafter to see whether he does get idiosyncratic reactions to other drugs, and then to warn him?

M. F. CUTHBERT: I follow the argument, but I have to try to think of the practicalities of doing it. It is an interesting question. It is obviously something one should do, but the practicalities would provide a great deal of work.

J. R. VANE: Do I take it that although the animal studies which are done on toxicology and so on still leave us relatively in the dark, the CSM are happy with them? Should they be increased, or in view of the possibility of monitored release, perhaps they could be decreased?

M. F. CUTHBERT: The way in which the major pharmaceutical companies submit their toxicological data on new anti-rheumatic drugs is entirely satisfactory. The problem that has been raised about monitored release is an important problem, and it is particularly important in relation to the approval for clinical trial certificates, because we are one of the few countries in the world that does a detailed scrutiny of data before a drug is allowed to go to clinical trial.

It may be, and it is a topic now under discussion, whether there is a mechanism for limited toxicology for limited clinical trial, say in one or two centres, with a very tight protocol, realizing that the most important thing that the company will want to know is whether the drug is effective. It is an area that could usefully be explored between industry and the regulatory authority.

The Quest for Anti-Rheumatic Drugs (Chapter 25)

I. F. SKIDMORE: Some comment on the steroidal anti-inflammatory drugs.

My experience is that these drugs appear to act primarily on cells, on inflammatory cells in particular, and on cells of the vasculature too; something that the non-steroidal anti-inflammatory drugs do not do very well.

We know that phospholipid turnover is a very early phenomenon in a variety of cell activation processes. Could not the steroids be working even earlier in the activation processes to switch them on, so that the end result is an inhibition of the release of arachidonic acid.

Secondly, the difference between the effect of steroidal and non-steroidal drugs in asthma is probably due to the involvement of cells in the chronic asthmatic response, the infiltration of eosinophils and of polymorphs that can be inhibited by steroids but cannot be inhibited by non-steroidal anti-inflammatory drugs.

J. R. VANE: It is an important point. Dr Moncada has mentioned that HETE which is an end-product oxygenase pathway of the arachidonic acid metabolism, is said to be highly chemotactic for cells, and it could be that by cutting this out by the use of steroids the chemotaxis is being cut out.

I. F. SKIDMORE: The use of inhibitors of the lipo-oxygenase in inflammatory systems where the alternate pathway of complement is involved strongly suggests that inhibition of HETE formation has very little effect on chemotaxis.

J. R. VANE: Has that been reported?

I. F. SKIDMORE: Not yet.

R. R. A. COOMBS: I must apologize if I gave any impression that we were putting this work forward as a possible model. That was just an apologia at the end. The real reason for the work is to investigate the pathogenesis of the disease, and *that only* at this stage.

J. R. VANE: And I must apologize if I gave the impression that that was what Professor Coombs and his colleagues were doing. I did not mean to do so. I wanted to say that it is out of such fundamental studies that the new screens will possibly arise.

S. ORLOFF: Was it Dr Vane's intention to speak only of animal models. Are there perhaps possibilities in cell cultures or eventually in organ cultures from humans that could provide a new vista into the studies in pharmacology?

J. R. VANE: Certainly. In my own research many of the models are enzymes in the PG system, and many of the research directions are now moving towards the individual cells, cell cultures, and so on.

M. F. CUTHBERT: Dr Vane made a passing reference to the generation of prostacyclin by healthy endothelium. I am not familiar with this. Is it smooth muscle endothelium, and if it is, what does prostacyclin do to smooth muscle, and does it do different things to different smooth muscles?

J. R. VANE: The vascular endothelium that we have looked at, aortic strips from rabbit and pig, has the highest concentration of prostacyclin synthetase in the whole of the vessel wall. About 60% of the prostacyclin synthetase is contained in the endothelial cells which represent about 5 per cent of the total weight of the vessel wall. The enzyme then decreases in occurrence as one gets further out of the vessel.

Prostacyclin itself causes vasodilatation in animals. It relaxes arterial smooth muscle and seems to have little or no substantial effect on intestinal smooth muscle.

I had hoped that Professor Buchanan or Dr Dick would respond to the idea of a multitude of drugs in arthritis.

W. CARSON DICK: We should be terrified at the thought. On the other hand, drugs in leukemia and certain proliferative situations have been used together, and the sequence is so different from any one given alone that it has to be considered. The present philosophical bias is to give only one drug at a time, then we know that whatever happens with efficacy, with lack of effect, or with side effects was attributable to that drug. We are frightened by the present prescribing cocktails, but it would be well worth thinking about at a research level.

P. A. BACON: Not all of us are quite such therapeutic nihilists as the Glasgow School. As has been well-demonstrated here, the majority of anti-rheumatic drugs are already given in combination, and more rational combinations would be greatly welcomed.

W. WATSON BUCHANAN: Might it be possible to produce blockers to the enzymes that are causing the cartilage and bone destruction? If it were not for the cartilage and bone destruction, RA would not be a serious disease. Patients would have painful and swollen joints, but as long as their cartilage and their bone ends were intact, they would function reasonably well.

Is it possible to look at mechanisms whereby inhibitors might be found to neutral proteases, lysosomal enzymes? Is this feasible? This is where the damage is being done.

J. R. VANE: If there is an enzyme, then it is feasible to inhibit it. Whether it is feasible to inhibit it selectively is a different question. Certainly that is *an* idea and I am sure that it is being followed up.

W. CARSON DICK: The other possibility is not to confine work to these enzymes and mediators. Rheumatoid arthritis has a metabolic component, and there is a disturbance of calcium metabolism in this disease (*Curr. Med. Res. Opinion,* **3**, 345; 1975). Perhaps we should be widening our view, to look at that side of the disease that we have not yet studied.

I. F. SKIDMORE: Rather than inhibiting enzyme action, as Professor Buchanan suggests, it may be more efficient, and biologically more feasible, to inhibit the release of these enzymes. We are referring to specific cell processes in specialized cells. There is already an example in the drug disodium chromoglycate, and several other drugs like it, that specifically inhibit the release of histamine from mast cells charged with antigen. It points the way to the potential for inhibiting inflammatory cells selectively, and selective functions of those inflammatory cells.

J. R. VANE: I would agree. If there was a way of rounding off the polymorph so that it would accept the substances that it must digest without vomiting them out again along with the enzymes, that would be fine.

Section VIII:
Round Table Discussion

Pharmacologists and Rheumatoid Arthritis

M. K. JASANI

In the course of his excellent presentation, Dr. Vane mounted a vigorous defence of pharmacologists but still left room for me to expand a little further on their role in the search of not only anti-rheumatic drugs but also of an understanding of the inflammatory process characteristic of rheumatoid arthritis.

In my introduction I mentioned that the advances in the art of testing drugs would ultimately depend on advances in scientific knowledge. Although Dr. Vane has outlined the possibilities that already exist, knowledge concerning rheumatoid inflammation itself has yet to evolve. Pharmacologists have provided us with useful data, some of it negative, but that negativity is also helpful.

I should stress that when people report data on the negative aspects of their test systems, we need not throw up our hands in desperation, but we should instead re-examine the theory concerning the probable physiological and immunological basis for the disease under consideration. We may then deductively arrive at knowledge which we could not have anticipated, nor reached, otherwise. I should like to illustrate this point using two sets of observations that have profoundly influenced my own standpoint concerning the pathogenesis of rheumatoid inflammation.

The first concerns the fact that contrary to observations made in experimental models of inflammation (*Arch. Int. Pharmacodyn.* **178,** 115; 1969), in rheumatoid arthritis the anti-inflammatory potency of ibuprofen was not found to be higher than that of aspirin (*Ann. Rheum. Dis.*, **27,** 457; 1968). The disparity between the results of pharmacological and clinical evaluation was even more pronounced with regard to the effect of ibuprofen (750 mg/day) and prednisolone (15mg/day). Finally, joint tenderness and swelling largely persisted despite the use of each drug for a week and even though the patients subjectively felt relieved of pain and stiffness. The scientific developments which have enabled me to rationalize these observations are: (i) the discovery in 1971 by Dr. Vane of the inhibition of PG synthetase by aspirin-like drugs including ibuprofen (*Ann. Rev. Pharmacol.*, **14,** p60; 1974), (ii) the observations of Dr. Ferreira that the PGs are responsible for hyperalgesia, and not for pain production (*Nature New Biol.*, **240,** 200; 1972), and the consequent realization that aspirin-like drugs can dull the pain but not eliminate tenderness, and (iii) the fact that drugs such as indomethacin which are potent inhibitors of PG synthetase are not as effective against swelling caused by lymphocyte-initiated inflammation as against that caused by non-specific inflammation (Chapter 14).

In the clinical world there is not yet universal recognition of these facts, as we have discovered today, even though the data (Chapter 16) support them.

The second concerns the lysosomal hypothesis (*Arthr. Rheum.*, **9,** 834; 1966) which attributed a very important role to immune complexes and the lysosomal hydrolases released by phagocytic cells in the pathogenesis of rheumatoid arthritis. Results of clinical as well as experimental investigations which I conducted, between 1966 and 1971 (*Ann. Rheum. Dis.*, **28,** 497; 1969 and *J. Physiol.*, **219,** 525; 1971), in collaboration with Professor Lewis proved, on the whole, to be most discouragingly negative. Yet, it was that negative experience which gave rise to the series of experiments reported in Chapter 14 and which alerted us to the possible role of non-lysosomal enzymes or other mediators that may control the development of joint swelling in RA through fibrin-induced blockage of lymphatics (Chapter 11).

Finally, as yet we do not know the inter-relationship between lymphocytes, macrophages and polymorphonuclear leukocytes. My own personal feeling is that with time we shall find that macrophages moderate immune responses — not exacerbate immune responses — and that it is the polymorph which is the real culprit: what Professor Humphrey has called, 'the reluctant bystander', but which might nevertheless prove to be full of punch. The best strategy for future development of anti-rheumatic drugs might well turn out to be the identification of key events which could be pharmacologically moderated without affecting the lymphocytes; but the possibility of selectively inactivating activated lymphocytes, leaving the immune surveillance mechanisms intact, should not be altogether dismissed.

Inter-relationship between Immunology and Virology and their possible Consequences in Rheumatoid Arthritis

C. M. PEARSON

It is entirely possible that the discussion I have planned could have been given earlier in the symposium, but since that did not happen, hopefully I can shed some light on the complexity of the mechanisms that are involved in rheumatoid arthritis and some of the models that have been discussed, although admittedly I am no pharmacologist but a rheumatologist and an experimentalist.

Although viruses cannot as yet be incriminated for rheumatoid arthritis, the idea that the immune response to viral infections, rather than the infection itself, might be responsible for the disease manifestations has received much experimental support in the past few years. For instance infection of adult mice with lymphocytic choriomeningitis (LCM) virus results in death, but not when the animals are immunosuppressed as for example with the use of cyclophosphamide (*Proc. Soc. Exp. Biol. Med.*, **92,** 194; 1956).

IMMUNE RESPONSE TO VIRAL ANTIGENS

The nature of immune response to viral antigens varies depending upon whether the animal encounters infectious (live) or non-infectious (killed or attenuated) virus. Rabbits innoculated with herpes simplex virus (HSV) show the presence of circulating specifically sensitized (immune) lymphocytes within 3–5 days after innoculation (*Proc. Natl. Acad. Sci.*, **69,** 756; 1972). The lymphocytic response reaches a maximum between 7 and 10 days and then abruptly falls remaining at 2–3-fold above normal for the duration of the experiment. In contrast, neutralizing antibody is not detected until several days after the appearance of immune lymphocytes, but then persists long after the cellular immune response has declined. When animals are innoculated with u.v.-inactivated virus, only the cellular immunity is observed; whereas neither humoral nor cellular immunity develop in animals innoculated with virus complexed with neutralizing antibodies (*J. Immunol.*, **112,** 1019; 1974).

The interaction of antibody with the virus may also influence the responsiveness of immune lymphocytes to viral antigens, and the effect may depend upon the class of immunoglobulin bound to the virion (*J. Exp. Med.*, **139,** 902; 1974). The ability of viral antigens to stimulate lymphocytes is also dependent upon the way in which the antigens are presented to the lymphocyte. In the case of subacute sclerosing panencephalitis virus and cytomegalovirus, infected cells are more effective in activating lymphocytes than free virus (*J. Exp. Med.*, **138,** 839; 1973). Antibodies can interfere, however, with such activation by shielding the virions present on the infected cells from the lymphocytes.

THE ROLE OF BIOLOGICAL MEDIATORS RELEASED FROM IMMUNOLOGICALLY STIMULATED LYMPHOCYTES AND THE ROLE OF ANTIBODIES IN THE DEVELOPMENT OF INFLAMMATION

In vitro studies show that inflammation associated with viral infection may be caused by both immunological and non-immunological factors. It has been found that destruction of cells by HSV can result in the release of enzymes (? lysosomal) which can cleave C5 into C5a; the latter is chemotactic for both polymorphonuclear and monocytic leukocytes (*Science,* **170,** 1104; 1970). Secondly, in certain circumstances, virus-infected cells can release a factor which in the absence of complement is chemotactic for leukocytes (*J. Exp. Med.,* **135,** 1095; 1972). Thirdly, the interaction of anti-viral antibody with virus can fix complement (Figure 1) and so activate C5a (*J. Infect. Dis.,* **126,** 207; 1972). Fourthly, interactions between the virus and immune lymphocytes (Figure 1) results in the release of a variety of soluble factors including chemotactic factors, migration inhibition factor, lymphocytotoxin and interferon (*J. Exp. Med.,* **140,** 764; 1974).

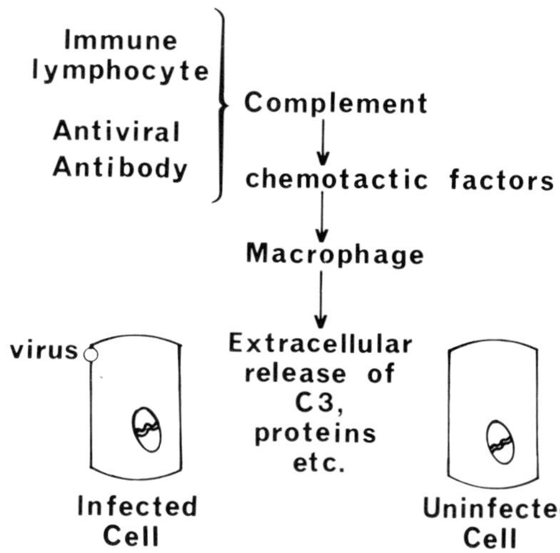

Figure 1 Defence mechanisms against virus infection. Complement and other agents can prevent cell-to-cell spread of viruses.

In vivo studies show that the induction of the inflammatory response in mice infected with Sindbis virus is lymphocyte mediated and immunologically specific (*J. Exp. Med.,* **136,** 216; 1972), and that its full expression in mice infected with Semliki Forest virus requires T cells (*Am. J. Pathol.,* **73,** 607; 1973).

Antibodies rather than immune lymphocytes play an all important role in the initiation of the inflammatory response characteristic of animals infected with lymphocytic choriomeningitis virus (*J. Exp. Med.,* **131,** 1; 1970), aleutian disease virus (*J. Immunol.,* **109,** 1; 1972), Langat virus (*J. Hyg. Camb.,* **66,** 343; 1968) and Venezuelan equine encephalitis virus (*J. Immunol.,* **87,** 509; 1961).

THE ROLE OF IMMUNE RESPONSE IN THE PREVENTION OF VIRAL SPREAD

Viral spread can be prevented either by anti-viral antibody neutralizing the extracellular virus or by destruction of the virus-infected cells. Not only antibodies, but immune lymphocytes and even the non-immunological factors such as complement, macrophages and various types of enzymes released from polymorphonuclear and monocytic leukocytes have an important role in the destruction of virus infected cells (Figure 1). The relative importance of these factors largely depends upon the mode of spread of the virus.

Of the three ways in which viruses can be transmitted from one cell to another (Figure 2), anti-viral antibodies readily prevent dissemination of the virus via the extracellular method, type

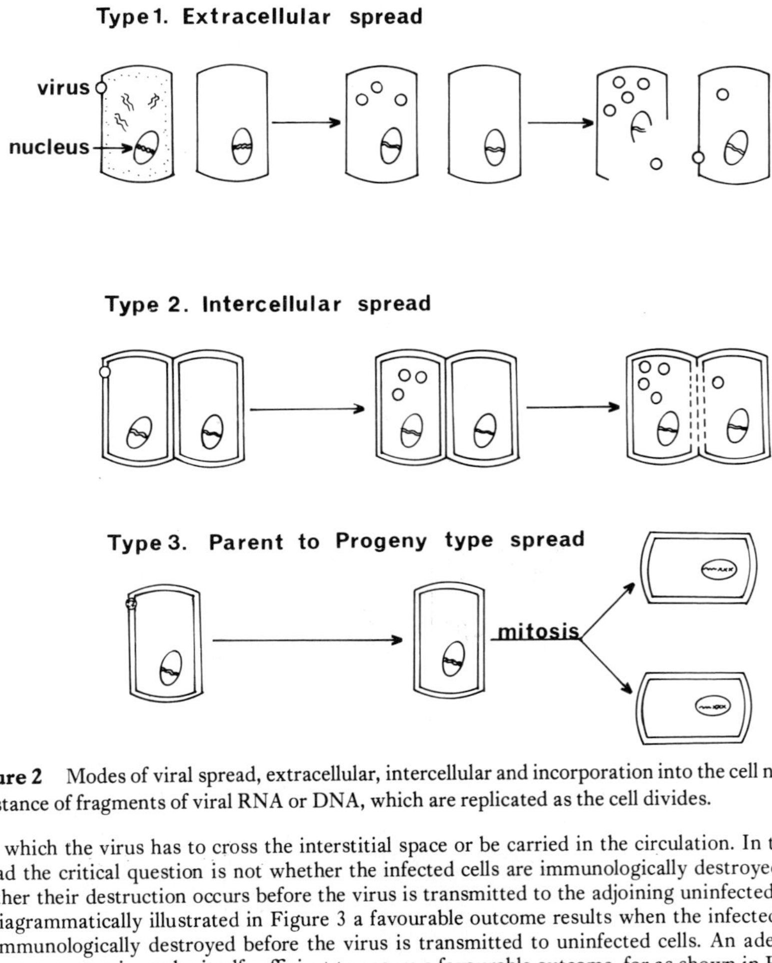

Figure 2 Modes of viral spread, extracellular, intercellular and incorporation into the cell nuclear substance of fragments of viral RNA or DNA, which are replicated as the cell divides.

1, in which the virus has to cross the interstitial space or be carried in the circulation. In type 2 spread the critical question is not whether the infected cells are immunologically destroyed, but whether their destruction occurs before the virus is transmitted to the adjoining uninfected cells. As diagrammatically illustrated in Figure 3 a favourable outcome results when the infected cells are immunologically destroyed before the virus is transmitted to uninfected cells. An adequate immune response is not by itself sufficient to ensure a favourable outcome, for as shown in Figure 3 an unfavourable outcome can ensue, e.g. as in the case of HSV infection (*J. Exp. Med.*, **137,** 706; 1973), even if the virus-induced new antigens on the surface of infected cells permitted cytolysis by anti-viral antibody and complement; because the viral spread occurred one step ahead of the immune attack.

The unfavourable outcome could, however, be favourably influenced by non-immunological factors such as enzymes and other macromolecules that can either disrupt connections between contiguous cells or inhibit viral replication in adjacent cells (*Progr. Immunol.*, **II (4),** 141; 1974).

Destruction of virus-infected cells can also be brought about by immune lymphocytes. It may be all important in the prevention of spread of infection by mumps virus (*J. Immunol.*, **101,** 409; 1968), measles (*J. Infec. Dis.*, **129,** 233; 1974), rubella (*J. Immunol.*, **110,** 1502; 1973), Sindbis (*J. Immunol.*, **113,** 173; 1974), LCM (*J. Exp. Med.*, **139,** 1329; 1974) and ectromelia virus (*J.*

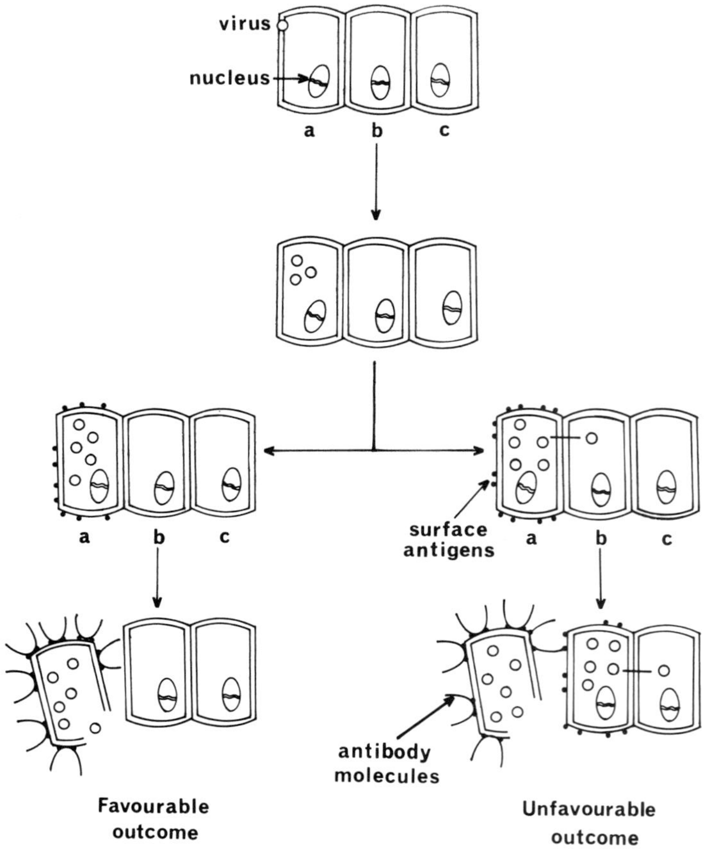

Figure 3 Critical factor for a favourable outcome against type 2 virus infection requires the immune attack on the virus-infected cell to precede the viral spread.

Exp. Med., **133**, 1090; 1971). Evidence in support of, and factors governing destruction of virus-infected cells by immune lymphocytes have been well reviewed (*Progr. Immunol* **II (4)**, 141, 1974).

BASIS FOR ANTIBODY AND CELLULAR IMMUNE RESPONSE TO VIRAL INFECTION

Figure 4 shows how the common precursor cell from which both the immune lymphocytes (T cells) responsible for cellular immunity and the antibody-producing B lymphocytes responsible for humoral immunity against the virus stem from the pool of bone marrow cells from which arise also the formed elements of the blood such as platelets, granulocytes, erythrocytes and monocytes. The critical factor which governs the behaviour of the progeny of the lymphoid stem cell would appear to be whether they pass through the thymus or the lymphoid bursa in the chick or its human equivalent. Presumably on passage through these organs the cells become differentiated under the influence of local hormones, ?thymosin, etc. to respond to viral antigen either by

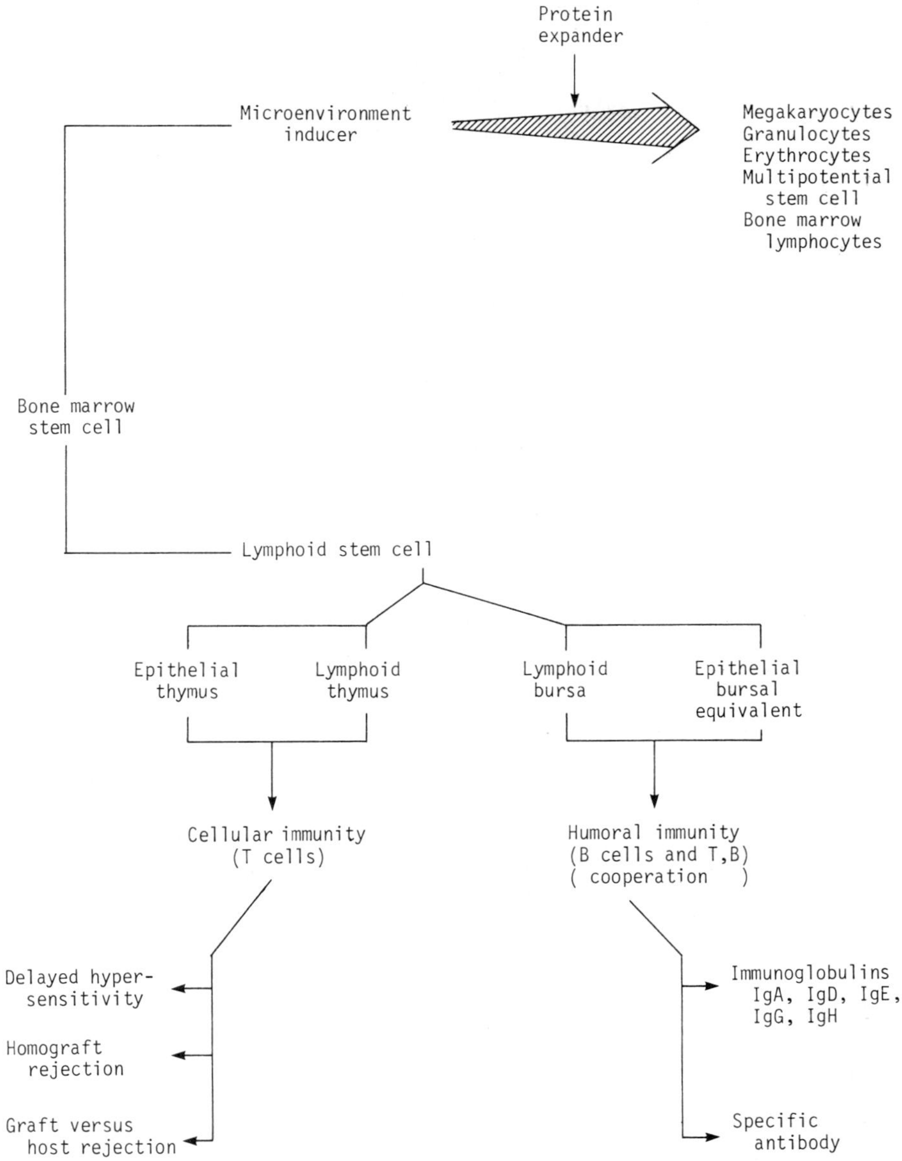

Figure 4 Origin and role of T and B lymphocytes.

proliferation and secretion of lymphokines (T cells) or by proliferation and the synthesis of antibody molecules (immunoglobulins; B cells). Although depicted as acting in isolation, in reality the T and B cells may interact to bring about this development of antibody synthesizing cells, and even to inhibit the T cell or B cell response (Chapter 12). Besides the lymphokine secreting cell, T cells may differentiate into cytotoxic cells, suppressor cells, K cells or remain as null cells.

Lymphocytes which can proliferate and become differentiated into lymphokine-secreting or antibody-producing cells continuously circulate as schematically shown in Figure 5. This fact may explain why depletion of circulating lymphocytes, as for example by continuous drainage of thoracic duct lymph of patients with rheumatoid arthritis, results in the rapid (5–10 days) improvement in their joint pain, swelling and stiffness (*Ann. N.Y. Acad. Sci.*, **256,** 150; 1975). We have observed similar benefits to result also in patients with scleroderma and SLE.

ROLE OF LYMPHOCYTES IN THE IMMUNOPATHOLOGY OF SLE

Figure 6 outlines the manner in which a virus-induced immune response could initiate the

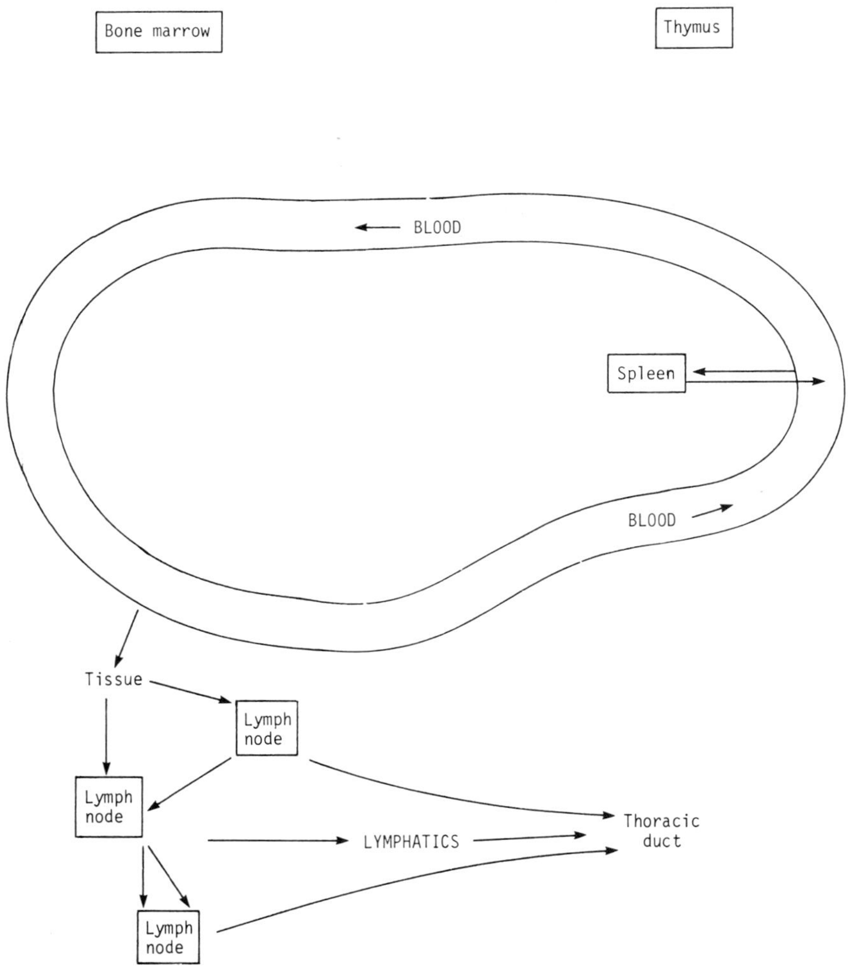

Figure 5 Anatomy of lymphocyte circulation in laboratory animals and man.

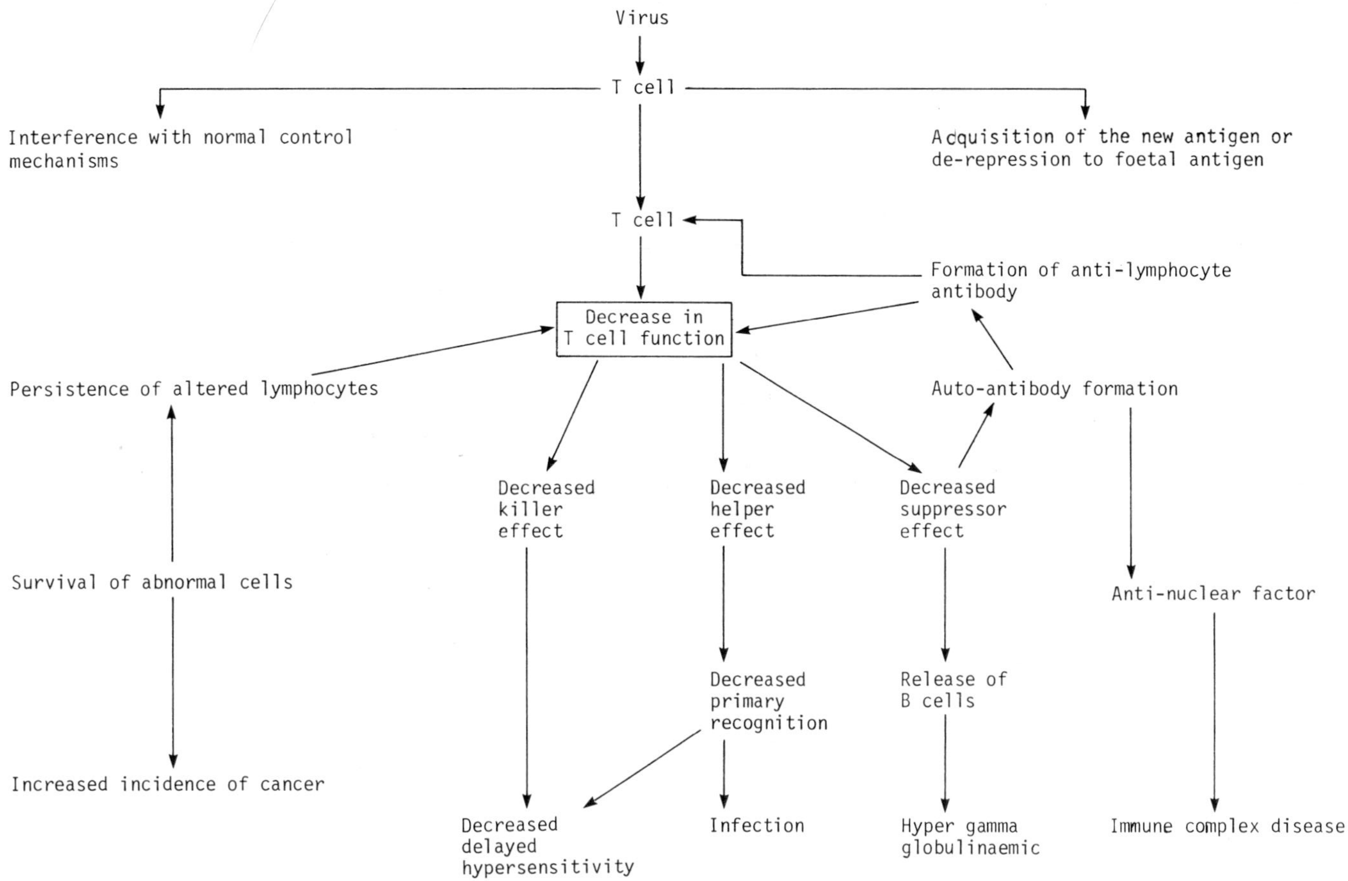

Figure 6 Hypothetical outline of the immunopathologic basis for five clinical manifestations of SLE: increased incidence of cancer, decreased delayed hypersensitivity, increased incidence of infection, hypergammaglobulinaemia and immune complex disease of the skin and kidney.

development of five clinical manifestations of SLE; namely, increased incidence of cancer, decreased delayed hypersensitivity, increased incidence of infection, hypergammaglobulinaemia and immune complex disease of the skin or kidneys and other tissues.

CONCLUSION

I believe that not only pharmacologists but also many other scientific investigators must assist us in the search for (a) viruses that may be responsible for the complex disease manifestations of SLE, rheumatoid arthritis and other immunological rheumatic diseases, and (b) means to control some subset(s) of T-cells or B-cells, or their interaction.

Pharmacological agents that are available at present include:

1 Those that control the inflammatory response, which is way down the line from what I have discussed.
2 The slower-acting pharmacologic agents, e.g. penicillamine, gold salts and levamisole, that seem to have other types of effects that we do not understand as yet.
3 The so-called immuno-suppressives which suppress only some of the immune mechanisms that are outlined above.

We must search for systemically tolerable anti-viral agents if at all possible, so that if a virus will move from one cell to another it may be possible to affect it and to effectively neutralize it.

On the other hand, there are ways now, using, for instance, DMSO and so forth, to get agents into cells, to cross cell membranes without damaging them, and theoretically it is possible that anti-viral agents could be introduced into cells, much the same way as specific hydrolytic enzyme inhibitors such as the relatively simple polypeptides (pepstatin, leupeptin) and some endogenous, recently discovered peptidases which may regulate the action of various hormones (Marks, N., In *Peptides in Neurobiology* (H. Gainer, ed.) New York: Plenum Press, 1977), can be introduced into cells, to effectively inhibit cell destruction that may occur in diseases such as muscular dystrophy, thyrotoxicosis, etc.

Finally, we must learn more about the macrophage monocyte system and how to pharmacologically manoeuvre these complicated systems.

How to Test Anti-Rheumatic Drugs?

G. P. LEWIS

Since we started our meetings people have been giving me 5 minutes notice and a title. I intend to relate some of the notes that I have jotted down, as a kind of summary.

It is getting more and more difficult — following on the previous speakers — to find new things to say and there is bound to be some overlap.

The aetiology of inflammatory joint diseases is pretty well unknown. Diagnosis of rheumatoid disease seems to be totally unsatisfactory and there appears to be little correlation between laboratory tests and the patient's condition. In lupus erythematosus, for instance, we are told that rather than making laboratory tests, it is better to see the patient every day and to test kidney function. The clinical rheumatologists tell us that they can tell more about their patients than any statistical analysis.

The mechanisms which underlie the diseases are anything but clear. It seems likely that immune complex formation plays a role, and even more likely that cell-mediated immune responses occur in chronic inflammation and that their mediators produce some of the signs of chronic inflammation, and perhaps even perpetuate the disease.

It seems difficult to develop models of single individual immunological pathways, although it does appear that certain pathways in the complement system offer an interesting possibility for a therapeutic approach. In addition to adjuvant arthritis there are two models which seem to have potential usefulness in the development of new drugs: the Dumonde–Glynn model and the new model of immune complex formation in rabbits described by Professor Coombs. The model of Professor Coombs is relatively new and it will be interesting to see the results after it has been used for some years. The Dumonde–Glynn model is novel, and unlike adjuvant arthritis, it seems to be much less sensitive to what we now call anti-inflammatory rather than anti-rheumatic agents which are used in the clinic, and this might lead on to drugs that are truly anti-rheumatic. On the other hand, the immunological stimulus in the model might be so great that no useful drug may ever be found in it.

When we look at the pharmacology from a therapeutic point of view, firstly we see that most experimental models used at present allow the development of anti-inflammatory agents rather than anti-rheumatic drugs. Secondly, we are told by the clinical rheumatologists that the best treatment for a rheumatoid patient is bed rest. Well perhaps. If, however, that really is true, then the anti-inflammatory agents whose main action is analgesic, might allow the patient a greater mobility, thereby making the disease itself worse.

Finally, with the delayed onset of action drugs — gold, D-penicillamine, chloroquine, levamisole — there are two difficulties, their toxicity and the fact that only a certain type of patient responds. A third difficulty with this series of drugs is that the pharmacologist has no model suitable for the measurement of this type of activity.

The main message that I take from this — and the earlier part of this meeting is this: The clinical rheumatologists are at a loss as to how to assess or treat their patients. The immunologists, the geneticists and the microbiologists have little factual knowledge of the aetiology of this group of diseases, and the pharmacologists do not yet know which model should be used to develop really useful anti-rheumatic drugs.

The message is that starting from now there should be much more contact between basic scientists, pharmacologists, immunologists and so on and clinical rheumatologists.

I have jotted down seven main points that I regard as practical points coming out of these discussions that might be followed through. Some of them have been mentioned by Dr. Vane. They are in no specific order (but I have jotted them down throughout the meeting).

— To examine the remaining metabolic pathway of the arachidonic acid and perhaps other unsaturated fatty acids.
— To use the Dumonde–Glynn model of joint disease in rabbits after intra-articular challenge and also Coomb's model of immune-complex disease formation after intravenous challenge.
— A more detailed study of the chronic mediators, lymphokines, because it is not until they have been characterized that we shall be able to attempt to assess their importance.
— To examine potential anti-rheumatic drugs on various pathways in the complement system.
— To define the mechanism of action of drugs having a delayed onset of action: D-penicillamine, gold, chloroquine, levamisole.
— To examine patients in such a way that we might be able to determine why some patients respond to treatment and some not.
— To find out why patients have remission of the disease — although I can make no suggestion as to a practical approach.

The last two items fall into a clinical rheumatological area rather than a pharmacological area.

On Statistics and Toxicology

W. W. BUCHANAN

We have had a long discussion on the progress, the pitfalls and the clinical evaluation of the drugs that we now have. It was quite clear from what Mr. Seldrup said that our knowledge of statistics is of a meagre kind. Indeed, he challenged many of the standard methods that we use for evaluating drugs. He did make one offer, which should be taken up. He has offered to work closely with the clinicians, and that is something to be pleased about.

Mr. Patterson's review of how doctors are actually using these drugs is of fundamental importance. Very little seems to be known of how doctors learn about drugs, how they are taught to prescribe them. We do not know what influences a doctor when he prescribes a drug. Is the general practitioner more influenced by social factors, for example, than medical reasons. Very little is known about how to educate doctors, and if they are educated do they learn, or are their prescribing habits so built into their psyche that little can be done to change those habits once established.

Dr. Cuthbert has told of how the Committee for the Safety of Medicines assesses toxicity to anti-rheumatic drugs, and this brings up the whole question of monitoring the release of new compounds. It will be a Herculean task because a very large denominator will be needed to find a rare complication.

We need to know, too, the background noise to any drug toxicity. We need to know how many people not taking drugs have the various side effects that would be attributed to drugs. We need controls.

The clinician will take away the conclusion that there is still a great deal of tidying up to do. Plenty is being done to improve what we are doing, and this will keep us busy for a few years, until we get a really effective drug.

Effect of Immune Complexes and Neutrophil Leukocytes

H. Z. MOVAT

As Dr. Jasani has just pointed out, the neutrophil or PMN-leukocyte may be the real culprit in tissue injury and perpetuation of an inflammatory reaction in a number of rheumatic diseases. Immune complexes have also been mentioned repeatedly. These complexes are inert *per se*, but by fixing complement, chemotactic substances are generated, which attract neutrophils. These phagocytose the immune complexes and during this process lysosomal enzymes, including proteases, are released by the neutrophils into the surrounding tissue. In this manner injury could be elicited by enzymes such as collagenase and elastase, the latter having been shown to attack cartilage. It is well known that in rheumatoid arthritis exacerbations are associated with an increase in the number of neutrophils in the joint fluid. In addition to the direct action of proteases, some of these enzymes can generate vasoactive sustances, i.e. kinins and cleavage products of complement by acting on appropriate substrates in plasma.

In vitro when immune complexes are incubated with neutrophils, one finds in the cell pellet neutrophils that have phagocytosed immune complexes. Evidence of degranulation and thus lysosomal enzyme release can be demonstrated ultrastructurally (Figure 1). When the supernatant of such an incubate is examined, one finds in it, among other things, an exzyme which hydrolyses proteins, such as casein and synthetic esters, such as butyloxycarbonyl *p*-nitrophenol. These are highly basic proteins and are adsorbed to a column packed with the cation exchanger SP-Sephadex. An aminopeptidase is excluded from such columns. It hydrolyses leucylnaphthylamide (Figure 2). The protease cleaves purified kininogen, giving rise to a kinin-like peptide, which is further degraded to bradykinin by the aminopeptidase. The protease also cleaves C3a from C3. Figure 3 shows the protease (elastase) in highly purified form. It consists of five bands, which represent charge isomers and migrates as a single band by SDS disc gel electrophoresis. Human neutrophil lysosomes also contain a chymotrypsin-like enzyme (cathepsin G), a third neutral protease, of higher molecular weight, as yet not well characterized and small amounts of an acid protease (cathepsin D).

Figure 4 shows the events which follow deposition of immune complexes. The antibody in such complexes is of the IgG class and fixes certain components and activates other components of complement via the classical pathway, generating C3a, C5a and the trimolecular complex C567. All these are chemotactic towards leukocytes, which are phagocytosed. Phagocytosis of the antigen–antibody–complement complexes by the neutrophils is associated with the release of the above described phlogistic substances, which together with C3a and C5a act on the microcirculation. By interacting with antigen on the surface of mast cells, antibody of the IgE class brings about release of vasoactive amines, which also act on the microcirculation, facilitating the deposition of immune complexes.

The described findings and detailed references are described in two recent reviews (*Fed. Proc.*, **35**, 2435, 1976; *Molecular and Biological Aspects of the Acute Allergic Reaction*, 391 (Plenum Press)).

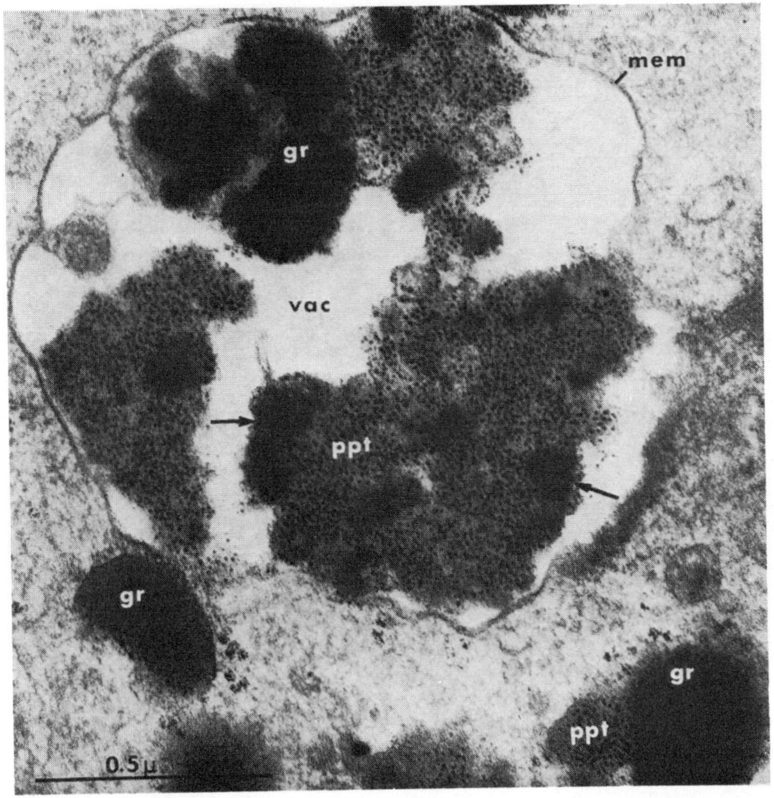

Figure 1 Electron micrograph of a neutrophil leukocyte containing immune precipitates (ppt). The precipitates are in a large digestive vacuole in the centre of the cell and in smaller vacuoles. Lysomes or granules (gr), devoid of their limiting membranes and partially lysed are present in the vacuoles. nuc = nucleus; gly = glycogen; mit = mitochondrion (from Movat *et al., Int. Arch. Allergy,* **40,** 197, 1971)

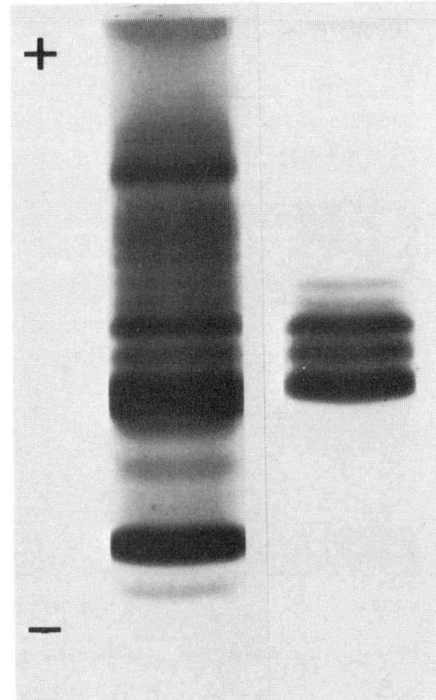

Figure 2 Chromatography of released lysosomal lysate (175 ml; total O.D. 280 nm = 118) on a 12 × 2.5 column of SP-Sephadex C-50, equilibrated with 0.01M phosphate buffer (pH 6.0), containing 0.2M NaCl. Elution was carried out by raising the NaCl concentration stepwise to 0.28 and to 0.4M. Aminopeptidase eluted in the excluded peak and protease (elastase) in the last peak

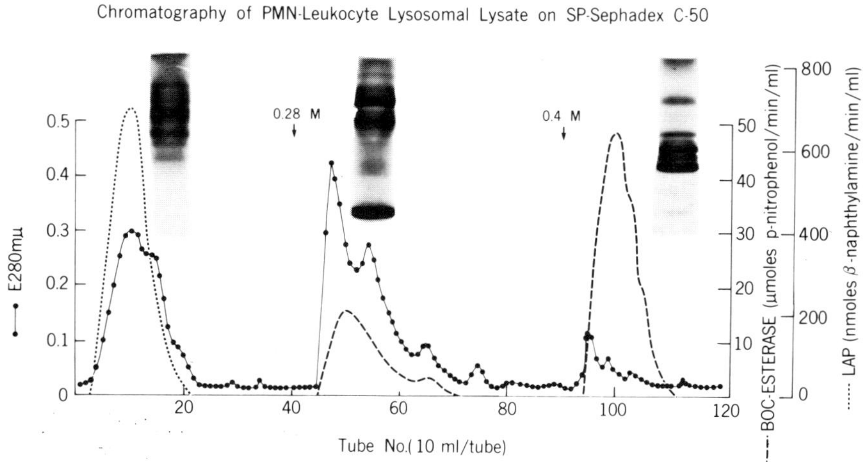

Figure 3 Alkaline disc gel electrophoresis of whole lysosomal lysate and of the protease (elastase)

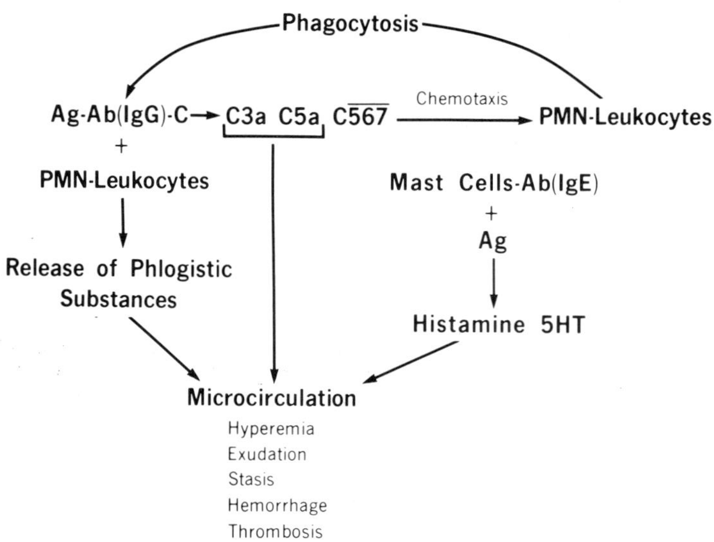

Figure 4 Diagram representing events which follow deposition of antigen-antibody complexes. For details see text (from Movat *et al.*, *Fed. Proc.*, **35**, 2435, 1976)

Discussion

W. CARSON DICK: We cannot close this meeting on a totally nihilistic tone.

Yes we are working in an area of 90% uncertainty, but we should not forget that rheumatology has advanced as much as, or possibly more than, any other speciality in internal medicine as a result of the work of basic scientists, immunologists, pharmacologists, surgeons and physicists. I should be very upset if we were to go home feeling completely nihilistic about the proceedings.

A. T. A. DOBLE: Might I ask for comments on a paper by MANSON and OHLHAGEN (*Bull Office Int. Epizoot.* **67,** 1319; 1967) describing the production of polyarthritis in pigs — large pigs — purely by changing their diet from normal to one rich in protein. They found that the normal gut flora changed in that the amount of *Clostridium perfringens* type A greatly increased. This was followed by the development of systemic immunity to this organism in the pigs and the chronicity of the joints was maintained while there was this change in the diet. By changing the diet back to the normal, they managed to get rid of the chronic arthritis.

The significance is that if rheumatoid arthritis is due to some persisting antigen, then one which derives from the gut is one which might be overlooked.

Is that work still considered valuable, or has it been discounted and I have missed the reference?

D. C. DUMONDE: This work has not been discontinued to my knowledge, and I am told that it is still being carried on.

Dr. Doble raised five points. Firstly, the change in gut flora might produce a change in entero-bacterial antigens. Secondly, the newly emergent antigens might produce changes in the response of susceptible pigs in terms of cross-reactive autoimmunity about which the genetic control is not much known.

Thirdly, a change in the pattern of endotoxin production in the bowel might lead to action at a distance, as it were, on susceptible sites in the micro-circulation, or on the potential of inflammatory cells for participating in inflammatory reaction.

Fourthly, a possibility that has not yet been considered and has only briefly been touched upon. There is increasing interest in the extent to which lymphocyte migration patterns might be affected by reactions that take place within the gastro-intestinal tract. It is known that there is a supplementary pathway of lymphocyte dumping, or even recirculation, in some animals, such as the sheep, and possibly also the pig, into the gut, and some upset in the homeostatic mechanisms of lymphocyte recirculation might be produced by a change in diet which in some animals leads to a change in bowel flora, and therefore to some local alteration in the emigration of lymphocytes into the gut.

There is no suggestion that the peripheral joints of these pigs have entero-bacterial antigen in them, and attempts to isolate related clostridia, such as *Clostridium perfringens*, from the joints of patients with rheumatoid disease have been entirely negative.

Ohlhagen has claimed that there are serological responses to clostridia of the *Clostridium perfringens* type in some patients with rheumatoid disease, but the immunotaxonomy of this particular group of enterobacterial organisms is up for sale.

Finally, there has been some unconfirmed evidence that cellular hypersensitivity to clostridial antigens could be detected in the rheumatoid subject as compared with the normals. This report was made by Manson and Ohlhagen at the Brighton Meetings in 1971, but has since remained unconfirmed.

At present, the diet itself is obtained from some Norwegian grass, or meal source and there have been no attempt to reproduce the model by veterinarians in the UK, nor — I believe — in the US.

R. R. A. COOMBS: If we neglect such observations we neglect them at our peril.

D. C. DUMONDE: I would endorse that wholeheartedly.

C. M. PEARSON: And I would too.

H. Z. MOVAT: A comment on what Dr. Dick said earlier.

Proteases of neutrophils are inactivated by a number of proteolytic enzymes, including natural proteinase inhibitors such as α-1-antitrypsin which is a normal component of plasma. Somebody made a comment about it and Dr. Skidmore then remarked that one could try to prevent the release, as we know, *in vitro* at least by raising cyclic nucleotides, or cyclic AMP, thus preventing the release from neutrophils, mast cells, etc. It remains to be ascertained, of course, how to make clinical use of these observations.

Index